Management of Open Fractures

Edited by

Charles M. Court-Brown MD FRCS Ed (Orth)
Consultant Orthopaedic Surgeon
Edinburgh Orthopaedic Trauma Unit
Royal Infirmary of Edinburgh
Edinburgh, UK

Margaret M. McQueen MD FRCS Ed (Orth)
Consultant Orthopaedic Surgeon
Edinburgh Orthopaedic Trauma Unit
Royal Infirmary of Edinburgh
Edinburgh, UK

Awf A. Quaba FRCS Ed (Plast)
Consultant Plastic Surgeon
Edinburgh Orthopaedic Trauma Unit
Royal Infirmary of Edinburgh
Edinburgh, UK and
St John's Hospital
Livingston, UK

With a foreword by

Augusto Sarmiento MD
Professor and Chairman Emeritus
Department of Orthopaedics and Rehabilitation
University of Miami School of Medicine
Miami, Florida, USA

MARTIN ■ DUNITZ

First published in the United Kingdom in 1996
by Martin Dunitz Ltd
The Livery House
7–9 Pratt Street
London NW1 0AE

A CIP record for this book is available from the British Library.

ISBN 1 85317 114 X

Composition by Scribe Design, Gillingham, Kent, UK
Printed and bound in Spain by Grafos, S.A. Arte sobre papel

CONTENTS

LIST OF CONTRIBUTORS

Nigel Brewster MB ChB FRCS Ed (Orth)
Senior Orthopaedic Registrar
Edinburgh Orthopaedic Trauma Unit
The Royal Infirmary of Edinburgh
Lauriston Place, Edinburgh EH3 9YW, UK

George C. Cormack MB ChB FRCS Ed
Consultant Plastic Surgeon
Addenbrooke's Hospital
Hills Road
Cambridge CB2 2QQ, UK

**James D. Frame MB BS FRCS Ed
FRCS (Plast) MRCS LRCP**
Consultant Plastic Surgeon
Burns and Plastic Surgery Unit
St Andrew's Hospital
Stock Road
Billericay
Essex CM12 0BH, UK

Ramon B. Gustilo MD
Professor of Orthopaedic Surgery
University of Minnesota and
President, Minneapolis Orthopaedic and Arthritis Institute
Minnesota MN 55415, USA

Geoffrey Hooper MB ChB FRCS Ed (Orth)
Consultant Orthopaedic and Hand Surgeon
Hand Unit
St John's Hospital at Howden
Livingston
West Lothian EH54 6PP, UK

John Keating MPhil FRCS Ed (Orth)
Consultant Orthopaedic Surgeon
Edinburgh Orthopaedic Trauma Unit
The Royal Infirmary of Edinburgh
Lauriston Place, Edinburgh EH3 9YW, UK

**Kwok-Sui Leung MBBS MD FRCS Ed
FHKAM (Ortho. Surg) Dip. Biomechanics**
Professor, Department of Orthopaedics and
Traumatology
Chinese University of Hong Kong
Prince of Wales Hospital
Shatin, New Territories, Hong Kong

Stephen P. Makk MD
Department of Orthopaedic Surgery
University of Louisville School of Medicine
530 South Jackson Street
Louisville
Kentucky 40292, USA

Clayton R. Perry, MD
Associate Professor
Department of Orthopaedic Surgery
Washington University School of Medicine
One Barnes Hospital Plaza
Suite 11300 West Pavilion
St Louis, Missouri 63110, USA

James N. Powell MD FRCS(C)
Foothills Hospital
Room AC144F
1403 29th Street North West
Calgary, Alberta T2N 2T9
Canada

James E. Robb MB ChB FRCS Ed FRCS Glas
Consultant Orthopaedic Surgeon
Royal Hospital for Sick Children
9 Sciennes Road
Edinburgh EH9 1LF, UK

M.J. Salahuddin MB ChB
Locum Consultant Plastic Surgeon
Department of Plastic Surgery
Odstock Hospital
Salisbury SP2 8BJ, UK

David Seligson MD
Professor and Vice Chair
Chief, Fracture Service
Department of Orthopaedic Surgery
University of Louisville School of Medicine
530 South Jackson Street
Louisville
Kentucky 40292, USA

Dean T. Tsukayama MD
Assistant Professor of Medicine
University of Minnesota Medical School and
Department of Infectious Disease
Hennepin County Medical Center
701 Park Avenue, Minneapolis
Minnesota 55415, USA

Markku Vornanen MD
Department of Orthopaedic Surgery
University of Louisville School of Medicine
530 South Jackson Street
Louisville
Kentucky 40292, USA

James D. Watson MB ChB FRCS Ed FRCSG (Plast)
Consultant Plastic Surgeon
St John's Hospital
Howden Road West
West Lothian EH54 6PP, UK

Gregory A. Zych DO
Chief, Orthopaedic Trauma and
Associate Professor
University of Miami
PO Box 016960 (D-27)
Miami, Florida 33101, USA

FOREWORD

Unless unanticipated radical developments alter the current treatment and prognosis of open fractures, this book will be the 'classic reference' for a long time to come.

The authors have succeeded in making clear the enormous differences that exist between closed and open fractures and the need to avoid hasty extrapolations between the two. In a systematic and organized fashion, they have described the epidemiology of the various fractures, the basic sciences aspect of them, and their diagnosis, treatment and prognosis.

The text reinforces my views that perhaps too often extreme efforts to salvage severely mangled extremities are unwise. In spite of great improvements in plastic reconstructive surgery and in the prevention of infections, over time many of those limbs that are preserved following multiple procedures become, in effect, less functional and more problematic that amputated limbs. Sometimes heroic attempts to preserve limbs are the result of the natural desire on the part of the surgeon to 'do every possible thing' and 'not to give up', as well as a lack of clear understanding of the true disability associated with amputation surgery. It is not widely recognized that the disability of a below-knee amputation can be minimal, particularly when compared to that created by a shortened and deformed limb with partially ankylosed and painful joints. Economic and psychological factors also need to be considered, particularly at a time when our society finds itself burdened with financial problems not anticipated even in the recent past.

I found the reading of this superb book a most enjoyable and extremely profitable educational experience.

Augusto Sarmiento MD
Professor and Chairman Emeritus
Department of Orthopaedics and Rehabilitation
University of Miami School of Medicine

PREFACE

The problems surrounding the management of open fractures have taxed the minds of surgeons for centuries but until recently they could do little except basic wound toilet and hope for the best! A success was defined as a patient that survived without needing amputation. However, the sequential introduction of antisepsis, antibiotics and improved fixation techniques, combined with an improved understanding of the vascular anatomy of the skin and the introduction of microvascular techniques has allowed surgeons to treat open fractures with a much greater certainty of success. The measurement of this success is that amputation and even infection are now poor arbiters of the efficacy of open fracture treatment.

It is important to realize that good results can only be achieved through close cooperation between orthopaedic and plastic surgeons. We have attempted this in this book, and we hope that readers will find this approach instructive. Although much of this book has been written in Edinburgh, and inevitably reflects our philosophy of management, we are very grateful for the expert contributions received from surgeons in other parts of the world.

C.M. Court-Brown
M.M. McQueen
A.A. Quaba
February 1996

1
History of the management of open fractures

C.M. Court-Brown

Man's desire to wage war has ensured a steady supply of open fractures over the centuries. The treatment of these fractures has exercised many of the world's greatest surgeons and has been instrumental in drawing together a number of medical and surgical disciplines. A study of the history of the management of open fractures provides us with considerable insight into much modern orthopaedic and plastic surgical practice.

Nowadays optimal management of an open fracture means that the surgeon must consider many different aspects of the problem. The size, location and degree of contamination of the wound must be determined, as must the extent of the associated bony damage. Consideration must be given to the optimal method of stabilizing the fracture and to the timing and type of soft-tissue cover that needs to be carried out. The surgeon must also consider whether the patient would benefit more from amputation or limb reconstruction. Modern surgeons often lose sight of the fact that their predecessors wrestled with many of these problems and that the philosophy of open-fracture management, as well as many of the currently used techniques, was suggested many years ago. Even early forms of currently used internal and external fixation methods were devised almost 150 years ago.

The major differences in the treatment of open fractures nowadays are the criteria by which successful management is judged. Most orthopaedic traumatologists would expect to achieve bone union and soft-tissue cover in a very high proportion of open fractures. Infection rates should now be low and amputation reserved only for fractures associated with catastrophic soft-tissue injury. Even from the early days of management, the surgeon's prime consideration should be the restoration of maximal limb and patient function.

The goals of surgery of previous generations were very different. Until comparatively recently, the main objective in treating a severe open long-bone fracture was to avoid death and amputation was commonly used for this reason. More recently, surgeons have taken the avoidance of infection as their yardstick for success, but the evolution of modern orthopaedic and plastic surgical techniques, as well as the introduction of asepsis, antibiotics and improved anaesthetic techniques, has allowed surgeons to minimize the complications of open fractures and improve their results.

There is evidence that amputation was practised in Neolithic times and in Pre-Columbian America although it is likely that this was either carried out as a punishment or as part of a religious ritual, rather than for the treatment of long-bone fracture (Kirk 1944, Aldea and Shaw 1986). The earliest known reference to an open fracture is presented in case 37 of the Edwin Smith papyrus. This papyrus was written about 2800 BC and was acquired by Edwin Smith, the American Egyptologist, in Luxor about 1867. Forty-eight case reports of various medical conditions are presented and the words for open and comminuted are introduced for the first time. Case 37 concerns a fractured humerus in association with an overlying soft-tissue wound. The author states that if the skin wound communicates with the fracture, the ailment should not be treated because of its poor prognosis (Breasted 1930).

As with many other aspects of medicine, the first surgeon to document his philosophy of the management of open fracture was Hippocrates working about 2500 years after the author of the Edwin Smith papyrus. He also felt that open fractures had a poor prognosis, particularly if they occurred in the larger bones close to the trunk, death usually resulting from infection. However, he had a more positive outlook than the ancient Egyptians and he did treat open fractures. He advocated the use of occlusive dressings using pitch or balsam for cleaning and sealing the wounds and then wrapping the limb in wine-impregnated dressings. He felt strongly that fracture reduction should be delayed, and in particular the wound should not be disturbed on the third and fourth days, these being the days which gave rise to inflammation, purulent discharge or fever. He advocated the use of levers to reduce the fracture, but this was delayed for 7–10 days (Adams 1939). The writings of Hippocrates were very influential and the other great surgeons of the period such as Galen and Celsus did not alter his philosophy.

The fact that most open fractures became infected presumably influenced the early physicians and surgeons to believe that purulent discharge was inevitable, a belief that persisted for over 1000 years. Paul of Aegina (AD 652–690), the last of the great Graeco-Roman physicians, suggested that the wounds associated with open fractures should be treated with ointments and encouraged to suppurate (Adams 1844). The legacy of the Graeco-Roman surgeons was handed down to the European surgeons of the 12th and 13th centuries by way of the Arabic literature. The works of Paul of Aegina and his contemporaries were translated into Arabic and their teachings were supplemented by Arabic physicians and surgeons of this period. The best known of these was Albucasis (AD 936–1013) who appears to have been the first surgeon to challenge Hippocrates' teachings. He disagreed with the multiple-bandage changes that Hippocrates suggested for the management of closed fractures and suggested instead that stiffened bandages should be applied for a prolonged period (Peltier 1990). Albucasis was a remarkable man, being credited with the first successful thyroidectomy as well as the introduction of both catgut and cotton sutures. He also accomplished successful small intestinal anastomoses by amputating the bodies of horned ants from their locked pincers which were left applied to the seromuscular layers of

the bowel. Albucasis was described as a 'Bold and, one might say, venturesome operator' (Harrison 1977). Interestingly, the work of Albucasis does not appear to have had much influence in the Muslim world, although there is little doubt that following the translation of his work into Latin it influenced surgeons in Western Europe to a considerable extent.

Following the fall of the Roman Empire, the Church became the controlling force behind medicine and its development for about 500 years. During this time, remarkably little progress was made and the philosophy of Paul of Aegina, that open wounds should be encouraged to suppurate, remained unchallenged. It was advocated by the influential surgical school of Salerno and one of their principal surgeons Ruggiero Frugardi of Palermo (Graham 1956). However, at about the same time, a number of innovative surgeons appeared to challenge the establishment view. Bruno of Longoburg, Hugh of Lucca and Theodoric all suggested that 'laudable pus' was not required to promote wound healing and they demonstrated that some wounds could be cleaned and primarily closed thereby allowing healing *per primum*. They realized that not all wounds could be closed and these larger wounds were allowed to suppurate. Unfortunately, their teachings do not appear to have been widely followed and suppuration with the formation of laudable pus continued to be established surgical practice until the time of Ambroise Paré (1510–1590).

Paré was another remarkable man. He was the first surgeon to describe an intracapsular femoral neck fracture and he also realized that metaphyseal fractures were often more difficult to treat than diaphyseal fractures, a fact that is frequently lost on modern trauma surgeons! He was an innovative surgeon, but as with other surgeons it was a fortuitous incident that altered his surgical practice. Paré began his surgical career in 1536 as a surgeon to General Montejean commanding the army of Francis I of France. He followed the prevailing opinion of the day and dressed open wounds with scalding oil. It is reported that when his supply of oil became exhausted he was forced to dress the wounds with a paste containing oil of roses, turpentine and egg yolk. He discovered that the wounds fared much better without oil and he abandoned its use (Paré 1575).

Paré also gave a remarkable account of the treatment of his own open tibial fracture. He was kicked by a horse and received an open fracture of the left tibia and fibula four fingers' breadth above the ankle. An excellent translation of the account of his fracture and its treatment is published by Peltier (1990) and makes fascinating reading. A review of a number of the extracts from this account illustrates Paré's understanding of the management of open fractures and give an insight into current treatment methods.

1. 'My bones thus broken and the foot distorted, I feared greatly that it would be necessary to amputate the leg.'
2. 'Moreover I admonished him [Monsieur Richard Hubert, the surgeon] to pull the foot straight and that if the wound was not large enough, to open it with his razor and let him easily put the bones in their normal positions, and that he searched the wound carefully with his fingers, which are better than any instrument. For the sense of touch is more certain than any instrument for removing the fragments and pieces of bone that can be widely separated.'
3. 'Rose ointment was applied around the wound and its neighbouring parts. This is strongly praised by the ancients for fractures, since it quiets pain and prevents inflammation. It repels humours from the injured part, since it is quite cold, astringent and repressive. It is made of oil of omphacin, rose water, a little viniger and white wax. Its use is continued to the sixth day.'
4. 'The compresses and bands were treated with Oxycrat in some coarse astringent wine to strength the part. This was especially recommended by Hippocrates for fractures with wound to dry and drive out the humours. When they are dry, I irrigated them with Oxycrat, alternating with Oxyrhodinun. For when they are too dry, pain and inflammation return to the part, since they squeeze more when moist. Some surgeons use only astringent medications and ointments from beginning to end in such a case. Unlike the method of Hippocrates and Galen. They consider that with astringent and ointment, they stop the skin pores of the part. This increases the strange heat, with severe pruritis and itching. This engenders under the skin a certain serous, acrid and morbid moisture which makes ulcers. This makes it well to remember not to continue such medications more than five or six days.'
5. 'Even such an exquisite regimen could not protect me against the fever that seized me on the eleventh day, with drainage which caused me an abscess which suppurated a long time. I believe all of this happened because of some humour retained in the part, as well as not having been able to stand having the wound tightly enough bandaged at first, as well as for some comminuted fragments separated from the ends of the bone, made both by the fracture and its reduction.'
6. 'This fever continued seven days, at the end of which it terminated partly by drainage, partly by profuse sweating. It was another month before I could get the foot to the ground without support. This was painful at first, because the callous held the muscles, for, before the movement can be free, it is necessary that the tendons and the membranes become loosened little by little where attached to the scar.'

These comments of Paré's illustrate the accepted treatment methods of the time and suggest that amputation was frequent following open tibial fracture. They also illustrate the importance of early Graeco-Roman teaching and highlight that Paré understood many of the basic principles of the management of open wounds that are accepted today. He obviously appreciated the need for adequate surgical exposure of the wound as well as the need for removal of devitalized bone fragments. He advocated soothing dressings rather than the astringent fluid that many of his contemporaries poured into wounds and it appears that he did not believe that infection was inevitable. He clearly felt that there was a reason for his purulent discharge and considered that it was in part associated with problems of the wound and bone ends. Finally, he appreciated the importance of early mobilization to avoid soft-tissue tethering, a philosophy that the modern AO group has propounded.

Paré's philosophy influenced succeeding generations of surgeons. The use of antiseptic fluids became widespread. Many different preparations were used. They often contained alcohol, pitch, oil of turpentine or various balsams. Many surgeons had their own preparation and it is recorded that Bilguer in 1764 reported good results using a mixture of frankincense, mastic, sarcocolla, finely powdered myrrh, true balsam of Peru, genuine essential oil of cloves and balsam of Fioraventi (Toledo-Pereyra and Toledo 1976). Surgeons at this time were beginning to realize the relationship between air contamination and infection and the use of improved antiseptic dressing improved the results of the management of open fractures.

The next major advance in the management of open fractures was the development of the concept of surgical wound cleansing. Hippocrates had advised that loose bone fragments should be removed from open fractures and it is clear from Paré's description of his own tibial fracture that he also understood that this was important. Leonardo Botallo (1560) emphasized the removal of all foreign matter from open wounds along with bone fragments, bits of contused and lacerated tissue and blood clots (Gurtl 1898).

The concept of surgical wound cleansing, however, was not accepted for a further two centuries and it is Desault (1744–1795) and his pupil Larrey (1766–1842) who are credited with popularizing the procedure and introducing the term 'debridement'. This term has given rise to some controversy in the literature. The word 'debridement' is derived from the French *débrider* meaning 'to unbridle' and strictly speaking it means 'to release constriction and tension by incision'. The word has, however, come to mean the surgical cleansing of a wound with removal of dead and devitalized tissue. Desault was an innovator who revolutionized the clinical teaching of surgery in Paris. Possibly, however, his greatest contribution was the influence that he had on Dominique-Jean Larrey, who rose to become the chief surgeon of the French army in the time of the Napoleonic wars. Like his mentor Desault, Larrey was a great innovator and introduced an ambulance service to Napoleon's army. His surgical skills were legendary and his practice was fashioned by the carnage that occurred during the Napoleonic wars. By his own account, Larrey practised debridement as we understand the term today. However, other authors have suggested that modern wound excision was not really practised until the First World War, crediting Desault and Larrey merely with the concept of opening up or decompression of the surgical wound. Milligan (1915), a surgeon with the British Expeditionary Force in the First World War, was probably the first surgeon to describe the method of wound excision. Later, Trueta (1944) described the operation of wound excision in considerable detail.

By the early 19th century it had become evident to all surgeons that the introduction of air and contaminated materials such as earth and bullet debris into a fracture site led to both systemic and local sepsis. As has already been detailed, surgeons since the time of Hippocrates had been using antiseptic agents, but by the time of the Napoleonic wars surgeons had begun to understand the need for early excision of devitalized tissues in salvageable limbs and early amputation in those that could not be salvaged. There was widespread use of antiseptic agents and occlusive dressings to exclude air from wounds. Pasteur (1822–1895) developed the germ theory of disease (Pasteur 1861) but Lister (1827–1912) is credited with developing antisepsis. In 1864, he became aware of the effects of carbolic acid on the sewage of Carlisle. A small proportion of this agent abolished all sewage odours and also rid the local cattle of parasitic bacteria. By 1865 he had used carbolic acid clinically. The air around the surgical wound was sterilized with carbolic acid as were the surgeon's hands and the instruments. He published results of 11 open fractures in *The Lancet* (Lister 1867) and reported only one death, a considerable achievement at that time.

Lister's work revolutionized the management of open fractures, and by the late 19th and early 20th centuries successful application of the principles of antisepsis, surgical debridement, early wound closure and immobilization of the wounds had been adopted by many surgeons. There were, however, a number of problems that still required a solution. There is little doubt that, despite early wound closure in selected open fractures, there remained a high infection rate, presumably because of inadequate wound excision coupled with skin closure under tension. There was also the problem of how to treat large soft-tissue wounds which could not be closed, this being a particularly common problem in war time. Lastly, surgeons were having to grapple with the problem of what to do with the fracture as internal and external fixation techniques were developing quickly.

The problem of the management of large wounds associated with bullet or shrapnel injuries taxed trauma surgeons in the early part of the 20th century. Surgeons followed three different philosophies. Many surgeons such as Trueta became convinced by the Winnett-Orr philosophy of occlusive dressings. Winnett-Orr (1877–1956) devised his regime of surgical wound excision with the use of occlusive dress-ing as a treatment of osteomyelitis, but it quickly became used for the management of severe open fractures (Winnett-Orr 1941). The technique was later adapted by Trueta and used in the Spanish Civil War (Trueta 1944). The technique merely involved packing the wound open with Vaseline gauze and immobilizing the limb in a plaster of Paris dressing. Changes were made only at infrequent intervals and once sufficient wound healing had taken place the wound was closed.

The second method of treating large open wounds was by irrigation with an antiseptic solution. This was popularized by Carrel (1873–1944), who used Dakin's (1880–1952) solution of sodium hypochlorite. Carrel used perforated irrigation tubes which were placed in the wound. The fractures were reduced and immobilized by plaster and the wound irrigated every two hours. The basic principle was again that the wounds would be kept clean until they had closed enough for skin suture to be under-taken. The third method of dealing with large wounds was to merely expose them to the air through a window in the plaster. This method was particularly advocated by the German school.

The Winnett-Orr method of occlusive dressings appears to have been the most popular way of treating severe open fractures, but with the evolution of plastic surgery techniques, surgeons soon became aware that the ideal method of closing large open wounds was with split-skin grafts or flaps.

History of fracture fixation

As with the history of the management of the open wound, the management of fractures goes

back to the Ancient Chinese, Egyptian and Indian civilizations. Initially, supportive dressings and splints stiffened with external agents such as grease, honey and mud were used. Hippocrates introduced the concept of bandaging, the bandages being stiffened with cerate, an ointment consisting of lard or oil mixed with wax, resin or pitch. He also introduced the concept of tibial external fixation using external leather rings which fitted snugly above the malleoli and below the flare of the tibial condyles. Once in position, the rings were distracted by inserting wooden rods of the appropriate length to facilitate fracture distrac-tion. Between the time of Hippocrates and the 18th century, remarkably few advances were made in fracture fixation. Hippocrates had laid down the principles of fracture reduction and management using bandages and these were not altered until the time of Albucasis. The only major innovation between the time of Albucasis and the Napoleonic wars was the introduction of traction by Guy de Chauliac in the 14th century.

The Napoleonic wars coincided with the time of the Industrial Revolution in Europe and the combination of increasing urbanization of the population with large numbers of wounded soldiers meant that more efficient methods of fracture fixation which allowed early mobilization had to be developed. Although Larrey and others developed more effective bandage stiffeners, it was Mathijsen (1805–1878) and Pirogov (1810–1881) who introduced the use of plaster of Paris bandaging. These revolutionized fracture management as they dried quickly, conformed to the shape of the wound and could be windowed, bivalved and removed easily. Although internal fixation techniques are described as early as 1775, in reality external casting was the only widely available method of fracture management until the latter half of the 19th century. It was therefore applied to both closed and open fractures. The identity of the first surgeon to internally fix an open fracture is unknown, but it seems logical to assume that the operation occurred in France sometime before 1775. It is recorded that Lapeyode and Sicre, surgeons from Toulouse, successfully internally fixed open fractures (Venable and Stuck 1947). In 1775, Monsieur Pujol, a physician from Castres, casti-gated Monsieur Icart because the latter had unsuccessfully internally fixed an open humeral fracture, following which the patient had died of gangrene. Monsieur lcart defended himself (Icart 1775), but the argument concerning internal fixation of open fractures had commenced. To this day, there is still debate about whether internal fixation should be used in severe open fractures.

The first book detailing techniques of fracture fixation was published by Bérenger-Féraud (1870). He described six methods of fracture fixation, including both internal and external fracture-fixation techniques. Three of these methods are still in use today, these being wire cerclage, interosseous wire suture and external skeletal fixation. It is difficult to discern a philosophy for internal fixation of open fractures during this time. Opinion regarding its usefulness appears to have polarized very quickly and surgeons either viewed internal fixation with contempt or accepted it with enthusiasm. The latter group appeared to use the same indications for the internal fixation of open fractures as for closed fractures. The common indication for internal fixation was an inability to hold the fracture in alignment with a cast. Initially, the approach to the use of internal fixation in open fractures was somewhat fragmented, but the use and range of internal fixation increased considerably after the knowledge of Lister's work with antisepsis became widespread. Hansmann (1886) developed the first bone plate (Figure 1.1) and Bircher (1893) and Senn (1893) both introduced intramedullary pegs, these being made of ivory or de-ossified animal bone.

The two great pioneers of fracture fixation worked in the early part of the 20th century. William Arbuthnot-Lane (1856–1943) felt that 'the displaced fragments of a broken bone were never, or hardly ever, restored to the normal position' and that the so-called 'setting of fractures was a myth'. He was a great enthusiast for internal fixation, but as with previous authors he appeared to have the same approach to open fractures as closed fractures. He favoured the use of plates, but also used wires, screws and staples. The other great enthusiast for fracture fixation at this time was Albin Lambotte (1866–1956) who spent most of his working life in Antwerp. He was undoubtedly the father of fracture surgery in Europe. He not only devised plates, staples and intramedullary wires for internal fixation, but documented the use of external

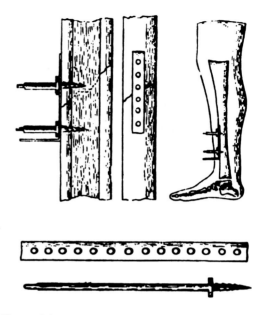

Figure 1.1

The original Hansmann plate. This had the interesting innovation of using percutaneous screws.

skeletal fixation using fixators which are not dissimilar to modern devices. More important, however, was the fact that he examined his results and detailed a substantive philosophy for fracture management. With regard to open fractures he, like many surgeons since, employed internal or external fixation to reduce unstable fractures which could not easily be handled by other methods. He did not advocate primary fixation of open fractures, as he believed that this was associated with an unacceptable infection rate, but he was enthusiastic about secondary fixation about ten days after the fracture. However, when maintenance of fracture position was very difficult he did employ primary fracture fixation successfully. He also defined the use of different types of fixation for diaphyseal and metaphyseal fractures, stressing, for example, the usefulness of plating for a proximal tibial diaphyseal fracture. His plates were made of aluminium as they were non-corrosive, did not oxidize and were malleable (Lambotte 1907).

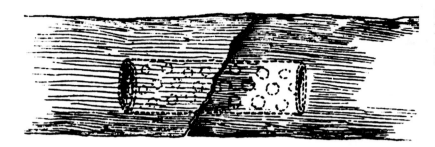

Figure 1.2

The original intramedullary cylinder, made from de-ossified animal bone, used by Senn.

In the United States, an internal fixation operation was undertaken by Rodgers in 1827 using silver wire loops. Later Nicholas Senn (1844–1908) was instrumental in encouraging American surgeons to adopt internal fixation techniques as was Beckman (1912) who was considerably influenced by Lane and published a paper on the repair of fractures with steel splints. Sherman (1912) developed vanadium steel bone plates and screws which were clearly superior to those of Lane and became a great advocate of internal fixation. He used his plates for the treatment of open fractures, but again the reason for operating was not because the fracture was open, but rather because it was unstable.

Lane's successor amongst British surgeons interested in the management of fractures was Ernest Hey-Groves (1872–1942). He was a great innovator and not only practised Lane's techniques, but also introduced intramedullary nailing in its modern form. He also carried out extensive work on external skeletal fixation, examining bone union in externally fixed cat tibiae. In his book entitled *On Modern Methods of Treating Fractures*, published in 1916, he devotes a chapter to the management of open fractures. He was a keen advocate of an adequate primary excision and described in detail how this should be done. He disagreed with the contemporary French philosophy from the Lyons school that the periosteum should be stripped from the bone and he was well aware of the necessity to remove dead bone but to retain vital bone. He did not agree with the increasing move towards primary internal fixation of open fractures. He felt that the wound enlargement that was necessary to allow plating encouraged sepsis and the requirement for drill

holes allowed infection to be carried into the medullary cavity. He advocated primary wound closure where this was possible and secondary internal fixation after the wound had healed. Hey-Groves' initial experiments with intramedullary nailing used small pegs made of bone or metal, but after the First World War he started to use long solid metal rods or fenestrated metal tubes. Although Hey-Groves used intramedullary nails not dissimilar to those used today, he was not the first to use intramedullary techniques—Senn had used intramedullary cylinders made from de-ossified animal bones in the 1890s (Figure 1.2).

Lambotte experimented with the use of intramedullary pins to fix metacarpal fractures in 1925, but the development of intramedullary nailing followed the work of the Rush brothers in the United States and Gerhardt Küntscher in Germany. The Rush brothers chose an unreamed intramedullary nail and Küntscher pioneered reaming. It is interesting to note that the two different philosophies have persisted until the present day. The Rush brothers initially used a thin unreamed intramedullary nail to immobilize a comminuted Monteggia fracture dislocation (Rush and Rush 1937). Subsequently, they developed their techniques considerably and produced an excellent book dealing with the use of Rush nails for many different clinical problems (Rush 1955). By the time the book was published, one of Rush's indications for intramedullary nailing was an open fracture, the rationale for this being to 'mitigate against infection'. In Europe, Küntscher developed reamed intramedullary nailing, the technique being used widely by German surgeons in the Second World War. There is little doubt that Küntscher did nail

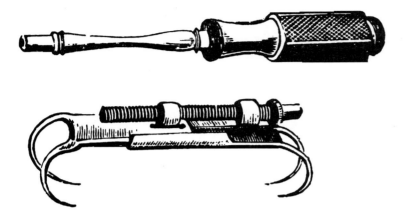

Figure 1.3

The first external fixator which resembled modern devices. It was devised by Malgaigne of Paris and used for the treatment of patellar fractures.

open long-bone fractures, but his philosophy was not dissimilar to that of Hey-Groves. He preferred secondary nailing as he felt that this would reduce the incidence of infection and felt that intramedullary nailing should be performed after 8–10 days when the soft tissues had healed (Küntscher 1967). He did, however, detail that a number of his colleagues had successfully nailed open long-bone fractures primarily.

By the time of the Second World War conditions were in place for increased interest in fixation of open fractures. Not only were there improved fixation devices, but sulphonamides and, later, antibiotics were available. There was a greater understanding of wound management and plastic surgical techniques were available to close large wounds. However, a review of the literature of this time shows that, although excellent results were obtained using primary plating (Davis and Fortune 1943, Davis 1948) and intramedullary nailing in open fractures (Street 1951, Bohler 1951, Lottes 1952), the surgical establishment did not accept the role of primary internal fixation in open fractures. In the 1960s and 1970s, the whole philosophy regarding internal fixation of open fractures changed. There were a number of reasons for this. The work of Rhinelander (1974) and other bone histologists showed that fracture fixation promoted capillary ingrowth and facilitated bone union. At the same time, the AO group (Müller et al 1965) provided the first organized approach to the management of fractures. They advocated primary internal

fixation, although stressing the need for absolute adherence to perfect technique. Their teaching, along with the improved instrumentation provided by the AO group, allowed surgeons to internally fix open fractures safely and also encouraged orthopaedic surgeons to audit their results and to devise new methods of fracture fixation. The last major innovation in internal fixation techniques was the introduction of the interlocking intramedullary nail (Klemm and Schellman 1972, Kempf et al 1978). This technique revolutionized the management of open long-bone injuries.

The other major fixation technique used for open fractures is external skeletal fixation. As already detailed, this was first used by Hippocrates, but the first modern external fixator was devised by Malgaigne in 1847. This was a clamp used for the rigid immobilization of patellar fractures (Figure 1.3). It was, however, Rigaud of Strasbourg who first inserted transcutaneous transfixion screws which were held by an external band, in this case string (Cucel and Rigaud 1850). The next milestones in the evolution of external skeletal fixation occurred in the 1890s when Keetley (1893) in London and Parkhill (1898) in Denver, Colorado, invented devices for stabilizing long-bone diaphyseal fractures. Keetley realized the potential flexibility of external fixation and that the bone ends could be held rigidly or elastically. He also experimented with different transfixion pin materials.

The major advance in external skeletal fixation was made by Albin Lambotte (1907). He used a single-bar fixator for many clinical injuries and reported excellent results with not only excellent union and low infection rates, but good patient function. The evolution of external skeletal fixation continued in North America and in Continental Europe, with no real interest being evident in Great Britain, apart from the work of Hey-Groves. He developed a rectangular frame similar in design to the later Charnley bone clamp and he applied it to osteotomized cat tibia. This was part of a study comparing different methods of fracture fixation. He commented that external fixation gave a more 'perfect union' than any of the direct fracture-fixation methods that he had tried (Hey-Groves 1916).

Although a number of different external fixators were devised in the 1920s and 1930s, the major innovation was that of Hoffmann (1938) who perfected a versatile external fixation device which has become widely used. This device had the merit of flexibility and could be made up into virtually any design. In addition, closed manipulation of the fracture with the device *in situ* was more easily performed with the Hoffmann than with previous unilateral frames. In the United States, there was considerable interest in external skeletal fixation from workers such as Anderson (1936), Stader (1937) and Haynes (1939). Bradford and Wilson (1942) reported that external fixation was of particular use in war surgery, as it was associated with a low incidence of infection and non-union. Despite the enthusiastic response of American orthopaedic surgeons to external skeletal fixation, a study undertaken by the American Academy of Orthopaedic Surgeons (Johnston and Stovald 1950) criticized the technique and the popularity of external skeletal fixation waned until it was re-introduced in the 1970s.

In Europe, however, the domination of the Hoffmann fixator continued, with early biomechanical investigations being undertaken by Lindahl (1962) and Vidal (1970). In particular, the Hoffmann–Vidal double frame with its increased rigidity stimulated orthopaedic surgeons to think about the role of rigidity in bone union and in the treatment of open fractures. In the 1970s, the trend was towards increasingly stiff external fixation frames in the belief that these would be advantageous in treating open fractures. More recently, interest in external skeletal fixation has centred round two areas. In the 1980s there was a move away from the bulky rigid double frames of the 1970s which tended to minimize soft-tissue access towards unilateral frames. The concept of micromovement of the fracture sites stimulating bone union resulted in the production of a dynamic external fixator (de Bastiani et al 1984). The other major innovation in external fixation work followed the invention by Ilizarov of a circular fixator employing multiple thin transfixion wires (Ilizarov 1954). The device was initially devised in Russia after the Second World War to deal with the large number of complications that followed open fractures sustained in the war. Later it became used for reconstructive procedures, mainly for the management of bone deformity, but its use in open and closed long-bone fractures is still advocated by many surgeons.

History of antibiotics

As has already been stated, surgeons have been using antiseptic fluids to treat open wounds since at least the time of Hippocrates. The first man-made drugs that were employed in an effort to lower the infection rate associated with open fractures were the sulphonamides. Although the first sulphonamides were synthesized in 1917, it was Domagk who introduced Prontosil, the first clinically used drug to contain sulphanilamide, in 1935. Surgeons were quick to adopt sulphonamides and a number of papers were written in the late 1930s and 1940s. Overall, surgeons were enthusiastic about the use of sulphonamides, stating that their infection rates were reduced. There was, however, debate about their usefulness. Meleney (1943) doubted their usefulness, but other workers (Jensen and Nelson 1942, Baker 1942) were enthusiastic. Bohler and Bohler (1966) stated that they had abandoned sulphonamide because the wound infection rate had risen as the surgeons had relied more on the use of antibiotics than on thorough wound excision.

Penicillin, the first antibiotic, became available in 1942 and was quickly used by war-time surgeons with considerable success. Initially there are reports of it being used in the same way as the sulphonamides, frequently as a topical agent. Smith-Peterson et al (1945) detailed the use of the Carrel technique to administer penicillin rather than Dakin solution. The clinical use of antibiotics in orthopaedics was studied by a number of authors. The consensus view was that antibiotics such as penicillin and chloramphenicol had little place in internal fixation of closed fractures (Schonholtz et al 1962). However, Godfrey (1962) in an American Academy instructional course lecture advocated the use of primary broad-spectrum antibiotics in the management of open fractures, the antibiotics being later modified according to the results of cultures. He again stressed that antibiotics should not be used instead of adequate debridement. Patzakis et al (1974) conducted the first prospective study of the efficacy of different antibiotics in open fractures. They showed a statistically significantly lower rate of infection following the use of a first-generation cephalosporin, cephalothin, when compared with a combination of penicillin and streptomycin or no antibiotic at all. Gustilo and Anderson (1976) confirmed the findings of Patzakis and his co-workers, showing that a combination of oxacillin and ampicillin lowered the infection rate in open fractures. Since these key papers were published, the numbers of antibiotics available to orthopaedic surgeons have increased markedly and a considerable amount of scientific and clinical research has been undertaken to investigate their usefulness in the management of open fractures.

The role of plastic surgery in open fractures

As with orthopaedic surgery, the origins of plastic surgery are ancient. However, it would appear that the origins of plastic surgery were more concerned with facial reconstruction than with the treatment of open fractures. In India, Sushruta (ca. 600 BC) described operations for reconstruction of the nose and ear lobes that continued to be used until the 15th century. At this time, the techniques of plastic surgery were handed down within families and it is probable that Branca in the 15th century used the first flap taken from the arm to repair facial defects

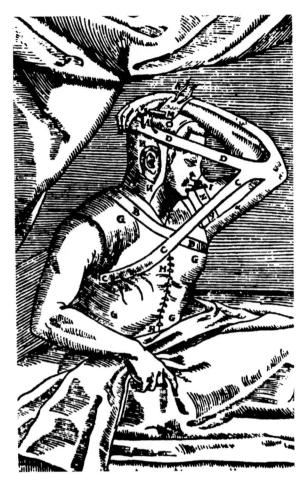

Figure 1.4

Much of the original plastic surgery literature dealt with nose reconstruction. In this illustration from the late 16th century an arm flap has been raised and the arm bandaged to the head. This type of pedicle flap was in use until relatively recently. The illustration is from the work of Tagliacozzi.

(Figure 1.4). These techniques were improved by Tagliacozzi (1545–1599) but in the 17th and 18th centuries, the practice of facial reconstruction declined somewhat. Given the fact that surgeons were exposed to large open wounds and that some techniques to raise flaps had been established by the 15th century, it is superficially surprising that they do not appear to have been used in the management of open wounds. However, the main purpose behind the treatment of open wounds at this time was to preserve life, and the preservation of limbs and their function was a secondary consideration. Thus, surgeons such as Verdun, Ravaton and Vermale contented themselves by designing better skin flaps following amputation in an effort to improve the stump (Aldea and Shaw 1986). In addition, the lack of adequate anaesthesia and asepsis meant that any form of plastic surgery more sophisticated than an amputation was almost certainly doomed to failure. The first recorded human skin graft was carried out by Sir Astley Cooper in 1817. It was, however, Reverda in 1869 who demonstrated the usefulness of small split-skin grafts. The technique of skin grafting was further developed when Ollier in 1872 and Thiersch in 1874 advocated the use of large split thickness skin grafts. Although available in the First World War, split thickness skin grafting did not appear to have been used much until the Second World War to close the large soft-tissue defects associated with open fractures.

The use of flaps in open fracture surgery followed the introduction of the tubed pedicle flap by Sir Harold Gillies during the First World War. Initially, orthopaedic surgeons used these flaps for the treatment of chronic osteomyelitis resulting from open fractures, with considerable benefit. Unfortunately, the methods for transferring a flap from one part of the body to another were not only slow and tedious, but somewhat uncomfortable for the patient. Waiting for a new blood supply to grow into a flap meant that an open wound might well be exposed for a prolonged period before flap cover was finally undertaken and therefore the technique was not readily applicable to open fractures.

There have been two recent major advances which have facilitated the use of flap cover in open fractures. These are the techniques of microsurgery and local flap cover. Microvascular surgery rose to prominence in the 1960s and 1970s. In 1962, the first successful implantation was performed in Boston (Malt and McKhann 1964) and by the 1970s the clinical use of re-implantation was widespread. At the same time, plastic surgeons began to use these techniques to allow for the transfer of free flaps to close large defects. In the 1970s and 1980s, there was

an explosion of interest in local flaps which were easier to use than free flaps and therefore carried a lower morbidity for the patient. Currently, both distant and local flaps are in widespread use and a combination of flap cover with modern orthopaedic techniques has revolutionized the management of open fractures.

History of amputation surgery

Amputations have been inextricably linked with the management of open fractures for several thousand years. It is probable that amputation practised in Neolithic times was punitive or part of a religious ritual, although it is quite possible that some were undertaken to treat badly injured limbs. As with other facets of the management of open fractures, Hippocrates was the first surgeon to discuss amputation in detail. He recognized that the amputation should be carried out through the devitalized tissue, so as to reduce pain and haemorrhage. The remaining gangrenous tissue eventually sloughed and the stump healed through the formation of granulation tissue. Amputation between healthy and gangrenous tissue was first recommended by Celsus in the 1st century. He stated that it was important that none of the diseased flesh should be left behind and that the bone transection should be more proximal than the soft-tissue transection. Both Hippocrates and Celsus used a sponge soaked in vinegar as an antiseptic dressing. Other improvements that were instituted by the Graeco-Roman surgical school were the use of ligatures to control major arterial bleeding and the use of a tight circular bandage above the amputation site to minimize bleeding. Although amputation surgery appeared to have been fairly sophisticated in Graeco-Roman times, just as the care of open fractures deteriorated during the early Middle Ages, there was also a decline in the standard of amputation surgery. Cautery replaced the use of ligatures and this may well have been in part due to the belief that suppuration was an important part of the healing progress. Albucasis also promoted cauterization, but suggested that this should only be undertaken for severe haemorrhage.

The requirement to practise adequate amputation surgery certainly increased in the early

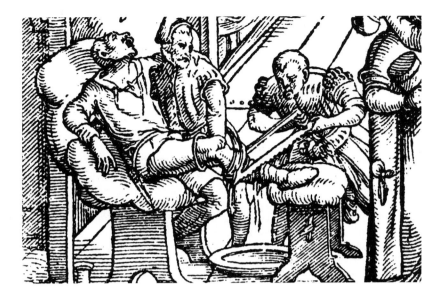

Figure 1.5

Part of an illustration by Paracelsus detailing the brutality of amputation in the 16th century. Little progress had been achieved since the time of Hippocrates.

Middle Ages. Gunpowder was introduced into warfare in 1338 and cannon shot was first used in the Battle of Crécy in 1346 with half-pound gunshot being used at Perugia in 1364. These new warfare techniques greatly increased the numbers of severe limb injuries and resulted in a major increase in amputations.

Many of the famous surgeons of the Middle Ages made their reputations in war surgery. Paré, in addition to his innovations in the management of open fractures, also devised new instruments to facilitate amputation as well as producing new prosthetic designs. At this time, ligatures were re-introduced instead of cautery for amputation work. By Paré's time, amputations had changed very little from those practised by Hippocrates and Celsus (Figure 1.5), but there was considerable progress in the 17th century. Surgeons such as Verdun (1696), Ravaton (1749), Alanson (1779), Vermale (1765) and Hey (1803) all devised improved flaps for bone coverage (Aldea and Shaw 1986). The Napoleonic wars provided surgeons with unprecedented exposure to severe limb injuries and surgeons such as Larrey became experts in amputations. Larrey was the first surgeon to disarticulate a hip joint in 1803. Such was the

requirement for the surgeon's craft that Larrey is reported to have carried out 200 amputations in one day at the Battle of Borodino. Although the surgeons were clearly hard-working enthusiasts, the morbidity and mortality of their work was colossal. Anaesthesia, antisepsis and analgesia were primitive, to say the least, and the surgeons relied on speed and dexterity. It is reported that the fastest amputation surgeon was Robert Liston (1749–1847). To save operative time, Liston held his amputation knife in his mouth! Soft-tissue division was rapid and was often achieved within a few seconds, the whole operation being frequently carried out within three minutes. The requirement for speed lessened in the middle of the 19th century when ether and chloroform anaesthesia were introduced. The rates of amputation in the middle of the 19th century were very high. Spencer-Wells (1864) detailed that amputation rates following major limb surgery in large city hospitals varied between 25% and 53%. Malgaigne (1858) noted that the mortality rate for major amputations carried out for trauma in Paris was 63%. Similar figures were published by McLeod (1858) who served in the Crimean War. He detailed an overall survival rate of 63% following gunshot wounds of the femur and an amazing 19% survival following gunshot wounds to the tibia.

The carnage continued through the American Civil War and the First World War. By the time of the First World War, the explosives were more powerful and the injuries were worse. However, surgeons were attempting to save more limbs than they had in earlier wars and the amputation rates were less. However, it is reported that in the 60 million men that were mobilized in the First World War, half a million underwent an amputation (Aldea and Shaw 1986). By the time of the Second World War, orthopaedic and plastic surgery techniques had improved, antibiotics had become available and there were improved ambulance services, anaesthesia and antisepsis. However, as the medical expertise increased, so did the destructive power of the weapons. The incidence of amputation actually rose in the Second World War to 5.3%, compared with an incidence of between 2% and 3% in the First World War. It is, however, interesting to note that the relative incidences of above- and below-knee amputations altered between the two wars, with more above-knee amputations being performed in the First World War and more below-knee amputations in the Second World War. In the Korean and Vietnam wars, the incidence of amputation was less than in the Second World War. However, as the solution to major soft-tissue loss, namely improved flap cover, did not materialize until the 1960s and 1970s, it has only been recently that the amputation rates following open fractures have declined dramatically. Recent interest in amputations has centred round trying to predict which patients are going to come to amputation, in a belief that these patients should have a primary amputation and therefore be spared prolonged periods of unsuccessful limb reconstruction. A number of predictive indices have been devised, but only time will tell whether these are in fact useful.

References

Adams F (trans) (1844–7) *Paulus Aeginata. The Seven Books of Paulus Aeginata* (The Sydenham Society: London).

Adams F (trans) (1939) *Hippocrates. The Genuine Works of Hippocrates* (Williams and Wilkins: Baltimore).

Aldea PA, Shaw WW (1986) The evolution of the surgical management of severe lower extremity trauma, *Clin Plast Surg* **13**: 549–69.

Anderson R (1936) An ambulatory method of treating fractures of the shaft of the femur, *Surg Gynecol Obstet* **62**: 865–73.

Baker LD (1942) Sulphonamides in traumatic and infected wounds, *J Bone Joint Surg* **24**: 641–6.

Beckman EH (1912) Repair of fractures with steel splints, *Surg Gynecol Obstet* **14**: 71–6.

Berenger-Feraud LJB (1870) *Traité de l'immobilisation directe des fragments osseux dans les fractures* (Adrien Delahaye: Paris).

Bircher H (1893) Eine neue Method unmittelbarer Retention bei Frakturen des Rohrenknochen, *Ann Klin Chir* **34**: 410–22.

Bohler J (1951) Results in medullary nailing of 95 fresh fractures of the femur, *J Bone Joint Surg (Am)* **33A**: 670–8.

Bohler L, Bohler J (1966) *The Treatment of Fractures* (Grune and Stratton: New York).

Bradford C, Wilson P (1942) Mechanical skeletal fixation in war surgery: report of sixty-one cases, *Surg Gynecol Obstet* **75**: 468–76.

Breasted JH (1930) *The Edwin Smith Papyrus* (University of Chicago Press: Chicago).

Cucel LR, Rigaud R (1850) Des vis métalliques enfoncés dans les tissues des os, pour le traitement de certaines fractures, *Rev Med Chir Paris* **8**: 115.

Davis AG (1948) Primary closure of compound fracture wounds, *J Bone Joint Surg (Am)* **30A**: 405–15.

Davis AG, Fortune CW (1943) Compound fractures, *J Bone Joint Surg* **25**: 97–120.

de Bastiani G, Aldegheri R, Brivio LR (1984) The treatment of fractures with a dynamic axial fixator, *J Bone Joint Surg (Br)* **66B**: 538–45.

Domagk G (1935) Ein Beitrag zur Chemotherapie den bacteriellen Infectionen, *Dtsch Med Wschr* **61**: 250–3.

Godfrey JD (1962) Major and extensive soft-tissue injuries complicating skeletal fractures, *J Bone Joint Surg (Am)* **44A**: 753–66.

Graham H (1956) *Surgeons All* (Rich and Cowan: London).

Gurtl EJ (1898) *Geschichte der Chirurgie und ihre Ausübung* Vol 2 (A. Hirchwald: Berlin) 403–14.

Gustilo RB, Anderson JT (1976) Prevention of infection in the treatment of 1025 open fractures of long bones, *J Bone Joint Surg (Am)* **58A**: 453–8.

Hansmann (1886) Eine neue Methode der Fixierung der Fragmentes bei komplizierten Frakturen, *Dtsch Ges Chir* **15**: 134–7.

Harrison TS (1977) The thyroid gland – historical aspects and anatomy. In: Sabiston DC, ed, *Davis Christopher Textbook of Surgery*, 11th edn (WB Saunders: Philadelphia).

Haynes HH (1939) Treating fractures by skeletal fixation of the individual bone, *South Med J* **32**: 720–4.

Hey-Groves EW (1916) *On Modern Methods of Treating Fractures* (John Wright: Bristol).

Hoffmann R (1938) Rotules à os pour la réduction dirigée, non sanglante, des fractures (ostéotaxis), *Helv Med Acta* 844–50.

Icart (1775) Letter in response to the memorandum of M. Pugol of Castre and of the Hôtel Dieu about a natural amputation of the leg together with reflection about some other cases relative to this operation, *J de Med Chir et Pharm de Roux* **44**: 164.

Ilizarov GA (1954) A new principle of osteosynthesis with the use of crossing pins and rings. In: *Collected Scientific Works of the Kurgan Regional Scientific Medical Society* (Kurgan Regional Medical Society: Kurgan, USSR) 145–60.

Jensen NK, Nelson MC (1942) Local sulfanilamide in compound fractures, *Surg Gynecol Obstet* **75**: 34.

Johnston HE, Stovald SL (1950) External fixation of fractures. *J Bone Joint Surg (Am)* **32A**: 460–7.

Keetley CB (1893) On the prevention of shortening and other forms of mal-union after fracture, *Lancet* **1**: 1377–9.

Kempf I, Grosse A, Laffourge D (1978) L'apport du verrouillage dans l'encloue centromédullaire des os longs, *Rev Chir Orthop* **64**: 635.

Kirk NT (1944) The development of amputation, *Bull Med Lib Assoc* **32**: 132.

Klemm K, Schellmann WD (1972) Dynamische und statische Verriegelung des Marknagels, *Monatsschr Unfallheilkunde* **75**: 568.

Küntscher G (1967) *The Practice of Intramedullary Nailing* (Charles C Thomas: Springfield, Ill).

Lambotte A (1907) *L'intervention opératoire dans les fractures récents et anciennes envisagée particulièrement au point de vue de l'ostéo-synthèse* (Lamertin: Brussels).

Lindahl O (1962) Rigidity of immobilisation of transverse fractures, *Acta Orthop Scand* **32**: 237–46.

Lister J (1867) On a method of treating compound fractures, abscess, etc., with observation of the conditions of suppuration, *Lancet* **1**: 326 and **2**: 95.

Lottes JO (1952) Intramedullary fixation for fractures of shaft of tibia, *South Med J* **45**: 407–14.

Malgaigne JF (1847) *Traite des fractures et des luxation* (JB Baillière: Paris).

Malgaigne JF (1858) *Études statistiques sur les résultats des opérations dans les hôpitaux de Paris* (Felix Locquin: Paris).

Malt RA, McKhann CF (1964) Replantation of severed arms, *J Am Med Assoc* **189**: 716–22.

McLeod GHB (1858) *News on the Surgery of the War in the Crimea with Notes on the Treatment of Gunshot Wounds* (John Churchill: London).

Meleney FL (1943) The study of the prevention of infection in contaminated accidental wounds, compound fractures and burns, *Ann Surg* **118**: 171.

Milligan ETC (1915) The early treatment of projectile wounds by excision of the damaged tissues, *Br Med J* **1**: 1081.

Müller ME, Allgöwer M, Willenegger H (1965) *Technique of Internal Fixation of Fractures* (Springer-Verlag: Berlin).

Paré A (1575) *Les Oeuvres. Aves les figures et portraits tant de l'anatomie que des instruments de chirurgie, et de plusieurs monstres* (Gabriel Buon: Paris).

Parkhill C (1898) Further observations regarding the

use of the bone clamp in ununited fractures, fractures with mal-union and recent fractures with a tendency to displacement, *Ann Surg* **27**: 553–70.

Pasteur L (1861) Mémoire sur les corpuscles organ-isées qui existent dans l'atmosphère, *Ann Sci Nat* **16**: 5.

Patzakis MJ, Harvey JP, Ivler D (1974) The role of antibiotics in the management of open fractures, *J Bone Joint Surg (Am)* **56A**: 532–41.

Peltier LF (1990) *Fractures: A History and Iconography of their Treatment* (Norman Publishing: San Francisco).

Rhinelander FW (1974) Tibial blood supply in relation to fracture healing, *Clin Orthop* **105**: 34–81.

Rush LV (1955) *Atlas of Rush Pin Technics* (Berivon: Meridian, Miss).

Rush LV, Rush HL (1937) A reconstructive operation for comminuted fractures of the upper third of the ulna, *Am J Surg* **38**: 332–3.

Schonholtz GJ, Borgia CA, Blair D (1962) Wound sepsis in orthopaedic surgery, *J Bone Joint Surg (Am)* **44A**: 1548–52.

Senn (1893) A new method of direct fixation of the fragments in compound and ununited fractures, *Trans Am Surg Assoc* **11**: 125–51.

Sherman WO (1912) Vanadium steel bone plates and screws, *Surg Gynecol Obstet* **14**: 629–34.

Smith-Peterson MN, Larson CB, Cochran W (1945) Local chemotherapy with primary closure of septic wounds by means of drainage and irrigation cannulae, *J Bone Joint Surg* **27**: 562–71.

Spencer Wells T (1864) Some causes of excessive mortality after surgical operations, *Br Med J* 384–8.

Stader O (1937) A preliminary announcement of a new method of treating fractures, *N Am Vet* **18**: 37–8.

Street DM (1951) One hundred fractures of the femur treated by means of the diamond-shaped medullary nail, *J Bone Joint Surg (Am)* **33A**: 659–69.

Toledo-Pereyra LH, Toledo MM (1976) A critical study of Lister's work on antiseptic surgery, *Am J Surg* **131**: 736–44.

Trueta J (1944) *The Principles and Practice of War Surgery*, 2nd edn (Hamish Hamilton: London).

Venable CS, Stuck WG (1947) *Internal Fixation of Fractures* (Blackwell Scientific Publications: Oxford).

Vidal J, Rabischong P, Boneel F (1970) Étude biomé-canique du fixateur externe d'Hoffmann dans les fractures de jambe, *Soc Chir Montpellier Séance* 20 January: 43–52.

Winnett-Orr H (1941) *Wounds and Fractures. A Clinical Guide to Civil and Military Practice* (Charles C Thomas: Springfield, Ill).

2
Classification of open fractures

C.M. Court-Brown

The need for a classification system for open fractures is accepted by most surgeons, although sometimes their usefulness is questioned. Many surgeons are of the opinion that if a classification system is to be sufficiently detailed to be useful it is, by definition, too complex to be remembered and is therefore of limited value. There is some truth in this statement but it does not alter the fact that excessively simple classification systems are often useless as they fail to fully define the fracture and its attendant problems. Over the last 30 years, classification systems have become more complex and it is likely that this trend will continue. The use of CT scans, MRI scans and other investigative modalities will allow surgeons to further subdivide fractures and soft-tissue injuries so that more and more extensive classification systems will probably be introduced.

The role of classification systems needs to be carefully defined. Many authorities state that the main purpose of any classification is to assist the surgeon in treating a fracture with the secondary goals being the prediction of fracture prognosis and assisting the surgeon in understanding the aetiology of the fracture. These beliefs are laudable but are asking a little too much of most classification systems. Fracture classifications may aid the surgeon in deciding on fracture management but the management of fractures is more likely to be dictated by surgical experience, available equipment and the patient's age and general medical condition. Surgeons may apply very different sets of therapeutic criteria when faced with fractures of similar types. There seems no doubt that prognosis is loosely related to fracture classification as most systems normally classify from the most simple fracture to the most complex. However, few useful classification systems have been subjected to rigorous analysis to see if they successfully predict patient outcome, this being the most important arbiter of management success. There is little doubt, however, that a good classification system is important in making the surgeon aware of the fracture or injury with which he or she is dealing. If the classification system has used appropriate criteria for characterizing each fracture, then the surgeon will gain insight into the different configurations of the fracture. In addition, the use of reproducible classification systems such as the AO system of long-bone fractures (Müller et al 1987) allows surgeons to compare results in a way which earlier surgeons could never do.

There are two basic types of classification system. The system may be aetiological in that it is based on the changing fracture patterns that are associated with increasing loading during the production of the fracture. The best example of this is the Lauge Hansen (1948–1954) classification system of ankle fractures. This was formulated from studies analysing the effect of different forces upon the ankle with the foot placed in different positions. The alternative type of classification system is morphological and is produced by merely studying a large number of X-rays and combining the fractures into an appropriate classification number. The best example of such a classification is the AO long-bone classification system in which all fractures are divided into 27 different groups and subgroups based on an alphanumeric system. There is no criticism implied in the suggestion that these classification systems are not based on aetiology in that if enough X-rays are studied and interpreted by experienced surgeons, then the fractures will be arranged in order of increasing severity and the net effect will be the same as an aetiological classification. Not all morphological classifications are as useful as the AO long-bone classification and many of the small classification systems in routine use which divide a particular fracture into three or more types are of little clinical value.

Classification of open fractures

Classification systems for open fractures are relatively new. Until the 1960s most surgeons merely classified fractures as open or closed, although authorities such as Ellis (1958) and Nicoll (1964) clearly understood the relationship of soft-tissue and bone damage to the prognosis of the fracture. However, even these authors only subdivided their fractures according to subjective criteria and Ellis referred to minor, moderate and severe fractures while Nicoll described wounds as being either 'nil or slight' or 'moderate or severe'. The first modern classification system which attempted to distinguish between different severities of open wound was devised by Cauchoix in 1965 and many later classification systems are based on it. He was most concerned with the size of the skin wound, dividing the skin wound into three types. Type 1 contained puncture wounds with little surrounding tissue damage. In the type 2 lesions he felt that there was a risk of skin necrosis secondary to the fracture and in the type 3 lesion there was loss of skin and subcutaneous tissue. He also realized the importance of the musculature as a source of infection and he further understood the relationship of the muscle blood supply to the prognosis of the fracture. It is interesting to note that Cauchoix in an analysis of 234 open fractures diagnosed type 1 lesions in 64.1% of all fractures. The type 2 lesion occurred in 24.8% of fractures and the type 3 lesion in only 11.1%. These data are very different from the more modern data presented in Chapter 3 but it should be remembered that Cauchoix analysed a number of fractures such as cranial fractures that modern orthopaedic surgeons would not normally be called on to deal with.

Cauchoix's initial classification system was followed by two very similar classifications from Allgöwer (1971) and Anderson (1971). Both recognized three grades of injury based on increasing soft-tissue damage. Allgöwer (1971) defined a grade 1 fracture as one where the skin was pierced from the inside by a spicule of bone. The grade 2 fracture occurred when the tissues

were contused by violence from without and grade 3 fractures were associated with extensive soft-tissue damage. Anderson's (1971) classification did not distinguish between soft-tissue injury from within or without. His type 1 injury was associated with minimal soft-tissue damage and the external wound was small. Type 2 status was conferred on larger wounds where there was little soft-tissue damage or contamination. The type 3 fractures had moderate or large wounds with devitalization or contamination.

These classifications were the forerunners of the Gustilo classification (Gustilo and Anderson 1976) that has become adopted worldwide. These authors divided open fractures into three types based on the size of the wound, the amount of soft-tissue damage or contamination and the type of fracture. Gustilo et al (1984) later subdivided the type III open fractures into three subtypes based on the degree of contamination, the extent of periosteal stripping and the requirement for operative revascularization. The complete Gustilo classification is shown in Tables 2.1 and 2.2 and illustrated in Figures 2.1–2.5. The Gustilo classification provides a workable system for defining the severity of open injuries. It recognizes the difference between low- and high-energy trauma, the importance of soft-tissue damage and in particular the effect of periosteal stripping. The prognostic value of this classification in terms of time to bone union has been highlighted in Edinburgh using one treatment method, namely the Grosse-Kempf intramedullary nail. The results for the different Gustilo types and subtypes are shown in Table 2.3. This shows that given a standardized treatment method as well as a consistent approach to soft-tissue cover and bone grafting, the Gustilo classification is of prognostic value as far as time to union is concerned. The prognostic value for non-union, requirement for bone grafting and joint function has also been examined and shown to correlate reasonably well with the Gustilo system (Court-Brown et al 1990, 1991). The prognostic value of the Gustilo classification system as regards final patient function is as yet unknown.

Other classification systems have been proposed. Oestern and Tscherne (1984) suggested a classification where the size of skin wound was of little importance and the main criteria were the degree of soft-tissue damage

Table 2.1 Definitions of the three Gustilo open fracture types (Gustilo and Anderson 1976)

Type	Definition
I	Open fracture with a clean wound <1 cm in length
II	Open fracture with a laceration of >1 cm long and without extensive soft-tissue damage, flaps or avulsions
III	Either an open fracture with extensive soft-tissue laceration, damage or loss; an open segmental fracture; or a traumatic amputation. Also: High-velocity gunshot injuries Open fractures caused by form injuries Open fractures requiring vascular repair Open fractures older than 8 hours

Table 2.2 Definition of the three Gustilo type III subtypes (Gustilo et al 1984)

Subtypes	Definition
IIIa	Adequate periosteal cover of a fractured bone despite extensive soft-tissue laceration or damage. High-energy trauma irrespective of size of wound
IIIb	Extensive soft-tissue loss with periosteal stripping and bony exposure Usually associated with massive contamination
IIIc	Associated with arterial injury requiring repair, irrespective of degree of soft-tissue injury

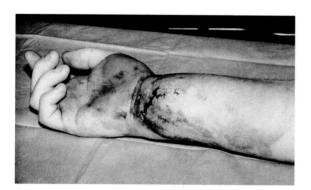

Figure 2.1

A Gustilo type I open fracture of the distal radius. The wound measured <1 cm and there was no contamination.

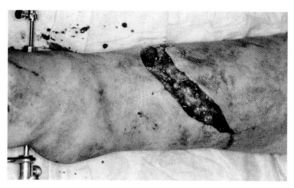

Figure 2.3

A Gustilo type IIIa open fracture of the distal tibia. Again there is no significant contamination or periosteal stripping.

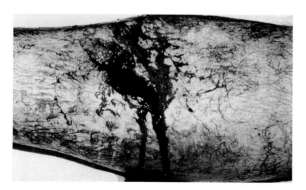

Figure 2.2

A Gustilo type II open fracture of the tibial diaphysis. The wound is longer but there is no significant contamination or periosteal stripping.

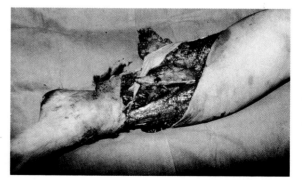

Figure 2.4

Gustilo IIIb wounds are very much more severe. This photograph illustrates the massive soft-tissue damage, bony comminution and periosteal stripping involved in this type of injury.

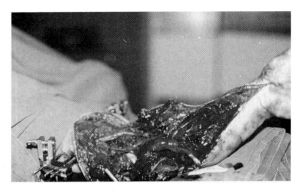

Figure 2.5

A Gustilo IIIc open fracture of the radius and ulna. The soft-tissue damage precludes adequate reconstruction. Vascular repair is essential and this fracture was treated by primary amputation.

Table 2.3 The time to union for the different Gustilo types and subtypes. IIIc fractures are rarely treated by primary nailing and are therefore not included. The amount of bone loss referred to is >2 cm and 50% bone circumference. Figures taken from Court-Brown et al (1990, 1991)

Gustilo type	Time to union (weeks)
I	14.7
II	23.5
IIIa	27.2
IIIb (no bone loss)	38.0
IIIb (with bone loss)	74.0

and the extent of muscle contusion. They emphasize that because of the importance of these criteria, a definitive classification may only be possible after the wound has been explored. In their grade I open fractures, there is an open wound with little or no skin contusion and negligible bacterial contamination. The fracture was generally of a mild configuration. The grade II fractures showed skin and soft-tissue contusion with moderate contamination and a fracture of variable severity. The grade III fractures include all open heavily contaminated wounds with extensive soft-tissue destruction often associated with vascular and nerve lesions. Any open

fracture with ischaemia and extensive comminution and all gunshot and contaminated farmyard injuries are included in this category. The grade IV open fractures consist of total or subtotal amputations. It is obvious that apart from the minor differences in Gustilo's failure to include a specific category for total or subtotal amputation the two classifications are very similar. The Tscherne grade IV, although it technically completes the classification, is of little practical value as nowadays many surgeons do not attempt re-implantation of severe lower limb injuries.

An important classification which should be mentioned was introduced by Byrd and his co-workers in the early 1980s (Byrd et al 1981, 1985). They modified the Gustilo classification, emphasizing the importance of the bony vasculature. They suggested four types (Table 2.4). The type I fracture was caused by low-energy forces. They emphasized that in type I fractures the fracture pattern allowed the periosteal and endosteal circulation to remain intact. In the type II injuries, they theorized that the endosteal circulation was disrupted and the wound was dependent on periosteal and soft-tissue circulation. In the type III injury, both the periosteal and endosteal circulations are disrupted and they suggested healing was dependent on vascular in-growth from the surrounding soft-tissue envelope. In the type IV injuries, the process of devascularization had extended to all of the surrounding soft tissues. The devitalized nature of the surrounding muscle precluded its use as a local muscle flap. They advocated microvascular free-tissue transfer for these injuries.

Comparison of Byrd's plastic surgery classification with the orthopaedic classifications of Gustilo and Tscherne is interesting. Byrd's interest in the vascular supply is well placed, particularly when considering flap cover. Gustilo and Tscherne are obviously more concerned with the problems of dealing with comminution or contaminated bone and soft tissue by primary debridement and thus the classifications are a little different. However, they are complementary and orthopaedic surgeons would do well to read Byrd's important contribution to this topic. The last classification system to be detailed is that of the AO group (Müller et al 1990). This very specialized classification is designed to be used in conjunction with the AO classification of the

Table 2.4 Classification of open tibia fractures according to Byrd and co-workers

Type	Definition
I	Low-energy forces causing a spiral or oblique fracture pattern with skin lacerations <2 cm and a relatively clean wound
II	Moderate energy forces causing a comminuted or displaced fracture pattern with skin lacerations >2 cm and moderate adjacent skin and muscle contusion but without devitalized muscle
III	High-energy forces causing a significantly displaced fracture pattern with severe comminution, segmental fracture, or bone defect with extensive associated skin loss and devitalized muscle
IV	Fracture pattern as in type III but with extreme energy forces as in high-velocity gunshot or shotgun wounds, a history of crush or degloving, or associated vascular injury requiring repair

Table 2.5 The AO classification of skin lesions, muscle/tendon injury and neurovascular injury

Type	Definition

Skin lesions IO (open fractures)
This grading of skin wounds fits well with the three-grade system for open fractures but adds a fourth grade for really extensive skin destruction

IO1	Skin breakage from inside out
IO2	Skin breakage from outside in <5 cm, contused edges
IO3	Skin breakage >5 cm, increased contusion, devitalized edges
IO4	Considerable, full-thickness contusion, abrasion, extensive open degloving, skin loss

Muscle/tendon injury (MT)

MT1	No muscle injury
MT2	Circumscribed muscle injury, one compartment only
MT3	Considerable muscle injury, two compartments
MT4	Muscle defect, tendon laceration, extensive muscle contusion
MT5	Compartment syndrome/crush syndrome with wide injury zone

Neurovascular injury (NV)

NV1	No neurovascular injury
NV2	Isolated nerve injury
NV3	Localized vascular injury
NV4	Extensive segmental vascular injury
NV5	Combined neurovascular injury, including subtotal or even total amputation

long bones (Müller et al 1987). It provides separate grading systems for skin injury, muscle and tendon injury and neurovascular injury. Each lesion is divided into four or five types of increasing severity (Table 2.5). The whole AO classification is designed to provide a definite description of a fracture and thereby allow comparisons. It is however a little unwieldy and of necessity will probably be used for scientific description and comparison rather than for everyday clinical activity. The Gustilo classification has become accepted worldwide and will be mainly used in this book. Its usefulness is therefore expanded a little further.

The Gustilo classification is based on a retrospective and a prospective study of 1025 open fractures of long bones carried out between 1955 and 1973 (Gustilo and Anderson 1976). The type III subtype classification was based on further analysis up to 1984 (Gustilo et al 1984). In 1987, Gustilo and his co-workers published a list of different fractures that they had classified using their classification. These included open fractures of the clavicle, humerus, radius and ulna, pelvis, femur, patella, tibia and fibula, and scapula. They did not apparently include ankle, foot and hand injuries. Despite this, the classification system is frequently applied to these injuries. The implication in Gustilo's papers is that the classification is based mainly on diaphyseal fractures and there is no literature as yet comparing its usefulness in diaphyseal and metaphyseal fractures. Open metaphyseal fractures generally have a better prognosis in terms of the incidence of infection and time to union than diaphyseal fractures because of their better blood supply, but the exact relationship between metaphyseal fractures and the Gustilo classification is unknown as yet. However, as the classification is based on sensible parameters, it has been used for both diaphyseal and metaphyseal fractures. As with all classification systems, the Gustilo system relies on subjective phraseology and terms such as 'extensive soft-tissue damage' or 'significant periosteal stripping' ensure a wide variation of interpretation between surgeons. There is as yet no solution to this problem and all classifications can be widely interpreted. Nicoll (1964) stated that minor degrees of a compounding of fractures did not interfere with the prognosis and this is undoubtedly true. The Gustilo type I fracture should only be applied to low-velocity fractures where the skin wound is almost an incidental problem (Figure 2.1). Many of these open wounds have been caused by bones coming out of the soft-tissue envelope. Many surgeons artificially distinguish between wounds that are 'compound from within' or 'compound from without', but the Gustilo classification does not and the distinction is in fact of no importance. All Gustilo type I wounds should be treated the same way regardless of the type of injury. The Gustilo type III fractures (Figures 2.3–2.5) can often be easily defined as strict criteria have been laid down for them. However, it can be difficult sometimes to distinguish between a type II and type III injury as the distinction may depend on a subjective assessment of the degree of soft-tissue damage. Again the distinction between a type IIIa (Figure 2.3) and type IIIb (Figure 2.4) fracture can be subjective as it is often based on the amount of periosteal damage. This may frequently be easy to assess as there may be a number of bone fragments that have no periosteal attachment whatsoever, but this may not always be the case and the surgeon may be confused as to what constitutes significant periosteal damage. The type IIIc (Figure 2.5) fracture should not be difficult to define as it strictly requires operative revascularization. I believe that the implication of the IIIc fracture is that the area of vascular damage is at the site of the fracture, but Gustilo and his co-workers do not actually say this. Thus, in theory, one could have the situation of a low-velocity tibial gunshot fracture where the second shot has divided the femoral artery and some surgeons have defined this as a IIIc fracture. I do not believe this is a correct interpretation of the Gustilo classification, but surgeons should be aware of the potential for confusion.

Some of the problems inherent in the Gustilo classification were documented by Brumback and Jones (1994). They presented a number of cases to 245 orthopaedic surgeons of different experience. They found that the average agreement among the observers was only 60%, there being very little difference between surgeons and trainees. They conclude that better classifications are required and there is little doubt that this is true. However, as already stressed, classification systems must be usable and until a straightforward system demonstrably better than the Gustilo system is devised it will continue to be used.

The mangled extremity severity score

The use of classification systems for open fractures has been extended recently to cover lower extremity trauma that may require an amputation. Chapter 23 deals with this subject in some detail, but the commonest of these scoring systems, the mangled extremity severity score ('MESS'), merits description. The MESS (Johansen et al 1990) is a relatively simple rating scale for lower extremity trauma based on the extent of the skeletal or soft-tissue injury, the extent of limb ischaemia, the degree of hypovolaemic shock and the patient's age. Table 2.6 shows the points given in the MESS system. If the points total is 7 or greater this indicates that an amputation may be required. Johansen and his co-workers undertook a retrospective

Table 2.6   MESS (Mangled Extremity Severity Score) variables

Type	Definition	Points
A.	Skeletal/soft-tissue injury	
	Low energy (stab; simple fracture; 'civilian' GSW)	1
	Medium energy (open or multiple fractures; dislocation)	2
	High energy (close-range shotgun or 'military' GSW; crush injury)	3
	Very high energy (above and gross contamination; soft-tissue avulsion)	4
B.	Limb ischaemia	
	Pulse reduced or absent but perfusion normal	1*
	Pulseless; paraesthesias; diminished capillary refill	2*
	Cool; paralysed; insensate; numb	3*
C.	Shock	
	Systolic BP always >90 mmHg	0
	Hypotensive transiently	1
	Persistent hypotension	2
D.	Age (years)	
	<30	0
	30–50	1
	>50	2

*Score doubled for ischaemia >6 hours.

study of 25 consecutive patients with 26 severely injured lower extremities, all associated with acute arterial insufficiency necessitating revascularization. Seventeen of the limbs were salvaged and nine required amputation. A retrospective analysis using the MESS system showed that all 17 salvaged extremities had scores of below 7, while the nine amputated extremities had scores ranging from 7 to 11. A subsequent prospective evaluation in 26 patients again showed good correlation between the score and the requirement for amputation. It is not suggested that scoring systems such as MESS should replace expert assessment of a severely injured extremity but such systems help to focus the surgeon's attention on the important parameters and provide a protocol which facilitates assessment. Further research into MESS and other scoring systems is required.

References

Allgöwer M (1971) Soft tissue problems and the risk of infection in osteosynthesis, *Lagenbecks Arch Chir* **329**: 1127–36.

Anderson LD (1971) Fractures. In: *Campbell's Operative Orthopaedics* (Mosby: St Louis).

Brumback RJ, Jones AL (1994) Interobserver agreement in the classification of open fractures of the tibia. The results of a survey of two hundred and forty-five orthopaedic surgeons, *J Bone Joint Surg (Am)* **76A**: 1162–6.

Byrd HS, Cierny G, Tebbets JB (1981) The management of open tibial fractures with associated soft tissue loss: external pin fixation with early flap coverage, *Plast Reconstr Surg* **68**: 73–82.

Byrd HS, Spicer TE, Cierney G (1985) Management of open tibial fractures, *Plast Reconstr Surg* **76**: 719–28.

Cauchoix J, Lagneau P, Boulez P (1965) Traitement des fractures ouvertes des jambe. Résultats de 234 cas observes entre le 1er janvier et le 12 juin 1964, *Ann Chir* **19**: 1520–32.

Court-Brown CM, Christie J, McQueen MM (1990) Closed intramedullary tibial nailing. Its use in closed and type 1 open fractures, *J Bone Joint Surg (Br)* **72B**: 605–11.

Court-Brown CM, McQueen MM, Quaba AA, Christie J (1991) Locked intramedullary nailing of open tibial fractures, *J Bone Joint Surg (Br)* **73B**: 959–64.

Ellis H (1958) Disabilities after tibial shaft fractures, *J Bone Joint Surg (Br)* **40B**: 190–7.

Gustilo RB, Anderson JT (1976) Prevention of infection in the treatment of 1025 open fractures of long bones: retrospective and prospective analysis, *J Bone Joint Surg (Am)* **58A**: 453–8.

Gustilo RB, Mendoza RM, Williams DM (1984) Problems in the management of type III (severe) open fractures. A new classification of type III open fractures, *J Trauma* **24**: 742–6.

Johansen K, Daines M, Howey T, Helfet D, Hansae ST (1990) Objective criteria accurately predict amputation following lower extremity trauma, *J Trauma* **30**: 568–72.

Lauge Hansen N (1948) Fractures of the ankle. Analytic historic survey as basis of new experimental roentgenologic and clinical investigations, *Arch Surg* **56**: 259–317.

Lauge Hansen N (1950) Fractures of the ankle. II. Combined experimental–surgical and experimental–roentgenologic investigations, *Arch Surg* **60**: 957–85.

Lauge Hansen N (1952) Fractures of the ankle. IV. Clinical use of genetic reduction, *Arch Surg* **64**: 488–500.

Lauge Hansen N (1953) Fractures of the ankle. V. Pronation-dorsiflexion fracture, *Arch Surg* **67**: 813–20.

Lauge Hansen N (1954) Fractures of the ankle. III. Genetic–roentgenologic diagnosis of fractures of the ankle, *Am J Roentgenol* **71**: 456–71.

Müller ME, Nazarian S, Koch P, Schatzker J (1987) *The Comprehensive Classification of Fractures of Long Bones* (Springer-Verlag: Berlin).

Müller ME, Allgöwer M, Schneider R, Willenegger H (1990) *Manual of Internal Fixation*, 3rd edn (Springer-Verlag: Berlin).

Nicoll EA (1964) Fractures of the tibial shaft, *J Bone Joint Surg (Br)* **46**: 373–87.

Osteren HJ, Tscherne H (1984) Pathophysiology and classification of soft tissue injuries associated with fractures. In: Tscherne H, Gotzen L, eds, *Fractures with Soft Tissue Injuries* (Springer-Verlag: Berlin).

3

Epidemiology of open fractures

C.M. Court-Brown and N. Brewster

The epidemiology of open fractures has received remarkably little attention in the orthopaedic literature despite its fundamental importance in allowing surgeons to plan the management of these difficult injuries and distribute their resources effectively. The apparent lack of interest in this topic is probably due to the difficulty that many orthopaedic trauma units face in compiling meaningful epidemiological data. Most hospitals in the United Kingdom and many other countries deal with a relatively small number of open fractures annually and those units that do treat larger numbers often concentrate on the more severely injured patient and therefore the more severe open fractures. This skewed distribution of patients is particularly seen in North America and in parts of continental Europe where better trauma systems exist and patients go to a hospital equipped to deal with their particular level of injury. It is therefore difficult for many hospitals to publish comparative epidemiological data about the incidence of open fractures of different bones.

In Edinburgh, the Orthopaedic Trauma Unit treats all in-patient and out-patient open and closed fractures for a catchment population of approximately 750 000. Thus the unit's database can provide information about the incidence of all open fractures. A study of all in-patient and out-patient fractures over the period between January 1988 and March 1994 was undertaken to examine which fractures were most commonly associated with open wounds. This particular period was selected to permit the assessment of 1000 consecutive open fractures. In addition, the age, Gustilo fracture type (Gustilo and Anderson 1976; Gustilo et al 1984), cause of accident and requirement for plastic surgery was also documented. Although the database is very comprehensive it must be stressed that in the study period there was only one gunshot open

fracture (of the forearm). Thus the relevance of the database to, say, a major urban hospital in the United States is questionable.

During the study, 31 575 fractures were dealt with in the Edinburgh Orthopaedic Trauma Unit. Of these, 1000 fractures were open, the average age of this open-fracture group being 42.4 years. The open fractures occurred in 933 patients: 875 presented with a single open fracture, 52 with two, 3 with three and 4 with four open fractures. Table 3.1 provides a breakdown of the 1000 open fractures, to highlight their relative frequency and indicate which open fractures surgeons will commonly be called on to treat. Open fractures

Table 3.1 The frequency and average age of open fractures in different body areas

Location	Number	Incidence (%)	Average age (years)
Hand phalanges	297	29.7	39.5
Tibial diaphysis	244	24.4	43.4
Distal radius/ulna	78	7.8	64.3
Femoral diaphysis	62	6.2	32.7
Foot phalanges	42	4.2	38.0
Forearm diaphyses	41	4.1	34.5
Ankle	40	4.0	47.8
Tarsus	30	3.0	35.2
Patella	27	2.7	41.3
Humeral diaphysis	18	1.8	47.4
Distal humerus	17	1.7	44.0
Proximal forearm	16	1.6	46.1
Metacarpus	16	1.6	42.8
Carpus	15	1.5	32.6
Tibial plafond	11	1.1	45.9
Metatarsus	11	1.1	38.5
Tibial plateau	10	1.0	48.1
Distal femur	10	1.0	41.6
Pelvis	6	0.6	29.3
Proximal humerus	5	0.5	31.8
Clavicle	2	0.2	32.5
Scapula	1	0.1	28.0
Proximal femur	1	0.1	40.0

Table 3.2 Relative frequency of open fractures in the upper limb

Location	Total fractures (n)	Open fractures (n)	Open fractures (%)
Proximal humerus	1568	5	0.3
Humeral diaphysis	314	18	5.7
Distal humerus	269	17	6.3
Proximal radius and ulna	1632	16	1.0
Radius and ulna diaphysis	442	41	9.3
Distal radius and ulna	3367	78	2.3
Carpus	764	15	2.0
Metacarpus	3992	16	0.4
Hand phalanges	3058	297	9.7
Total	15406	503	3.3

of the hand phalanges and the tibial diaphysis are by far the most common and such is their frequency that most surgeons will develop some experience in their management. Fractures of the distal radius and ulna, femoral diaphysis, foot phalanges, forearm diaphyses and ankle all occur with reasonable frequency but some open fractures, such as those of the pelvis, proximal humerus, clavicle, scapula and proximal femur, are extremely uncommon and many surgeons will have little or no experience in their management. Their rarity means that they are usually associated with severe high energy injuries and failure to understand the complexities inherent in their management may prove fatal.

Table 3.3 Relative frequency of open fractures in the lower limb

Location	Total fractures (n)	Open fractures (n)	Open fractures (%)
Proximal femur	4560	1	0.02
Femoral shaft	503	62	12.1
Distal femur	185	10	5.9
Patella	496	27	5.4
Tibial plateau	431	10	2.3
Tibial diaphysis	1131	244	21.6
Tibial plafond	188	11	5.8
Ankle	2898	40	1.4
Fibula	28	0	0
Tarsus	982	30	3.1
Metatarsus	1206	11	0.9
Foot phalanges	488	42	8.6
Total	13096	488	3.7

The British Orthopaedic Association recently estimated the average population served by a District General Hospital in Britain to be 241 360 patients, about a third of the population served by the Edinburgh Orthopaedic Trauma Unit. Assuming that these hospitals have a similar distribution of fracture types, interpolation of our data shows that each hospital will see about 13 open tibial diaphyseal fractures, 4 open distal radial fractures, 2 open ankle fractures and 1 open patella fracture each year. At the other end of the spectrum, staff in these hospitals are likely to see an open pelvic fracture only every three years and an open scapula or proximal femoral fracture only every eighteen years. If one assumes a 1:4 or 1:5 rota it is self-evident that many surgeons will have little experience in the management of certain open fractures.

Tables 3.2–3.4 show the comparative incidence of open fractures in different body areas, taking into account the total number of fractures treated. They indicate that open fractures of the tibial diaphysis are very common, comprising 21.6% of all tibial diaphyseal fractures. Open hand phalangeal fractures constitute 9.7% of all hand phalangeal fractures. Other fractures associated with a high incidence of open wounds are those of the femoral diaphysis, radius and ulna diaphyses and the foot phalanges.

The comparative incidence of open fractures of the upper limb is shown in Table 3.2. It can be seen that 48.8% of all fractures occurred in the bones of the upper limb, the most common fractures involving the metacarpus, distal radius and phalanges. In total, 3.3% of the upper limb fractures were open. Table 3.2 also shows that the most common open fracture in the upper limb is an open fracture of the phalanges, these representing 9.7% of all phalangeal fractures. The only other two areas with a relatively high incidence of open fractures were the diaphyseal forearm fractures showing an incidence of 9.3% and the diaphyseal humeral fracture which occurred in 6.3% of cases. The lowest incidences of open fractures in the upper limb were seen in the proximal humerus at only 0.3%, with low incidences also being recorded in the carpus, metacarpus, the proximal forearm and the distal radius.

Fractures of the lower limb accounted for 41.5% of all the fractures seen in the study period (Table 3.3). However, the incidence of

Table 3.4 Relative frequency of open fractures in the limb girdles and axial skeleton

Location	Total fractures (n)	Open fractures (n)	Open fractures (%)
Clavicle	1306	2	0.2
Scapula	142	1	0.7
Spine	683	0	0
Pelvis	942	6	0.6
Total	3073	9	0.3

Table 3.5 Frequency and average age of different Gustilo open fracture types in the tibial diaphysis

Gustilo type	Total number (n)	Percentage	Average age (years)
I	59	24.1	40.3
II	53	21.7	36.7
IIIa	55	22.5	54.5
IIIb	68	27.9	42.0
IIIc	9	3.7	44.9

open fractures was slightly higher than that of the upper limb, at 3.7%. The most common lower-limb fractures treated were those of the proximal femur and the ankle, with fractures of the tibial diaphysis, metatarsus and tarsus occurring with similar frequency. By far the highest incidence of open fractures was seen in the tibial diaphysis, with 21.6% of all tibial diaphyseal fractures being open. High incidences were also seen in the femoral diaphysis and the foot phalanges. Fractures of the distal femur, the patella and the tibial plafond all showed a similar, lower incidence. In contrast, open fractures of the proximal femur were very rare with an incidence of only 0.02%. Low incidences were also seen in fractures of the ankle, metatarsus and tibial plateau.

Open fractures of the limb girdles and axial skeleton are very rare (Table 3.4). A total of 3073 such fractures were seen, comprising 9.7% of the whole fracture group. Despite this, only nine open fractures of the limb girdles and axial skeleton were seen. Clavicular fractures accounted for 42.5% of the group, but only 0.2% were open. There were only six open pelvic fractures, one open scapular and no open spinal fractures.

In this chapter, epidemiology of different open fractures will be discussed. For the purposes of description the mode of injury has been divided into six different types, these being: simple falls; falls down steps, stairs or embankments; falls from a height to include any height; sporting injuries; direct blows or assaults; and road-traffic accidents. The only exceptions to this are in open hand phalangeal fractures, which are usually caused by cutting or crushing injuries (although a few are caused by animal bites).

Table 3.6 Fracture severity for different modes of injury in open tibial fractures

Mode of injury	Open fractures (n)	Average age (years)	I	II	Gustilo type (%) IIIa	IIIb	IIIc
Fall	31	59.4	41.9	22.6	32.2	–	3.2
Fall down stairs	3	48.0	66.6	33.3	–	–	–
Fall from height	20	37.0	30.0	35.0	15.0	20.0	
Sport	16	28.0	50.0	37.5	6.2	6.2	–
Blow/assault/crush	18	39.9	33.3	27.8	11.1	22.2	5.5
Road-traffic accident	156	42.9	15.4	17.3	25.0	37.8	4.5

Open fractures of the lower limb

Open fractures of the tibia and fibula

Open fractures account for 6.5% of all fractures involving the tibia and fibula. Table 3.3 shows that there is a considerable variation in the incidence of open fractures in different parts of the tibia and fibula. The commonest open fracture encountered by orthopaedic surgeons is that of the tibial diaphysis, 21.6% of all such fractures being open. The average age of the open diaphyseal fracture group was 43.4 years.

The Gustilo grading and average age of patients in the tibial diaphyseal group is shown in Table 3.5. This illustrates that the Gustilo type III fracture is the commonest open fracture of the tibial diaphysis with 54.1% being so classified. A breakdown of the data relating to the type III fracture shows that 51.5% were IIIb in severity, 41.7% IIIa and only 6.8% were IIIc. There was no significant difference in the average age of patients in the three Gustilo types, although there was an overall trend towards increasing severity with increasing age and the average age in the IIIa group was considerably higher than in other grades.

Table 3.6 illustrates the mode of injury for the open tibial diaphyseal fractures. It can be seen that 156 (63.9%) open tibial diaphyseal fractures were caused by road-traffic accidents. This mode of injury tends to be associated with the more severe Gustilo fracture types, in contrast to open fractures caused by falls, falls down stairs and sporting injuries which are generally less severe. The causes of open tibial diaphyseal fracture are somewhat different from closed fractures. A detailed analysis of the 523 closed and open tibial diaphyseal fractures admitted to the Trauma Unit between January 1988 and December 1990 has been prepared by Court-Brown and McBirnie (1995). Table 3.7 shows the average age and causes of both closed and open fractures during the period under study. Interestingly, the average age of the open-fracture group is considerably higher than that of the closed-fracture group, this probably being due to the relative infrequency of open sporting tibial fractures. Tables 3.6 and 3.7 also indicate that, in general, open tibial diaphyseal fractures

are caused by road-traffic accidents, falls from a height and simple falls, although it must be stressed that open fractures following simple falls occur in the elderly, the average age of this particular subgroup in the Court-Brown and McBirnie (1995) study being 71.3 years. Open tibial diaphyseal fractures are relatively rare in sporting injuries, direct blows and falls down stairs, steps or embankments.

The incidence of open fractures following road-traffic accidents is particularly high. Further analysis of the data relating to road-traffic accidents between 1988 and 1990 (Court-Brown and McBirnie 1995) shows that 37.8% of all tibial diaphyseal fractures were caused by this mechanism. Of these fractures, 58.6% occurred in pedestrians, 21.7% occurred in motorcycle drivers or passengers and 17.2% affected car, van or bus drivers or passengers. The remaining 2.5% of injuries occurred in bicycle riders.

Analysis of the severity of the open fractures in the three road-traffic accident subgroups shows that 33.6% of the pedestrian subgroup presented with open fractures, the average age being 52.2 years. The vehicle occupants' subgroup also showed a similar incidence of open fractures at 35.3% with an average age of 41.5 years. The highest incidence of open fractures relating to road-traffic accidents was seen in the motorcycle subgroup where 62.8% had open fractures, the average age of this subgroup being 31.6 years.

Table 3.7 Epidemiological differences between closed and open fractures of the tibia and fibula diaphysis

Parameter	Closed fractures	Open fractures
Number	400	123
Average age (years)	28.5	42.6
Causes		
Fall	20.7%	7.3%
Fall down stairs	3.0%	0.8%
Fall from height	3.7%	13.8%
Sport	38.5%	5.7%
Direct blow	4.0%	5.7%
Road-traffic accident	29.0%	66.7%

Table 3.8 Frequency of different Gustilo open fracture types in the femoral diaphysis

Gustilo type	Total number (n)	Percentage	Average age (years)
I	12	19.7	40.5
II	10	16.4	36.8
IIIa	12	19.7	32.3
IIIb	20	32.8	29.9
IIIc	7	11.5	36.1

Analysis of the grade of open fractures in the three road-traffic accident subgroups shows that pedestrians, vehicle occupants and motorcyclists tend to have severe open fractures, there being 74.3% of Gustilo type III fractures in the pedestrian subgroup with 66.6% in both the vehicle occupant and motorcycle subgroups.

Open fractures of the tibial plateau

Open fractures of the tibial plateau are surprisingly uncommon. This is probably because despite the relative vulnerability of the knees in road-traffic accidents, this mode of injury usually causes proximal diaphyseal tibial fractures rather than intra-articular fractures involving the plateau. Only 2.3% of patients with tibial plateau fractures had associated open wounds. These tended to be older patients with an average age of 48.1 years. All of the open tibial plateau fractures occurred as a result of road-traffic accidents, five being seen in elderly pedestrians (average age 64.6 years), four in vehicle drivers (average age 31.8 years) and one in a motorcyclist aged 31 years. Thus the bi-modal age pattern typical in most fractures is clearly seen. The open tibial plateau fractures were generally less severe than open tibial diaphyseal fractures, there being three Gustilo type I, four type II, two type IIIa and only one type IIIb open fracture.

Open fractures of the tibial plafond

After diaphyseal fractures the highest incidence of open fractures of the tibia and fibula occur in fractures of the tibial plafond. Table 3.3 shows that 5.8% of Pilon fractures were open. The average age of the eleven open Pilon fractures was similar to that of the diaphyseal group, at 45.9 years. However, Pilon fractures also demonstrate other differences from diaphyseal fractures. The majority of open pilon fractures (54.5%) were caused by falls from a height, with three (27.3%) occurring in road-traffic accidents and the remaining two (18.2%) in falls. There is a high incidence of Gustilo type III fractures with eight (72.7%) showing this degree of severity. The remaining three fractures comprised one type II and two type I fractures. As with the diaphyseal group the highest age was seen in the Gustilo type IIIa group at 53.4 years. This contrasts with an average age of 49.5 years for type I fractures and 35.7 years for IIIb fractures. Again this emphasizes the relative vulnerability of the elderly to type IIIa fractures with significant soft tissue damage and less severe bone damage.

Open fractures of the ankle

Review of Tables 3.2–3.4 indicates that ankle fractures are the fifth most common fracture seen by orthopaedic surgeons. Despite this, open ankle fractures are surprisingly uncommon accounting for only 1.4% of all ankle fractures. They show similarities to some open tibial plateau fractures in that they tend to occur in an older age group, the average age of the open fracture group being 47.8 years. In addition, Gustilo IIIb fractures are unusual with only two (5%) occurring in this series. Five (12.5%) were Gustilo type I in severity, eighteen (45%) were type II, the remaining fifteen (37.5%) being type IIIa. Ten (25%) of the open ankle fractures followed simple falls and as would be expected these tended to be in older patients, this subgroup having an average age of 58.7 yerars. Nineteen (47.5%) fractures occurred as a result of road-traffic accidents, ten of these being in pedestrians, six in motorcyclists and only two in vehicle drivers. Seven (17.5%) of the remaining fractures occurred after falls from a height with two (5%) being associated with falls down stairs and a further two (5%) with crushing injuries.

Open fractures of the fibula

Isolated fractures of the fibula that do not represent suprasyndesmotic ankle fractures are very rare and only 28 were diagnosed during the period of the study. All of these were low velocity injuries and no open fibula fractures were seen.

Open femoral fractures

If the femur is considered in its entirety then only 1.4% of fractures involving the femur are open. However, this figure disguises the fact that the femoral diaphysis is second only to the tibial diaphysis in its susceptibility to open fractures. The large numbers of proximal femoral fractures coupled with the extremely low incidence of associated open injuries accounts for the fact that the overall figure for open femoral fractures is much lower than the equivalent figure for the tibia.

The incidence of open fractures of the femoral diaphysis is about half that of the tibial diaphysis, this probably being caused by the relative protection provided by the bulky thigh muscles and the fact that the car bumpers tend to strike the proximal tibia. The average age of the open femoral diaphyseal fracture group was younger than the equivalent tibial group, at 32.7 years. A full breakdown of the femoral diaphyseal group according to their Gustilo group and average age is shown in Table 3.8. Comparison of Table 3.5 with Table 3.8 shows remarkable similarities between open femoral and tibial fractures. As with the tibial diaphysis type III open femoral diaphyseal fractures are relatively common, accounting for 63% of the group. Again IIIb fractures are the commonest subgroup and IIIc fractures are relatively unusual, although somewhat more common than IIIc tibial diaphyseal fractures. The major difference between open tibial and femoral diaphyseal fractures is that virtually all open femoral fractures occur as a result of road-traffic accidents or falls from a height. All but seven of the open femoral diaphyseal fractures occurred in road-traffic accidents, four of the others occurring in falls from a height with one each from a crush injury, a simple fall and an explosion. Further analysis of the road-traffic accident patients showed that 29.6% of open femoral fractures occurred in pedestrians, 42.6% in vehicle occupants and a further 27.8% in motorcycle drivers or passengers. Interestingly, 69.6% of the fractures sustained by vehicle occupants occurred to the driver rather than the passenger and it would appear that while the severe open tibial fracture occurs mainly in motorcyclists, it is car drivers who are more likely to sustain severe open femoral fractures.

Open fractures of the distal femur

Distal femoral fractures are very much less common than femoral diaphyseal fractures, but there is a comparatively high incidence of open fractures (Table 3.3). It is interesting to note that the incidence is very similar to that of open distal humeral fractures (Table 3.2). Eleven supracondylar and intercondylar open femoral fractures were treated during the study. This group of patients was older than the femoral diaphyseal group with an average age of 41.6 years. Three (27.3%) of the fractures were Gustilo type I, two (18.2%) were type II and the remaining six (54.5%) were type III, all being IIIb in severity. Two (18.2%) fractures occurred after a simple fall and two (18.2%) were caused by a fall from a height. However, the majority (63.6%) of open distal femoral fractures were caused by road-traffic accidents. Of these, only one occurred in a pedestrian and it would appear that vehicle drivers and motorcyclists are more at risk of open distal femoral fractures.

Open fractures of the proximal femur

Proximal femoral fractures are usually the most common fracture admitted to orthopaedic trauma wards, but open proximal fractures are extremely rare. The reason for this is obvious, as most proximal femoral fractures are low-velocity injuries occurring in the elderly after a simple fall. In the period under review, there was only one open proximal femoral fracture. This was a type I open intertrochanteric fracture in a

40-year-old car driver. There were no open subcapital or femoral head fractures.

Open fractures of the patella

As previously noted, open fractures of the distal femur and the patella have a similar incidence. They also have a similar average age, the 27 patients with open patella fractures having an average age of 41.3 years. However, the open patella fractures were less severe than the open distal femoral fracture group, there being nine (33.3%) Gustilo type III fractures, eight of these being IIIa in severity. A further five (18.5%) were type I and the remaining thirteen (48.1%) were type II. As with fractures of the tibia and femur, road-traffic accidents are an important cause of patella fractures, being responsible for 22 (81.4%) of the group. Three of the remaining fractures occurred after a fall from a height and two after a simple fall. Fifteen (68.2%) of the road-traffic accident fractures occurred in vehicle occupants with five (22.7%) occurring in motor-cyclists and two (9.1%) in pedestrians.

Open fractures of the foot

Table 3.3 indicates that fractures of the foot are remarkably common, 2676 being seen in the study period. Open fractures of the bones of the foot occurred in 3.1% of cases. Fractures of the metatarsus accounted for 45.1% of all foot fractures, but very few of these were open. Fractures of the phalanges were less common, accounting for 18.2% of foot fractures, but 8.6% of the phalangeal fractures were open. Tarsal fractures were relatively common, but again open fractures accounted for only 3.1% of all tarsal fractures.

Analysis of the 30 open tarsal fractures showed that there were three types of open fractures. Twelve of the fractures were open calcaneal fractures and a further five were open fractures of the talus. The remaining thirteen open fractures involved one or more of the other tarsal bones. The average age of the tarsal open fracture group was 35.2 years. The fractures tended to be severe in that no Gustilo type I

fractures were seen. Nine (30.0%) of the fractures were type II in severity and the remaining 21 (70.0%) were type III. Eleven (36.6%) of the latter fractures were IIIa, seven (23.3%) were IIIb and the remaining 3 (10.0%) were IIIc. Thus tarsal fractures have the highest incidence of type III open fractures of any of the body areas. Thirteen (43.3%) of the tarsal fractures occurred in road-traffic accidents, nine (30.0%) were caused by a fall from a height, five (16.7%) followed a blow or crushing injury and one fracture each was caused by a lawn mower injury, a fall and an animal bite.

Analysis of the open calcaneal fracture group showed that the average age was 34.9 years. Four fractures (33.3%) were Gustilo type II and the remaining eight (66.6%) were type III (five type IIIa, 3 type IIIb). Six (54.5%) were caused by falls from a height with three (27.3%) being caused by road-traffic accidents and the remaining two (18.2%) by a crushing injury.

The patients who had the five open talar fractures were the youngest group, with an average age of 30.6 years. There was one type II fracture and four type IIIa fractures. Three of the fractures resulted from road-traffic accidents, one from a fall and one from a crushing injury.

The thirteen other tarsal fractures occurred in a slightly older group with an average age of 36.1 years. Four (30.8%) were type II, the remaining nine (69.2%) being type III fractures. Two (15.4%) of the type III fractures were IIIa, four (30.8%) were IIIb and the remaining three (23.1%) were IIIc. Six (46.1%) were caused by road-traffic accidents, three (23.1%) by falls from a height, two (15.4%) followed crushing injuries with one fracture being caused by a fall and one by an animal bite.

The open metatarsal fractures predominantly involved the hallux metatarsal with seven (63.6%) of the eleven metatarsal fractures occurring in this bone. The remaining four (36.4%) occurred between metatarsals two and four. There were no open fractures of the fifth metatarsal. The average age of the metatarsal group was 38.5 years. Three (27.2%) of the fractures were Gustilo type I, four (36.4%) were type II and four (36.4%) were type III (two type IIIa, two type IIIb). Four (36.4%) occurred in road-traffic accidents, five (45.5%) in crushing injuries, one after an assault and one in an accident with a lawn mower.

Table 3.9 Gustilo types, average age and percentage of simple falls in open fractures of the distal radius and ulna

Gustilo type	Total (n)	Percentage	Average age (years)	Simple falls (%)
I	51	67.1	69.2	80.4
II	19	25.0	57.7	52.6
IIIa	6	7.9	50.8	0
IIIb	1	1.3	17.0	0

The commonest bones in the foot to sustain open fractures are the phalanges with 8.6% of these fractures being open. The average age of this group was 38 years. Twelve (28.6%) were Gustilo type I, twenty-two (52.4%) were type II and only eight (19%) were type III. Five of the type III fractures were IIIa in severity with relatively minor fractures and major soft tissue injuries, and the remaining three were IIIc fractures with gross tissue destruction. All of the IIIc fractures were treated by amputation. Twenty-two (52.4%) of the open phalangeal fractures occurred in crushing injuries and nine (21.4%) were caused by cutting or sawing accidents, often with lawn mowers. Seven (16.6%) followed road-traffic accidents and of the remaining four (9.5%) injuries two occurred in falls and two in falls from a height.

Open fractures of the upper limb

Table 3.2 indicates that fractures of the upper limb are more commonly seen than fractures of the lower limbs, although open upper-limb fractures occur less frequently. Many of the common upper-limb fractures are frequently treated on an out-patient basis and, as trauma statistics are usually centred around in-patient work, the surgeon may be unaware of the relative frequency of upper-limb fractures. There are certain similarities between the epidemiology of open fractures of the upper and lower limbs. Comparison of Tables 3.2 and 3.3 shows that the diaphyses of the long bones are more at risk of open fracture although the humerus and forearm

diaphyses show a lower incidence than those of the femur and tibia. Open distal humeral fractures occur with a very similar frequency to open distal femoral fractures. As in the lower limb, the phalanges of the upper limb have a high incidence of open fracture. Otherwise, the incidence of open fractures in the upper limb is remarkably low.

As in the lower limb, the overall incidence of fractures in the distal long bones is higher than in the proximal long bone, with an overall incidence of 2.5% open fractures involving the forearm bones compared with 1.9% in the humerus. Thus forearm fractures will be discussed first.

Open fractures of the radial and ulnar diaphyses

Table 3.1 shows that 9.3% of all fractures of the radial and ulnar diaphyses were open. Twenty-eight (68.3%) of the open fractures involved both the radius and the ulna with eleven (26.8%) only involving the ulna and two (4.9%) the radius. The average age of the whole group was 34.5 years, there being no significant difference in age between fractures involving both bones and those involving one bone. Overall the fractures tend to be less severe than the equivalent tibial fractures, with twenty (48.8%) being Gustilo type I, nine (21.9%) being type II and the remaining twelve (29.3%) being type III. Of the type III fractures, four were IIIa, seven were IIIb and there was one IIIc fracture which eventually resulted in amputation. Comparison of the open fractures involving both bones with those only involving the radius or ulna showed that 32.1% of the former were type III compared to 23.1% of the latter. A review of the causes of open fractures in the complete forearm group shows that eighteen (43.9%) were the result of road-traffic accidents. Six (14.6%) occurred in sports injuries with six more following direct blows or crushes to the forearm. The remainder were caused by simple falls (4), cutting injuries (4), a fall down stairs (1) and a shotgun wound (1). It is not all that surprising that a comparatively high number of open fractures (36.4%) of the ulna followed a direct blow to the bone.

Open fracture of the proximal radius and ulna

These fractures are very uncommon. Most elbow fractures follow simple falls on the outstretched arm and the resulting fractures are usually closed. Of the sixteen open proximal radius or ulna fractures seen, none was associated with isolated radial head or neck fractures. Fifteen of the fractures were associated with the olecranon, this area of the ulna being subcutaneous and therefore at risk. The remaining fracture was a complex fracture of the proximal radius and ulna and was grade IIIa in severity. The average age of this group was older than the diaphyseal fracture group at 46.1 years. Five of the open olecranon fractures were Gustilo type I in severity, seven were type II and three were type IIIa fractures. Thus it is clear that open olecranon fractures follow relatively low energy injuries. As with other fractures, the IIIa fractures tend to occur in older patients with more vulnerable soft tissues and often less severe fracture patterns. The average age for the type IIIa olecranon fracture group was 59 years. Eight (50%) of the fractures occurred in road-traffic accidents, three (18.7%) in assaults, two (12.5%) each in simple falls and falls from a height with the remaining one being a sporting injury.

Open fractures of the distal radius and ulna

Table 3.1 shows that, in numerical terms, open fractures of the distal forearm are the third most common open fracture that surgeons will encounter, after fractures of the tibial diaphysis and fractures of the hand phalanges. However, as distal radial fractures are so common the relative incidence of open fractures is comparatively low, being only 2.3% of all distal forearm fractures. As expected, these are mainly fractures in older patients with an average age of 64.3 years. Thirty-six (46.7%) of the 77 fractures occurred in patients of 70 years or older. The relative incidence of the different Gustilo fracture types is shown in Table 3.9. Open fractures of the distal radius are rarely severe, often representing laceration of the skin from within by a bone fragment. Thus, 66.2% of the series were Gustilo type I in severity and 24.7%

were type II. Only 9.1% were type III, all but one being IIIa fractures. Table 3.9 also indicates that the more severe open distal radius and ulna fractures were seen in younger patients and the simple falls which account for 66.2% of the injuries virtually always produced less severe open fractures. The remaining open distal radial fractures resulted from road-traffic accidents in fourteen (18.2%) patients, falls from a height in seven (9.1%) patients, falls down stairs in two patients and one patient each sustained their fracture as a result of an animal bite, a crushing injury and an assault.

Open fractures of the humerus

Humeral fractures are much less common than fractures of the radius and ulna, accounting for only 6.8% of all the fractures in the series. Both the humeral diaphysis and the distal humerus show a significant incidence of open fractures, with both areas having a similar frequency (Table 3.1). The proximal humerus is relatively protected from open injury.

Open fractures of the humeral diaphysis

Eighteen open humeral diaphyseal fractures were seen during the period of the study. The average age of this group was 47.4 years. The humerus is relatively protected from severe open injury and twelve (66.6%) of the open fractures were Gustilo type I. A further four (22.2%) were type II and there were only two (11.1%) type III fractures, one of these being a IIIa fracture and the other a IIIb. Ten (55.5%) of the fractures occurred in road-traffic accidents, five (27.8%) followed a simple fall in elderly patients (the average age of this subgroup was 72.4 years), two (11.1%) followed a direct blow or crushing injury and the remaining fracture was a sporting injury.

Proximal humeral fractures

Open fractures of the proximal humerus are as rare as open fractures of the proximal femur.

Only five were seen in the study period, giving an incidence of 0.3%. Closed proximal humeral fractures frequently occur in the osteoporotic bone of the elderly, but the open proximal humeral fractures in this series followed road-traffic accidents and the average age was comparatively young at 31.8 years. Three fractures were Gustilo type II in severity, the other two being type IIIa fractures.

Distal humeral fractures

Open distal humeral fractures occur with an incidence similar to that of the humeral diaphysis (Table 3.2) and the distal femur (Table 3.3). Seventeen open distal humeral fractures were seen in the study period. The average age was 44.0 years. As with other open upper limb fractures open distal humeral fractures tended not to be severe. Eight (47.1%) were Gustilo type I, seven (41.2%) were type II and the remaining two (11.8%) were type III (one IIIa and the other IIIb in severity). There were two basic modes of injury: road-traffic accidents and falls. Six (35.3%) of the fractures followed road accidents with a further six (35.3%) being associated with simple falls. Four (23.5%) occurred in a fall from a height and the remaining one followed a fall down stairs.

Open fractures of the hand

The spectrum of open fractures of the hand has changed considerably in many areas over the past 15–20 years. The decline of heavy industry and improved safety regulations have greatly reduced the incidence of severe hand injuries and open carpal and metacarpal fractures are much less common than in the past. Table 3.2 indicates that open fractures comprise 4.2% of all hand fractures, with the incidence of open phalangeal fractures greatly outweighing the incidence of open carpal and metacarpal fractures.

Open carpal fractures

Fifteen open carpal fractures were treated in the study period. These tended to involve younger

patients, the average age of the open carpal fracture group being 32.6 years. The carpus appears to be protected from severe open fractures and it is interesting to observe that 12 (80%) of the fractures were type III in severity. Ten of these were IIIa with the remaining two being type IIIb fractures. There were two (13.3%) type I fractures and one (6.7%) type II fracture. The majority of the open carpal fractures were caused by a direct blow or crushing injury with seven (46.7%) occurring this way. A further four (26.7%) occurred in road-traffic accidents, three (20%) were caused by cutting injuries with circular saws and the remaining fracture was caused by an explosion.

Open metacarpal fractures

Sixteen open metacarpal fractures were treated. For the purpose of this study, impaction fractures of the metacarpal head caused by a tooth indentation secondary to a punch were excluded. The average age of the open metacarpal group was 42.8 years. None of the open metacarpal fractures were severe with seven (43.7%) being Gustilo type I and the remaining nine (56.3%) being type II. There were no type III fractures. Predictably in many cases the patient was the aggressor in a fight and nine (56.3%) of the fractures were sustained in an assault or a fight; two (12.5%) each occurred in simple falls, falls from a height and road-traffic accidents and one was caused by a power saw.

Open phalangeal fractures

Open fractures of the finger phalanges were the most numerous open fractures treated in the study period: 297 fractures were seen, representing 9.7% of all finger phalangeal fractures. The average age was 39.5 years. The Gustilo classification is particularly difficult to apply to phalangeal injuries, especially as many of the fractures are associated with non-viable fingertips. It was considered that as vascular reconstruction of the fingertip is not feasible these should not be classified as IIIc fractures. Rather they were classified according to the size of the skin wound and the extent of contamination with the IIIc description being reserved for severe fractures of the finger rather than just the tip. Ninety-five (32%) of the open phalangeal fractures were Gustilo type I, 157 (52.9%) were type II and the remaining 45 (15.1%) were type III. Not surprisingly, these open fractures showed the highest incidence of type IIIc fractures with eighteen (40%) of the type III fractures having significant vessel damage. Thirteen (51.1%) of the type III fractures were IIIa, the remaining two (8.9%) being IIIb fractures. The aetiology of open phalangeal fractures is different from other open fractures. Most open phalangeal fractures are either caused by crushing in a machine or car door or by being struck by a sharp object such as a saw. It may be difficult to distinguish between the two as industrial machines frequently both crush and cut, but it was considered that 184 (61.9%) of open phalangeal fractures followed a crushing injury and 75 (25.2%) were caused by a cutting or sawing mechanism. Fourteen (4.7%) followed simple falls, seven (2.4%) occurred following direct blows or in assaults, four (1.3%) were associated with sports activities, five (1.7%) were caused by dog bites and only eight (2.7%) were caused in road-traffic accidents.

Open fractures of the limb girdles and axial skeleton

Fractures of the limb girdles and axial skeleton are relatively common with 9.7% of all fractures occurring in the clavicle, scapula, pelvis or spine. However, open fractures are extremely rare and many surgeons may never encounter one. In the study period, there were two open clavicular fractures; one was a Gustilo type I mid-shaft fracture occurring in a 27-year-old car driver following a road-traffic accident and the other was a type III fracture sustained in a game of ice hockey. There was one type I open scapula fracture which occurred in a 28-year-old patient involved in a road-traffic accident.

Six open pelvic fractures were seen in the study period. Open pelvic fractures carry a poor prognosis as they only occur in severe high velocity injuries and are frequently associated with massive soft-tissue damage. The open pelvic fractures in this series were all associated with extreme pelvic ring damage and were all type III fractures, four being technically type IIIa and one being IIIb in severity. The average age of the patients was 29.3 years and all were injured in road-traffic accidents. There were no open spinal fractures.

References

British Orthopaedic Association (1992) The management of skeletal trauma in the United Kingdom.

Court-Brown CM, McBirnie J (1995) The epidemiology of tibial fractures, *J Bone Joint Surg (Br):* **77B**: 417–21.

Gustilo RB, Anderson JT (1976) Prevention of infection in treatment of 1025 open fractures of long bones: retrospective and prospective analysis, *J Bone Joint Surg (Am)* **58A**: 453–8.

Gustilo RB, Mendoza RM, Williams DM (1984) Problems in the management of type III (severe) open fractures: a new classification of type III open fractures, *J Trauma* **24**: 742–6.

4
Microbiology of open fractures

D.T. Tsukayama and R.B. Gustilo

Intact skin is an important mechanical barrier to potential microbial pathogens. When this crucial host defence is breached in an open fracture, bacteria are introduced into the injured site. The soft tissue adjacent to the fracture has suffered significant, often extensive, injury, providing a favourable environment for growth of bacteria and establishment of infection. It has been shown that the risk of infection in open fractures is proportional to the extent of injury to the soft tissue.

When cultures are obtained from the open wound prior to any surgical or antibiotic therapy, most will grow bacteria which contaminate the wound at, or shortly after, the time of injury. However, most infections following open fractures are caused by bacteria which are acquired after hospitalization, most commonly *Staphylococcus aureus* and facultative Gram-negative bacilli. The management of open fractures requires knowledge of the bacteria which are most likely to cause infection, and of the antibiotics which are most useful against these pathogens.

The risk of infection in open fractures correlates with the degree of soft-tissue injury associated with the fracture. Open fractures can be classified into three major types (Gustilo and Anderson 1976).

1. A type I open fracture has a wound that is relatively clean and <1 cm long.
2. A type II open fracture has a laceration >1 cm long without extensive soft-tissue damage, flaps, or avulsions.
3. A type III open fracture has extensive soft-tissue damage. Included in this category are open segmental fractures, fractures with arterial injury, high-velocity gunshot wounds, shotgun injuries and untreated injuries >8 hours old. Type III open fractures can be

further classified into three subtypes (Gustilo et al 1984):

(a) Type IIIa open fractures have adequate soft-tissue coverage of the fractured bone despite extensive laceration or flaps. Open fractures resulting from high-energy trauma are also considered type IIIa, even when the wound is relatively small, because of the extensive damage to the underlying soft tissue.

(b) Type IIIb open fractures have extensive soft-tissue injury with periosteal stripping and bone exposure.

(c) Type IIIc open fractures have an associated arterial injury requiring repair.

Infections in type I and type II open fractures are infrequent. Infection rates in type I fractures range from 0 to 2% and in type II fractures, 2–7%. The overall rate of infection in type III fractures is often quoted as 10–25%, but can be as high as 50% in types IIIb and IIIc (Gustilo et al 1990).

The bacteria which cause infections in open fractures come from two major sources. First, bacteria may contaminate the wound at, or shortly after, the time of injury. Studies have shown that bacteria are present in 60–70% of open fractures in cultures obtained prior to treatment (Gustilo and Anderson 1976, Lawrence et al 1978, Patzakis and Wilkins 1989). Most of these isolates are normal skin flora such as coagulase-negative staphylococci, *Proprionibacterium acnes*, *Corynebacterium* species and *Micrococcus*, or environmental contaminants such as *Bacillus* or *Clostridium* (Lawrence et al 1978). These bacteria rarely cause infection. When more virulent pathogens such as Gram-negative bacilli gain access to the open wound, the risk of infection is greater. Patzakis and Wilkins (1989) reported that organisms isolated from the initial cultures were present in 66% of open fracture wound infections. Benson et al (1983) reported that, although Gram-negative bacilli were infrequently recovered in initial cultures, 50% went on to cause clinical infection. A pathogenic role for bacteria which colonize the wound soon after injury is suggested by studies which show that early presumptive antibiotic therapy is effective in decreasing the infection rate in open fractures (Patzakis et al 1974, Worlock et al 1988). In a prospective, double-blind, randomized study of the efficacy of early antibiotic therapy in the management of open fractures, Patzakis et al (1974) reported an infection rate of 2.3% in the group treated with cephalothin in contrast to a 13.9% rate in the placebo group. Specific pathogens are associated with certain types of environmental exposure (Tsukayama and Gustilo 1990). Gas gangrene caused by *Clostridium perfringens* can follow farm-related injuries. Exposure to fresh water is associated with infections by *Pseudomonas aeruginosa* and *Aeromonas hydrophila*. Salt-water contamination is associated with infection by *Aeromonas*, *Vibrio* and *Erysipelothrix*.

The second major source for bacteria which cause infections in open fractures is the hospital. The most frequently cultured pathogens causing infection after open fracture are bacteria such as *Pseudomonas*, *Staphylococcus aureus* and *Enterococcus* which are acquired after hospitalization (Roth et al 1986, Dellinger et al 1988). We found that only 7% of the bacteria isolated in the initial culture taken from the wound prior to treatment are recovered in subsequent infections (Tsukayama and Gustilo 1990). In a study of type IIIb open fractures, we found that bacteria which were recovered in the initial cultures were never implicated in later infection unless they were Gram-negative bacilli (Fischer et al 1991). Lawrence et al (1978) found that 64% of patients with open fractures had positive initial cultures, but only 3% subsequently became infected. The number, as well as the type, of bacteria present may be an important risk factor for infection. Both Moore et al (1989) and Cooney et al (1980) found that bacterial counts >10^5 colony-forming units per gram of tissue were associated with an increased risk of infection. We found no such correlation in a limited study of type III open fractures (Gustilo and Gruninger 1987). Merritt (1988) has reported that high bacterial counts in cultures taken after surgical debridement, but not before, are associated with a higher risk of infection. Antibiotic therapy also influences the microbiology of infections in open fractures (Antrum and Solomkin 1987). Open wounds become colonized with bacteria which are resistant to the antibiotics which are administered to the patient. Following the institution of antistaphylococcal antibiotic therapy, investigators noted an increase in the incidence of infections caused by Gram-negative bacilli. The addition of Gram-negative antibiotic coverage was associated with a decrease in the infection rate from 29.1% to 8.8% in type III open fractures at our institution (Gustilo and Gruninger 1987), but highly resistant pathogens such as *Pseudomonas aeruginosa* and *Enterococcus* continue to pose a significant problem. It is becoming increasingly clear that antibiotics alone will not prevent bacterial colonization of open wounds, but may exert a selective pressure favouring resistant organisms.

Table 4.1 Microbiology of osteomyelitis. Hennepin County Medical Center, 1986–1991

Bacterial group	n
Gram-positive cocci and bacilli	
Coagulase-positive *Staphylococcus*	81
Coagulase-negative *Staphylococcus*	28
Beta-haemolytic *Streptococcus*	18
Viridans *Streptococcus*	4
Enterococcus	11
Corynebacterium	4
Bacillus	4
Gram-negative bacilli	
Pseudomonas aeruginosa	21
Enterobacter	11
Escherichia coli	8
Serratia	7
Proteus	7
Acinetobacter	6
Klebsiella	3
Morganella	3
Aeromonas	2
Achromobacter	1
Pasteurella	1
Haemophilus	1
Anaerobes	
Bacteroides	3
Peptostreptococcus	9
Clostridium	2
Other	3
Miscellaneous	
Mycobacterium	1
Candida	2

Table 4.1 shows the microbiology of osteomyelitis at Hennepin County Medical Center (Minneapolis, Minnesota) from 1986 to 1991. There were 152 patients; 54 had polymicrobial infections. Coagulase-positive *Staphylococcus* was the single most frequently recovered pathogen, comprising 34% of all isolates. Gram-negative bacilli, when considered in aggregate, accounted for 30% of the total. *Pseudomonas aeruginosa* was the most frequently recovered Gram-negative bacillus. Other commonly recovered pathogens included *Enterobacter* and *Enterococcus*. The most frequently recovered anaerobe was *Peptostreptococcus*. A review of the recent literature on the microbiology of infections following open fractures shows similar results (Patzakis et al 1985, Roth et al 1986, Caudle and Stern 1987, Dellinger et al 1988). Gram-negative pathogens show an even greater predominance, accounting for 45% of a combined total of 155 isolates. Coagulase-positive staphylococci were found in 23% of cases and *Enterococcus* in 15%.

Common pathogens

Coagulase-positive staphylococci

These bacteria are the most important pathogens of musculoskeletal infections. The only significant coagulase-positive staphylococcus for humans is *Staphylococcus aureus*. Humans are the natural reservoir for *S. aureus*, carrying organisms in the nasopharynx and transiently on the skin, especially when skin is traumatized. Infections with this bacteria are characterized by purulence and abscess formation at the site of infection. Bacteraemia leading to metastatic foci of infection, and systemic toxicity including septic shock, also occur. Most coagulase-positive staphylococci are now resistant to penicillin, but remain sensitive to nafcillin, oxacillin and most cephalosporins. The combination of a penicillin with a beta-lactamase inhibitor such as clavulanate or sulbactam is also active against these organisms. Third-generation cephalosporins such as cefotaxime and ceftriaxone are less active against staphylococci than first- or second-generation cephalosporins, but have sufficient activity to be effective when given at maximal

doses. Alternative antibiotics include vancomycin, clindamycin, imipenem–cilastatin and trimethoprim–sulphamethoxazole. Although treatment of *S. aureus* has been relatively straightforward since the introduction of antistaphylococcal penicillins and first-generation cephalosporins, the emergence of methicillin-resistant *Staphylococcus aureus* (MRSA) has changed the management of these infections, especially in areas where there is a high prevalence of methicillin resistance. Methicillin-resistant staphylococci are resistant to all penicillins, cephalosporins and other related beta-lactams. Vancomycin is the only antibiotic with proven clinical efficacy against MRSA. For patients unable to tolerate vancomycin, there is no alternative agent of comparable efficacy. We have used quinolones and trimethoprim–sulphamethoxazole in these patients with some success.

Streptococci

There are several classification schemes for streptococci, resulting in some confusion in the naming of these bacteria. Major pathogens include *Streptococcus pyogenes* (also commonly referred to as group A *Streptococcus*), *Streptococcus agalactiae* (group B *Streptococcus*), *Streptococcus pneumoniae* and alpha-haemolytic (or viridans) streptococci.

These bacteria are normal inhabitants of the mouth, pharynx and skin, and also of the gastrointestinal and genito-urinary tract. Infections associated with these pathogens include endocarditis, pneumonia, abscesses, upper-respiratory infections and bone-and-joint infections. Streptococci are susceptible to many antibiotics including beta-lactams, vancomycin, clindamycin and erythromycin. Quinolones and trimethoprim–sulphamethoxazole are somewhat less active. Penicillin G remains the antibiotic of choice for streptococcal infections.

Enterococci

Formerly classified as group D streptococci, these bacteria, which are part of the normal flora of the gastrointestinal tract, are implicated in urinary-tract infections, endocarditis and intra-abdominal infections. Orthopaedic infections with this pathogen include cellulitis, infected ulcers, prosthetic joint infections and wound-and-bone infections following trauma. They are more resistant than streptococci to most antibiotics. Of the penicillins, only ampicillin, penicillin G and ureidopenicillins such as piperacillin are effective agents. Imipenem is active against *Enterococcus faecalis* but not *Enterococcus faecium*. Vancomycin is an effective alternative in penicillin-allergic patients. Recent reports suggest that enterococcal resistance to multiple antibiotics, including ampicillin and vancomycin, may be increasing (Herman and Gerding 1991). Enterococci are not susceptible to cephalosporins or clindamycin. It is possible that one may encounter an enterococcal infection for which there is no effective antibiotic therapy. Another issue in the treatment of enterococcal infections is whether bactericidal activity is needed. Bactericidal activity can only be achieved with a combination of aminoglycoside plus either a penicillin or vancomycin. Some infections such as enterococcal endocarditis appear to require bactericidal therapy to eradicate the infection, but whether combination therapy is needed for other sites of infection such as the bone is not clear. Our practice has been to treat with one systemic antibiotic (either a penicillin or vancomycin) and place aminoglycoside-impregnated beads at the site of a bone infection.

Enteric Gram-negative bacilli

As the name implies, enteric Gram-negative bacilli are colonizers of the gastrointestinal tract. Rarely seen as pathogens in community-acquired infections (other than urinary-tract infections), they assume a more prominent role as a nosocomial cause of bacteraemia, pneumonitis, urinary-tract infection, and wound infection. The musculoskeletal infections associated with these pathogens include post-operative wound infections, soft-tissue infections secondary to bacteraemia, infected ulcers secondary to vascular insufficiency or pressure

necrosis and wound-and-bone infections following open fractures. The introduction of many highly effective antibiotics of relatively low toxicity has greatly enhanced our ability to treat these pathogens. Beta-lactams such as extended spectrum penicillins, penicillins combined with a beta-lactamase inhibitor, imipenem and aztreonam have become the agents of choice in the treatment of Gram-negative bacilli infections.

Quinolones and trimethoprim-sulphamethoxazole are two alternative agents that have the advantage of oral administration. Although aminoglycosides have excellent *in vitro* activity against Gram-negative bacilli, we rarely administer these antibiotics systemically because of the potential for serious adverse reactions in patients who generally require prolonged, high-dose treatment.

Pseudomonas aeruginosa

This organism can be associated with water-related infection, but is primarily acquired in the hospital. The spectrum of disease which it causes is similar to enteric Gram-negative bacilli, but *Pseudomonas aeruginosa* can be more difficult to treat. It is susceptible to fewer antimicrobial agents, and even when susceptible, requires a higher concentration of drug to inhibit its growth. Resistance to antibiotics being used for treatment may develop rapidly. The antibiotics which can be used to treat *Pseudomonas* infections include ceftazidime, imipenem, aztreonam, ureidopenicillins (piperacillin, mezlocillin, azlocillin) aminoglycosides and quinolones. Among the presently available quinolones, ciprofloxacin appears to have the best *in vitro* activity. Reports of treatment failure utilizing a single antibiotic have led to the recommendation that combination therapy be used in the treatment of serious *Pseudomonas* infections (Korvick and Yu 1991). The combination of an aminoglycoside and a beta-lactam results in synergistic *in vitro* activity. We treat *Pseudomonas* infections with one systemic agent, usually of the beta-lactam class, and place tobramycin beads at the infection site.

Anaerobes

In some reports, anaerobes are recovered in more than 20% of cases of osteomyelitis (Lewis et al 1978, Hall et al 1983, Templeton et al 1983). The most commonly recovered anaerobes are *Peptostreptococcus* and *Bacteroides*. *Clostridium* should be suspected when there is a possibility of faecal contamination such as injuries that occur in a farm setting. Anaerobic infections most often occur as part of a polymicrobial infection. Penicillin is considered the drug of choice for *Clostridium* and *Peptostreptococcus*, although clostridial resistance to penicillin has been reported. Metronidazole has excellent activity against *Bacteroides* and *Clostridium*, but may be less active against anaerobic Gram-positive cocci. Clindamycin usually is active against both *Bacteroides* and anaerobic Gram-positive cocci, but some clostridia are resistant. Imipenem, and beta-lactamase inhibitor combinations are usually active *in vitro* against all these pathogens, but clinical experience with these agents in clostridial infections is limited.

References

Antrum RM, Solomkin JS (1987) A review of antibiotic prophylaxis for open fractures, *Orthopedic Rev* **16**: 246–54.

Benson DR, Riggins RS, Lawrence RM, Heoprich PD, Huston AC, Harrison JA (1983) Treatment of open fractures: a prospective study, *J Trauma* **23** 25–30.

Caudle RJ, Stern PJ (1987) Severe open fractures of the tibia, *J Bone Joint Surg* **69A**: 801–6.

Cooney WP, Fitzgerald RH Jr, Dobyns JH, Washington JA (1980) Quantitative wound cultures in upper extremity trauma, *J Trauma* **22**: 112–17.

Dellinger EP, Miller SD, Wertz MJ, Grypma M, Droppert B, Anderson PA (1988) Risk of infection after open fracture of the arm or leg, *Arch Surg* **123**: 1320–7.

Fischer MD, Gustilo RB, Varecka TF (1991) The timing of flap coverage, bone-grafting, and intramedullary nailing in patients who have a fracture of the tibial shaft with extensive soft-tissue injury, *J Bone Joint Surg* **73A**: 1316–22.

Gustilo RB, Anderson JT (1976) Prevention of infection in the treatment of one thousand and twenty-five open fractures of long bones, *J Bone Joint Surg* **58A**: 453–8.

Gustilo RB, Gruninger RP (1987) Classification of type III (severe) open fractures relative to treatment and results, *Orthopedics* **10**: 1781–8.

Gustilo RB, Mendoza RM, Williams DN (1984) Problems in the management of type III (severe) open fractures: a new classification of type III open fractures, *J Trauma* **24**: 742–6.

Gustilo RB, Merkow RL, Templeman D (1990) Current concepts review the management of open fractures, *J Bone Joint Surg* **72A**: 299–304.

Hall BB, Fitzgerald RH Jr, Rosenblatt JE (1983) Anaerobic osteomyelitis, *J Bone Joint Surg* **65A**: 30–5.

Herman DJ, Gerding DN (1991) Antimicrobial resistance among enterococci, *Antimicrob Agents Chemother* **35**: 1–4.

Korvick JA, Yu VL (1991) Antimicrobial agent therapy for *Pseudomonas aeruginosa*, *Antimicrob Agents Chemother* **35**: 2167–72.

Lawrence RM, Hoeprich PD, Huston AC, Benson DR, Riggins RS (1978) Quantitative microbiology of traumatic orthopedic wounds, *J Clin Microb* **8**: 673–5.

Lewis RP, Sutter VL, Finegold SM (1978) Bone infections involving anaerobic bacteria, *Medicine* **57**: 279–305.

Merritt K (1988) Factors increasing the risk of infection in patients with open fractures, *J Trauma* **28**: 823–7.

Moore TJ, Mauney C, Barron J (1989) The use of quantitative bacterial counts in open fractures, *Clin Orthop* **248**: 227–30.

Patzakis MJ, Wilkins J (1989) Factors influencing infection rate in open fracture wounds, *Clin Orthop* **243**: 36–40.

Patzakis MJ, Harvey P Jr, Ivler D (1974) The role of antibiotics in the management of open fractures, *J Bone Joint Surg* **56A**: 532–41.

Patzakis MJ, Wilkins J, Wiss DA (1985) Infection following intramedullary nailing of long bones, *Clin Orthop* **212**: 182–91.

Roth AL, Fry DE, Polk HC (1986) Infectious morbidity in extremity fractures, *J Trauma* **26**: 757–61.

Templeton WC III, Wawrukiewicz A, Melo JC, Schiller MG, Raff MJ (1983) Anaerobic osteomyelitis of long bones, *J Bone Joint Surg* **5**: 692–712.

Tsukayama DT, Gustilo RB (1990) Antibiotic management of open fractures. In: Greene, WB, ed, *Instructional Course Lectures*, Vol XXXIX (American Academy of Orthopaedic Surgeons: Chicago) 487–90.

Worlock P, Slack R, Harvey L, Mawhinney R (1988) The prevention of infection in open fractures, *J Bone Joint Surg* **70A**: 1341–7.

5

Pre- and per-operative wound assessment and management

C.M. Court-Brown and G.A. Zych

In current usage, the word 'debridement' is used to describe the operative removal of devitalized, contaminated or dead tissue from a wound. Some surgeons do not approve of the term as it is derived from the French word *débrider* meaning 'to unbridle' and therefore strictly does not describe the surgical procedure that it has come to mean. However, unbridling or incising of the wound is an essential component of the operation of debridement and given this fact and the acceptance of the term in modern surgical practice, it—rather than its synonym 'wound excision'—will be used. Until comparatively recently, surgeons could only carry out a thorough debridement of a Gustilo IIIb or IIIc wound if they accepted that there would be considerable difficulty in reconstructing both the bone stock and soft-tissue envelope. It has only been in the last 15–20 years that advances in plastic surgery techniques have allowed for early closure of large soft-tissue defects. Additionally, the techniques of bone transport, allografting and vascularized bone grafting are also of comparatively recent origin. It is therefore understandable that there is a legacy of conservative debridement and many surgeons still remain concerned about removing large quantities of skin, muscle or devitalized bone. However, if dead or devitalized tissue remains in the wound, the prognosis is poor; there is a high incidence of infection and its attendant problem of non-union. Haury et al (1978) showed that devitalized skin, fat and muscle enhanced infection to a comparable degree. This occurred because of direct bacterial contamination but also because the devitalized tissue inhibits leukocyte function. Thus debridement is very important and the adequacy of its performance on the day of injury

may dictate the prognosis of the fracture. The operation of debridement is essentially straight-forward. It consists of the surgical removal of all dead, devitalized or contaminated tissue. This is supplemented by the use of antibiotics and by mechanical aids such as tissue lavage.

Pre-operative assessment

Much has been written about the pre-operative assessment of polytraumatized patients, many of whom will present with open fractures. This topic has been well covered in other texts (McMurty and McLellan 1990, Border et al 1990) and discussion about the overall pre-operative evaluation of these patients will not be repeated. It is, however, important to remember that the treatment of open fractures may well be affected by the presence of other injuries which might take priority. The physical state of the patient may also influence the surgeon's perception of the open wound. A hypotensive patient who is peripherally shut down may have peripheral pulses that are difficult to palpate suggesting the presence of a Gustilo type IIIc fracture to the inexperienced examiner. Muscle colour may also be influenced by tissue oxygenation and the evaluation of the neurological state of the limb may be profoundly influenced by alteration of the patient's conscious level. Surgeons have become used to assessing the radiological features of the fracture pre-operatively to assist with planning bone fixation. Pre-operative planning may determine the type of implant to be used and where plates and screws are to be employed; pre-operative planning is particularly useful in deciding on the exact location of the implant (Müller et al 1987). However, pre-operative evaluation of the X-rays can also be useful in planning an adequate debridement. There are three principal aspects of pre-operative evaluation to be considered, these being the clinical history and examination, the radiological appearance of the fracture and the characteristics of the open wound.

Clinical history and examination

There are a number of factors to be assessed by the surgeon before debridement is performed. It is important that the surgeon appreciates whether the open fracture has occurred as a result of a high- or low-velocity injury as the former is likely to be associated with greater soft-tissue injury and more bone damage. The cause of the fracture should therefore be known. Open fractures occurring as a result of a road traffic accident, high-velocity gunshot injury, a fall from a height or a direct blow from a heavy object have a worse prognosis than fractures that have followed a simple fall or sporting injury. Where there is a potential for considerable soft-tissue injury, the surgeon should be aware that the debridement may be more extensive and complex soft-tissue and bone reconstruction may eventually be required. The surgeon should also be aware of the age and general health of the patient. Although age does not affect the type or adequacy of debridement performed, elderly bone is more osteoporotic (McCalden et al 1993) and subject to greater comminution than younger bone given an equivalent injury. Where possible, the pre-operative physical and mental state of the patient should also be known. Again the presence of active disease will not affect how the debridement is performed but in the presence of a severe open lower limb fracture, amputation may be more readily considered in a demented patient whose walking ability was markedly restricted pre-operatively. This should not, however, be interpreted as encouraging the use of amputation rather than limb reconstruction in all elderly patients as it should be remembered that these patients are least likely to ambulate with a prosthesis. The surgeon must base the decision regarding amputation or limb reconstruction on the clinical findings taking into consideration the overall state of the patient.

Pre-operative clinical examination is also very important. As has already been suggested, the examining surgeon should be aware of the overall physical state of the patient as well as the nature and distribution of all injuries. Chapter 3 shows that virtually all open fractures occur in the limbs and a thorough examination of the affected limb or limbs is important. Examination of the vascular supply of the limb will help to determine the overall prognosis and whether an amputation needs to be considered. Thus, the peripheral pulses should be palpated and the overall colour and presence of capillary refill assessed. The surgeon must always bear in mind that if the patient is hypotensive or peripherally shut down, an incorrect pre-operative assessment may be made. If there is dubiety about the vascular supply of a limb, a pre-operative angiogram should be obtained. It is also important to carefully examine the neurological status of the limb as abnormal sensation may represent occult intracranial or spinal damage. If there is a peripheral nerve injury associated with the fracture, this suggests the presence of considerable soft-tissue injury and the prognosis for the limb is usually poor. In the lower limb, the association of an open femoral fracture with sciatic nerve transection or an open tibial fracture with division of the posterior tibial nerve may convince the surgeon that an amputation is required. The surgeon should also observe the limb for other skin and soft-tissue problems. Any contamination, road tattooing or abnormal skin markings should be noted. Their presence may well help to define the severity of the open fracture.

Radiological examination

A detailed examination of the pre-operative anteroposterior and lateral X-rays of the fracture should be performed. This is not only important in assisting the planning of the surgical procedure but it also facilitates the performance of an adequate debridement. The purpose of examining the X-rays pre-operatively is to assess the degree of energy involved in the production of the fracture as well as the extent of the soft-tissue injury and the presence of contamination

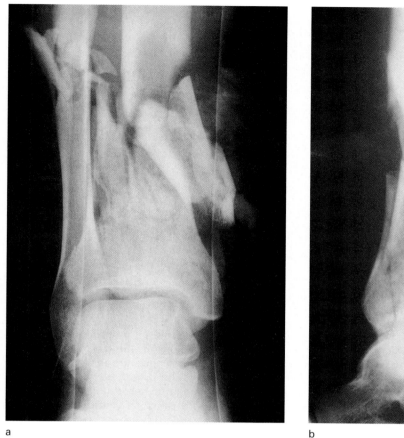

a

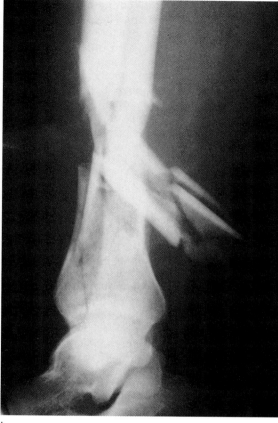

b

Figure 5.1

The anteroposterior (a) and lateral (b) X-rays of a Gustilo IIIb open distal metaphyseal fracture with an undisplaced intra-articular extension. There is considerable bony damage and displacement of bone fragments. The obvious inference is that there is also major soft-tissue damage and many of the loose bone fragments will be denuded of any soft tissue and therefore will be avascular. The fact that the intra-articular extension is undisplaced suggests that it is a relatively minor problem. The periosteum is likely to be intact around the intra-articular extension and the ankle joint does not require to be explored unless there is evidence of local contamination at the time of surgery.

or foreign bodies (Figure 5.1). The presence of air in the soft tissue following fracture may be a useful radiological sign for two reasons. It may indicate that an apparently innocent break in the skin does in fact communicate with an underlying fracture or it may demonstrate the extent of possible soft-tissue damage and contamination. Air may be seen at a considerable distance from the fracture site and the surgeon should always bear in mind that if there is air there may be other contaminants. The extent of the debridement may well therefore be influenced by the spread of air in the tissues on the pre-operative X-ray. Similarly, the appearance of foreign material such as bullets, shot, road dirt, glass or other radiopaque objects will influence the extent of the initial debridement. The degree of soft-tissue damage and associated bone avascularity may be inferred from the initial X-rays. Significant displacement of the bone ends, bone loss, significant bone comminution or the presence of more than one fracture in the bone are all strongly suggestive of a high-velocity injury associated with soft-tissue damage. Segmental fractures also occur in high-energy injuries, although these usually are associated with less muscle damage and periosteal stripping than comminuted fractures. More direct evidence of bone avascularity may be gained by assessing the amount of displacement of bone fragments from their original location within the bone (Figure 5.1). The elastic properties of muscle permit comminuted fracture fragments to displace to a certain extent with a degree of safety, but if the fragments are significantly displaced this suggests that their blood supply has been seriously compromised and they will need to be removed. The radiographic assessment of comminuted bone fragments differs between bones. Open fractures of the femur and tibia are the commonest high-velocity injuries. The muscle attachments in the tibia are such that there is frequently soft-tissue stripping from bone. In the femur, however, the soft-tissue attachment to the linea aspera is very strong and the attached bone fragment usually retains vascularity. As the size of this fragment is frequently large, the surgeon may well not have to remove too much of the femoral diaphysis following severe fracture. This can often be assessed in the pre-operative X-rays. There are a number of other features that may be looked for on the pre-operative X-ray. Extension of the fracture into an adjacent joint suggests possible contamination of the joint which will then require to be opened or examined arthroscopically to assess the degree of contamination. Old injuries may also be noted and the presence of any congenital or developmental anomalies which might confuse a surgeon during debridement will be seen.

Examination of the open wound

There is a tendency for open wounds to be examined by every member of the medical and nursing team prior to surgery. This is unnecessary and can be avoided by an adequate wound examination being carried out when the patient is initially reviewed by an orthopaedic surgeon.

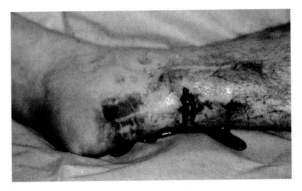

Figure 5.2

The fracture shown in Figure 5.1 was associated with two open wounds. Both were small but the presence of more than one wound suggests considerable local damage. The area between the wounds will be degloved and it is quite possible that the degloved area is much more extensive.

At that time a Polaroid photograph can be taken and other members of the team can subsequently examine the photograph. After the initial inspection the wound should be covered with an antiseptic dressing. Tscherne (1984) and his co-workers demonstrated a reduction in the incidence of sepsis if the wound is kept covered by an antiseptic dressing and not examined repeatedly. If this regime is to be followed, the initial wound inspection should be carried out by an experienced surgeon as much information can be gained. Wound inspection may allow the surgeon to determine the extent of the necessary debridement, to assess the need for a plastic surgeon and to give the patient a pre-operative prognosis if this is required. There is a tendency to use the length of the wound as a measure of the requirement for debridement and as an indicator of prognosis. There is a loose relationship between wound length and prognosis but it should never be assumed that the prognosis is always good if the wound is small. In addition to wound size, the surgeon should note the extent of skin contusion and in particular the area of skin degloving. The number of skin wounds should also be assessed as two or three small wounds close together suggest not only the presence of degloved skin between the wounds, but that the energy associated with the fracture

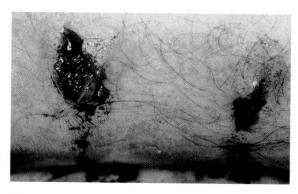

Figure 5.3

A close-up view of the open wounds. Bone is apparent in the lower wound. There does not appear to be significant contamination.

will have significantly damaged other soft tissues (Figure 5.2). The degree of wound and skin contamination should be noted as should the presence of bone fragments at the surface of the wound (Figure 5.3). It is also important to examine the apparently intact skin very carefully as not only may there be other open wounds but there may be skin marking suggestive of localized or generalized crushing injuries.

Operative procedure

To adequately perform debridement the surgeon should have a standardized approach to the procedure which facilitates the exposure of all the affected tissues and removal of all devitalized or dead material. There are a number of basic rules which should be followed.

1. With the exception of low-velocity gunshot wounds, all open fractures require surgical debridement. Failure to do this constitutes inadequate treatment.
2. All affected tissue planes should be opened.
3. The bone ends must be exposed and carefully examined for contamination and soft-tissue stripping.
4. All dead and devitalized tissue must be removed.
5. The wound should not be closed primarily.

There is debate about whether the operation of debridement should be performed under tourniquet to ensure a bloodless field. This may not be possible in treating femoral or humeral open fractures, but it certainly remains an option in open fractures of the forearm, hand, tibia and foot. Proponents advocate its use to ensure a bloodless field and opponents suggest that a bloodless field is contraindicated in an operation designed to examine tissue vascularity. In reality, adequate haemostasis can usually be achieved without a tourniquet but the surgeon should use whichever technique he or she is most comfortable with.

Surgery of the skin

Skin is very resistant to direct trauma but susceptible to shearing forces, the plane of the cleavage being outside the deep fascia. These forces produce degloving injuries which particularly affect the lower limb and may be very extensive or even circumferential. Elderly patients are particularly at risk of degloving injury. Isolated small skin wounds produced by direct trauma may be treated by local excision of the contused skin edge, this being performed prior to extension of the wound to allow for inspection of the underlying tissues. Where there are two or more adjacent wounds (Figures 5.2 and 5.3) these will communicate subcutaneously and they should be treated by connecting the excised wounds or by excising all wounds with an ellipse of skin (Figure 5.4). Where there are two skin incisions separated by a significant distance, it is likely that these will not communicate and usually they can be treated as two separate incisions with separate debridements. After the initial wound excision, it is important that the surgeon look for skin degloving (Figure 5.5). It is preferable to do this before the open wound is extended, as the presence of degloved skin may influence the placement of the wound extensions. Initially, skin degloving should be sought by careful subcutaneous digital examination. Intact tissue planes should not be broken but the surgeon should be

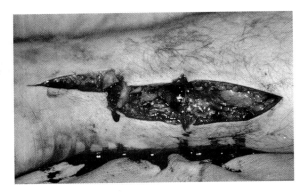

Figure 5.4

The initial incision has been made to include both open wounds. Longitudinal, rather than transverse, incisions should be used. The length of the wound is governed solely by the need to visualize the bone ends and all the affected soft tissues.

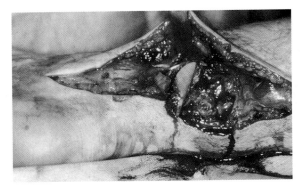

Figure 5.5

Predictably, the degloved area was more extensive than was initially obvious. However, there was excellent dermal bleeding and little more skin resection was required. Pieces of loose bone are seen in the wound.

able to palpate any degloved areas. The area of degloved skin to be removed at the initial debridement is often difficult to determine and will vary according to the location of the wound and the amount of direct skin damage associated with the degloving injury. The surgeon should resect degloved skin until dermal bleeding is encountered. In the lower leg, this may even require circumferential resection but it must be remembered that degloved skin without a blood supply will die and soft-tissue reconstruction will be required. If the appropriate area of degloved skin can be assessed and removed at the initial debridement then a split skin graft can be harvested from the degloved skin for later use. This is impossible once the degloved skin has died.

In an effort to accurately delineate degloved areas McGrouther and Sully (1980) used fluorescein and ultraviolet light. They gave a rapid intravenous infusion of 1 g of 5% fluorescein Na in 200 ml of 1 normal saline over 10 minutes. After a further 10 minutes, ultraviolet light was used in a darkened operating theatre to assess skin viability. A dark blue colour confirms skin death and yellow suggests well-vascularized skin. The significance of mottling is more difficult to determine, but the authors did find the technique to be useful. As with all ancillary techniques, it may

well be difficult to use fluorescein in the emergency situation particularly in the multiply injured patient and the surgeon will usually have to rely on dermal bleeding to determine the extent of degloving.

After skin excision has been performed the surgeon should extend the open wound to allow adequate exposure of the underlying bone and soft tissues. Some surgeons believe that open fractures that are 'compound from within' do not require thorough debridement. This is a misplaced belief, as such fractures may well be contaminated and associated with considerable soft-tissue damage. All open wounds with the exception of straightforward low-velocity gunshot wounds should be extended.

The skin extensions will depend on the location and size of the original wound but ideally extensions should be longitudinal and follow, where possible, normal surgical approaches. The surgeon should be aware of what local flaps might be used to close a soft-tissue defect and avoid planning extension incisions in these areas. This is particularly true of wounds associated with open fractures of the lower third of the tibia where fasciocutaneous flaps may be used to close the defect. If there is any doubt, a plastic surgeon must be consulted about the optimal skin extension incisions.

Transverse extension incisions should not be used and intact skin over the subcutaneous border of the tibia should not be breached as the resultant defect requires flap cover. The length of the skin extension incisions is governed by the twin requirements of opening all injured tissue planes and visualizing and cleaning the bone ends.

Fat and fascia

All devitalized fat should be removed. At surgery the extent of fat necrosis may well be greater than was apparent pre-operatively and the surgeon may well have to resect more overlying skin if there is significant subcutaneous fatty devitalization.

Fascial resection rarely presents a problem for the surgeon. The surgeon should, however, bear in mind that foreign material may spread between the deep fascia and the underlying muscles and if there is evidence of this, the subfascial space must be explored thoroughly.

It used to be thought that open fractures were not associated with compartment syndrome but this belief has been disproven (DeLee and Stiehl 1981, McQueen et al 1990). It is unlikely that the surgeon will encounter a compartment syndrome in association with a Gustilo type III fracture although it is theoretically possible. However, compartment syndromes associated with less severe open fractures do occur and the surgeon must be aware of this and be prepared to perform a fasciotomy at the time of initial debridement if this is required. Fasciotomy will either be performed on clinical grounds or not infrequently nowadays if there is a rise in intracompartmental pressure in relation to the diastolic blood pressure (Whitesides et al 1975, McQueen et al 1990). If a fasciotomy is to be performed it should be undertaken using the principles outlined in Chapter 20.

Muscle

It is important that all damaged muscle is surgically explored. The easiest way to assess the direction and extent of muscle damage is to digitally examine the wound after the skin has been excised. Palpation should be gentle to prevent the creation of tissue spaces but it will allow the surgeon to assess where there has been muscle damage. The area should then be opened to allow full muscle exposure.

All devitalized muscle should be removed. This is not always possible at the initial debridement as it is sometimes difficult to fully assess muscle viability. The classical signs of muscle viability are colour, consistency, contractility to mechanical stimulation and bleeding. These may obviously be affected by the overall condition of the patient and if the patient is hypotensive or peripherally shut down, muscle viability may be particularly difficult to assess.

Attempts have been made to estimate the oxygen saturation of the muscle and use this value as a predictor of viability, but the method is not in widespread clinical practice and often the time available to the surgeon is limited and he or she must rely on clinical judgement.

Muscle bleeding is probably the best test of viability. Colour may be difficult to evaluate if there has been local contusion or haemorrhage within the muscle belly and although normal muscles undoubtedly contract when pinched gently with tissue forceps, all surgeons will be aware that this test can be difficult to interpret in clinical practice. The surgeon should also be guided by the appearance and consistency of the muscle. Muscle that is shredded or disintegrates on touch should be excised.

The surgeon should not hesitate to excise a considerable amount of muscle if this is required. At the end of a successful debridement only viable muscle tissue should remain. In some injuries it is relatively easy to assess the degree of damage but in crushing injuries in particular the extent of muscle damage may be difficult to define at the first debridement and further debridements may be required.

When resecting muscle, it is particularly important to avoid damaging the neurovascular structures in the area. The nerves and larger vessels should be located and protected. Damage to local blood vessels should be minimized as the vessels may provide blood supply to a particular segment of muscle.

Tendon

Unlike muscle, tendon is resistant to direct trauma. However, the surgeon may find that there is superficial tendon contamination and this should be excised at the time of debridement. Rarely, there may be severe tendon damage necessitating tendon resection and later reconstruction. This is usually associated with considerable muscle damage.

Bone

The extent of bone resection in open fractures usually stimulates considerable debate amongst orthopaedic surgeons. However, bone resection should be treated in the same way as resection of the soft tissues and therefore all devitalized separate bone fragments should be removed regardless of their size (Figure 5.6). As with muscle, it may be difficult to assess bone viability in separated fragments, but the presence of attached periosteum or muscle will aid the surgeon. However, the surgeon must be wary of preserving bone attached by devitalized soft tissues and such fragments should also be discarded.

In the femur, surgeons will occasionally meet the problem of a length of diaphysis denuded of all soft tissues, but with bone continuity proximally. It is not recommended that this bone be excised as there may be, at least theoretically, preservation of the intramedullary circulation.

Swiontkowski (1989) has investigated the use of laser Doppler flowmetry (LDF) for the assessment of bone viability. He believes it to be a useful supplementary test in bone debridement but further confirmation of the clinical usefulness of the technique is awaited and as with other ancillary methods of assessing tissue viability it remains to be seen if it is a useful aid in the management of severely injured patients.

Lavage

Lavage with fluids such as isotonic saline, distilled water and antibiotic solutions is an essential part of the operation of debridement. The principle of lavage is simple. It is used to irrigate the wound and thereby remove all blood clots and extraneous matter. In addition, the lavage fluid will dilute the degree of bacterial contamination and the use of antibiotic solution may well further reduce the local bacterial counts. Commonly, surgeons use anything between 5 and 40 litres of fluid in wound lavage although a volume of approximately 10–15 litres is probably adequate. Ideally, the lavage fluids should be delivered under pressure through a pulsed lavage system to facilitate maximum tissue cleaning.

There is debate about the usefulness of antibiotics in the lavage fluid. If an adequate surgical debridement is performed and only vascularized tissue remains in the wound, then it is logical to assume that appropriate intravenous antibiotic administration will result in adequate tissue levels. However, there is some evidence that the addition of antibiotics to the middle 3 litres of a 9-litre lavage regime is associated with lower infection rates (Rosenstein et al 1989). Despite this work, it is likely that the main effect of lavage is mechanical and although the surgeon may reasonably add antibiotics to the lavage fluid, this should never be used to compensate for an inadequate debridement.

As far as the timing of lavage is concerned, many surgeons employ it pre-operatively to clean the wound of superficial debris. This is not

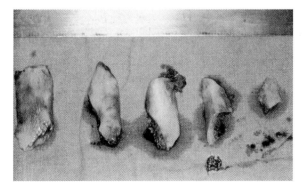

Figure 5.6

The bone fragments that were excised from the wound. None of these fragments had a viable blood supply.

unreasonable but the lavage should be continued once the whole extent of the wound has been opened. Lavage at this time has more chance of removing devitalized and contaminated material. It is sensible, therefore, to use lavage throughout the debridement, making certain that the whole of the wound is exposed to the irrigation fluids.

Wound closure

There are no indications for the primary closure of open wounds. It is impossible to close an open wound without some tissue tension. Even in small wounds, the surgeon will have undertaken skin edge resection and this combined with the associated local swelling ensures that the wound cannot be closed without tension. Theoretically, it is reasonable to close the surgical wound extensions but again only if this can be achieved without tension. There is no evidence that leaving small wounds open for 24–48 hours increases the infection rate and it is much safer to close the wound secondarily at this time either by secondary suture, split skin grafting or flap cover.

If the wound is going to require flap cover for closure and the surgeon is happy that there is no residual contamination or soft-tissue damage after debridement, a primary flap can be performed as this can be undertaken without tension. However, in larger open wounds it is a good policy to re-examine the wound at 24–48 hours after the initial surgery and if a primary flap is undertaken this is impossible. For this reason, it is probably wise to delay flap cover until the relook procedure is undertaken.

Post-operative treatment

Post-operatively, the open wound should be treated by the application of a sterile, moist, absorbent dressing. An antibiotic impregnated gelonet dressing with overlying gauze swabs and absorbent wool bandaging is appropriate although other dressings may be used. Some surgeons advocate the use of bead pouches with antibiotic-impregnated beads enclosed within a plastic

adhesive dressing (Henry et al 1993). Alternatively, the impregnation of the overlying dressings with iodine-containing solutions or antibiotics such as neomycin, bacitracin and polymyxin is advocated by some surgeons. These regimes are largely the result of a time when wounds had to be left to granulate and with modern wound closure philosophy advocating early flap cover, there is no need to use anything more than a simple dressing provided flap cover is carried out within a few days of the initial surgical procedure.

Subsequent debridement

It is suggested that all Gustilo type III fractures and any other open wound that gives rise to concern be re-explored 24–48 hours after the initial operation. If an adequate primary debridement has been performed then it is unusual to resect much more tissue at the second procedure. However, in cases of crushing injuries it is particularly difficult to assess the extent of the muscle damage initially and there may well be further resection at the second procedure. If a second debridement is performed then a further debridement must be performed after a further 24–48 hours. Sequential debridements must be carried out until the wound is completely clean. In reality if, despite aggressive debridement being carried out on a number of occasions, the wound cannot be adequately cleared, within a week it is likely that the extent of the muscle damage is such that the limb is not viable and amputation should be considered.

Debridement of joints

Surgical debridement of joints is essentially the same as for diaphyseal or metaphyseal fractures. If there is significant contamination the joint must be opened and carefully lavaged. The open wound must be extended to allow this to be performed. If the contamination of the joint is minimal the surgeon may choose to arthroscopically lavage the joint.

It is always advocated that if possible the synovium should be closed after a joint debridement to prevent dessication of the joint.

However, in cases of major soft-tissue loss, the articular open fracture will be treated in the same way as a long-bone fracture, the wound left open with a second debridement being carried out 24–48 hours after the initial procedure. Under these circumstances, a flap will be required to close the defect.

Debridement of gunshot fractures

Throughout this chapter, reference has been made to some differences in the debridement of wounds associated with fractures caused by gunshot injury. This is an increasing problem in many countries but in the United States fractures caused by gunshots are one of the most common mechanisms of injury that are seen in urban trauma centres. Gunshots can be divided into categories with the velocity of the bullet used to differentiate between the groups. Bullets with a velocity below 2000 ft/s are termed 'low velocity' and those above 2000 ft/s 'high velocity'. Treatment of the two groups is different and based on the amount of tissue damage produced by the bullet. The majority of handgun and civilian injuries are low velocity while rifle and military injuries are high velocity.

Low-velocity gunshots are characterized by small entrance and exit wounds. As the bullet penetrates, it tends to push the soft tissues aside until it impacts against the bone, causing a fracture (Figure 5.7). There is minimal necrosis or devitalization of the soft tissues as the bullet has low energy. The degree of bone comminution is variable and may vary from the fracture being a mere incomplete cortical fracture to significant segmental comminution. It is, however, not unusual for there to be little comminution as shown in Figure 5.7. Bullets have been shown not to be sterile (Demuth 1966) but these fractures have insignificant bacterial contamination.

Proper treatment of low-velocity gunshot fractures consists of minimal skin debridement and the administration of broad-spectrum antibiotics for between 24 and 72 hours as would be prescribed for other open fractures. Formal surgical debridement of the soft tissues and fracture is not required (Howland and Ritchey 1971). Fracture treatment should be carried out

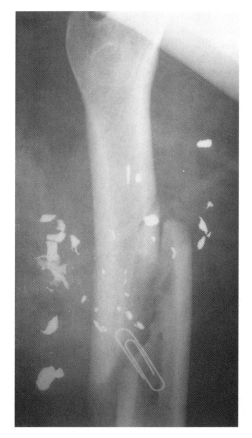

Figure 5.7

An anteroposterior X-ray of a low-velocity gunshot wound of the femur. There is no bony comminution and very little associated soft-tissue damage. The paper clip marks the entry wound.

using an appropriate technique regardless of the presence of bullet fragments in the fracture area.

High-velocity injuries are quite different from their low-velocity counterparts (Fackler et al 1988). Due to the high velocity of the bullet, there is a tremendous amount of energy transmitted to all tissues. This may result in tissue necrosis and devitalization for some distance from the actual pathway of the bullet. There may be a cavity of injured tissues extending all the way to the skin envelope. Generally, the entrance wound is not much larger than the bullet itself but the exit

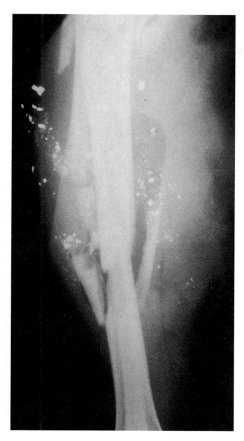

Figure 5.8

An anteroposterior X-ray of a high-velocity gunshot wound of the femur. In contrast to Figure 5.7, note the degree of comminution and the extent of the associated soft-tissue wound.

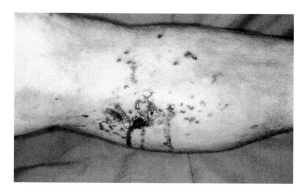

Figure 5.9

A shotgun wound of the calf. Most of the shot has entered in one area but there is significant scattering of the pellets. The main wound requires a standard debridement but it is unnecessary and undesirable to attempt to remove the individual pellets.

wound may measure 15 cm or more. There is, however, poor correlation between bullet velocity and the size of the entrance and exit wounds. The associated fractures are usually comminuted and there may be considerable bone loss (Figure 5.8). Knowledge of the type of weapon that caused the fracture is very useful.

It is best to consider high-velocity gunshot fractures in the same way as any Gustilo type III open fracture. Operative debridement is mandatory and must include a thorough exploration of the entire bullet path from entrance to exit wounds. The soft tissues should be explored some distance away from the projectile path and all devitalized tissue excised as already described. The fractures should be stabilized using an appropriate implant or external fixator.

Shotgun injuries are a special case in which the velocity is not important but the large mass of multiple pellets results in much soft-tissue damage particularly at close range (Figure 5.9). Acute treatment should proceed as in high-velocity gunshot injuries but removal of the multiple pellets is not indicated and may result in further damage to relatively intact soft tissues.

References

Border JR, Allgöwer M, Hansen ST, Ruedi TP (1990) *Blunt Multiple Trauma. Comprehensive Pathophysiology and Care* (Marcel Dekker: New York).

DeLee JC, Stiehl JB (1981) Open tibial fracture with compartment syndrome, *Clin Orthop* **160**: 175–84.

Demuth WE (1966) Bullet velocity and design as determinants of wounding capability: an experimental study, *J Trauma* **6**: 222–32.

Fackler JL, Bellamy RF, Malinowski TA (1988) The wound profile: illustration of the muscle–tissue interaction, *J Trauma* **28**: 521–9.

Haury B, Rodeheaver G, Vensito J, Edgerton MT, Edlich RF (1978) Debridement: an essential component of traumatic wound care, *Am J Surg* **135**: 238–42.

Henry SL, Ostermann PAW, Seligson D (1993) The antibiotic bead pouch technique: the management of severe compound fractures, *Clin Orthop* **295**: 54–62.

Howland WS, Ritchey SJ (1971) Gunshot fractures in civilian practice, *J Bone Joint Surg (Am)* **53A**: 47–55.

McCalden RW, McGeough JA, Barker MB, Court-Brown CM (1993) Age-related changes in the tensile properties of cortical bone, *J Bone Joint Surg (Am)* **75A**: 1193–205.

McGrouther DA, Sully L (1980) Degloving injuries of the limbs: long-term review and management based on whole-body fluorescence, *Br J Plast Surg* **33**: 9–24.

McMurtry RY, McLellan BA (1990) *Management of Blunt Trauma* (Williams and Wilkins: Baltimore).

McQueen MR, Christie J, Court-Brown CM (1990) Compartment pressures after tibial nailing, *J Bone Joint Surg (Br)* **72B**: 395–7.

Müller ME, Allgöwer M, Schneider R, Willenegger H (1987) *Manual of Internal Fixation: Techniques Recommended by the AO Group*, 3rd edn (Springer-Verlag: Berlin).

Rosenstein BD, Wilson FC, Funderburk CH (1989) The use of bacitracin irrigation to prevent infection in postoperative skeletal wounds. An experimental study, *J Bone Joint Surg (Am)* **71A**: 427–30.

Swiontkowski MF (1989) Criteria for bone debridement in massive lower limb trauma, *Clin Orthop* **243**: 41–7.

Tscherne M (1984) The management of open fractures. In: Tscherne M, Gotzen L, eds, *Fractures with Soft Tissue Injuries* (Springer-Verlag: Berlin) 10–32.

Whitesides TE, Haney TC, Morimoto K, Harada H (1975) Tissue pressure measurements as a determinant of the need for fasciotomy, *Clin Orthop* **113**: 43–51.

6
Management of open femoral fractures

J. Keating

Open femoral fractures are uncommon injuries, and until recently the literature contained few reports dealing specifically with their management. The success of locked intramedullary nailing in the last decade for treatment of closed fractures of the femur has also stimulated considerable interest in use of the method for open femoral diaphyseal fractures. Although some authors still advocate a cautious approach with regard to early fixation (Green and Trafton 1991), there is an emerging consensus of opinion that open femoral fractures are best treated by locked intramedullary nailing. There is still debate regarding the suitability of the method for all grades of open femoral fractures, the current role of external fixation and the optimal timing of fixation. The potential risks of the reaming process have also been under close scrutiny.

Open metaphyseal injuries of the femur are even rarer than open diaphyseal fractures. Metaphyseal fractures have most commonly been treated with rigid internal fixation but there has been a recent trend away from former techniques of anatomical open reduction and rigid internal fixation. Newer designs of locking nail for the proximal and distal femoral metaphysis are now available and may represent a very useful addition to the surgical armamentarium for dealing with difficult fractures in this region. This chapter reviews the literature on open femoral fractures and assesses the current role of the various treatment alternatives available to the orthopaedic surgeon in the management of these challenging injuries.

Epidemiology

There is a limited amount of information regarding the incidence of open femoral fractures. Over a six-and-a-quarter year period in the trauma unit in Edinburgh, a total of 62 open femoral fractures in 55 patients were treated, or 10 per year on average (see Chapter 3). Since the catchment area served by the unit is 750 000, this gives an annual incidence in a UK population of 1.3 per 100 000 per annum. Green and Trafton (1991) reported on 62 open femoral fractures over a seven-year period from a catchment population of 1.5 million, giving an annual incidence of 0.6 per 100 000 per annum in a North American population. Tertiary referral centres will naturally see a higher proportion of these injuries. In a series of 469 femoral fractures treated at a level I trauma unit, Brumback et al (1989) reported that 108 (23%) were open. Road traffic accidents are the single most common cause and account for 60–83% of these fractures in larger studies (Lhowe and Hansen 1988, Brumback et al 1989, O'Brien et al 1991). The victims have usually been drivers or passengers in the vehicle, with motor cyclists also comprising a significant proportion. Pedestrians struck by vehicles are less prone to sustain this injury. In societies where gun ownership is common, gunshot injuries are also a frequent mechanism of injury (Wiss et al 1991).

Because of the violence involved, it is unusual for open femoral fractures to occur in isolation. In the Edinburgh series, all of the patients had an injury severity score in excess of 16. Lhowe and Hansen (1988) reported that 60% of their patients had multiple injuries, while O'Brien et al (1991) had an incidence of 83%. In another series, the mean Injury Severity Score was 23 points (Brumback et al 1989). The commonest associated injuries are other long-bone fractures, but pelvic and acetabular fractures were also frequent and 10–20% of these patients will require a thoracotomy or laparotomy to deal with visceral injury (Lhowe and Hansen 1988). Mortality rates reported in association with this injury vary from 1.5% to 8.3% (O'Brien et al 1991, Lhowe and Hansen 1988) and in almost all cases are due to head or visceral injuries incompatible with survival.

Classification

Classification systems used to describe these injuries have been based either on the severity of soft-tissue injury or the fracture morphology. The most commonly used classification of the soft-tissue injury associated with open long-bone fractures is that of Gustilo and Anderson (1976), and the subsequent modification of the grade III category by Gustilo et al (1984). This classification remains the most widely used system in the UK and North America. It has been well documented particularly for the description of open tibial fractures and has been considered to be a reproducible prognostic indicator in terms of both complication rates and functional outcome (Caudle and Stern 1987, Court-Brown et al 1990a, 1991). As might be expected, however, the level of interobserver agreement is variable. Brumback has shown that for open tibial fractures, the overall rate of interobserver agreement using the classification was only 60% (Brumback and Jones 1994).

Although it is also generally used in the description of open femoral fractures, the number of type III injuries in most series is small, and there is not a clear difference in outcome between type I and type II injuries in most reports. Moreover, in the subsequent elaboration of the type III classification, Gustilo indicates that high-energy injuries and any segmental fracture should properly be classified as type IIIa (Gustilo et al 1984, 1990). Since virtually all open femoral fractures occur as a consequence of high-energy trauma, this implies that the vast majority of these fractures should be regarded as being at least IIIa injuries. The corollary is that few if any open femoral fractures can be considered to be type I or type II injuries. It is unclear whether the subdivisions of the type III group have the same prognostic value as for tibial fractures and a classification specifically designed for open femoral fractures might be of more value. Despite these shortcomings, the Gustilo system is widely used, has the benefit of simplicity and will remain the standard classification until an alternative method is shown to be superior.

The most widely used classification of the femoral fracture morphology is that of Winquist and Hansen (1980) which divides diaphyseal fractures into four groups based on the degree of comminution and circumference of cortical contact between the two major fragments. This system was developed specifically for use with intramedullary nailing and correlates with the violence of the initial injury. For fractures classified having grade III or IV comminution, proximal and distal locking is considered mandatory (Brumback et al 1988a).

The only other commonly used classification is that proposed by the AO group (Müller et al 1990). This provides a comprehensive means of description of all degrees of fracture comminution with division into 27 different subtypes. It has the drawback of being complex and to date it has not been widely used in published literature. Although it has its advocates (Colton 1991), its adoption awaits validation that such a detailed classification is justified in terms of being a useful guide to either prognosis or treatment.

Treatment

Initial assessment and management

Since up to 80% of these cases will have multiple injuries, the early assessment and management usually requires a multidisciplinary team approach. This implies that these patients are best managed in a unit with the relevant personnel and facilities to rapidly assess and deal with the associated life-threatening injuries that are commonly present. Major intrathoracic or abdominal haemorrhage clearly will take precedence but the most crucial initial step in management of an open femoral fracture is an early and adequate debridement of the wound. This may necessitate different surgical teams operating simultaneously on the combination of injuries present.

The key steps in debridement need not be reiterated here but it is mandatory to visualize the bone at the fracture site and in the femur this usually requires extension of the open wound to allow adequate access. It is common to encounter butterfly fragments and other portions of bone with no soft-tissue attachment in these high-energy injuries and these must all be excised even if this means leaving a segmental defect. Once debridement is complete, irrigation of the wound with 10 litres of normal saline solution is performed. The wound is left open at the end of the procedure.

Broad-spectrum antibiotic treatment should be commenced as soon as possible after arrival of the patient, and antitetanus measures taken in all patients with contaminated wounds or in those patients who have a history of inadequate or uncertain immunization. A notable feature of the infections reported in association with open femoral fractures has been the high number of Gram-negative organisms, particularly *Enterococcus*, *Enterobacter*, *Klebsiella*, *Pseudomonas*, and Gram-negative *Bacteroides* (Murphy et al 1988, Lhowe and Hansen 1989, Brumback et al 1989). These are at least as common as more conventional pathogens such as *Staphylococcus aureus*. For this reason a third-generation cephalosporin is recommended as the initial antibiotic (Gustilo et al 1990). Anaerobic cover should also be given for type III open fractures. Antibiotic treatment should be maintained for 3 days. There is no evidence that prolonging therapy beyond this time prevents the development of infection (Gustilo and Anderson 1976, Dellinger et al 1988a,b). Soft-tissue coverage is usually straightforward in open femoral fractures. Flaps are rarely required and most wounds can be treated by delayed primary closure or split-skin grafting.

Open fractures with vascular injury

Type IIIc open femoral fractures are fortunately rare. Salvage of the limb with these injuries is a formidable surgical problem. Amputation rates for type IIIc long-bone fractures vary from 25% to 90% (Lange et al 1985, Caudle and Stern 1987, Gustilo et al 1987). Bad prognostic signs are a major soft-tissue injury, ischaemic times in excess of 6 hours, the presence of a significant neurological deficit and other major organ injuries (Lange et al 1985, Schlickewei et al 1992). The optimum sequence of vascular repair and skeletal fixation, and the role of pre-operative angiography, remain a source of debate since few centres have adequate experience with large numbers of these injuries.

There is an emerging consensus that pre-operative angiography in type IIIc fractures of the lower limb is unnecessary in most cases and merely wastes valuable time (Schlickewei et al 1992). The site of vessel injury is seldom in doubt and intra-operative angiography can be performed in doubtful cases. With regard to the sequence of revascularization and stabilization, a rational approach is to initially perform a temporary shunt at the site of vessel injury. This will allow time for a thorough debridement which is facilitated by the limb reperfusion which enhances the distinction between viable and non-viable tissue. Blood from the limb distal to the vessel injury will have a low pH and toxic metabolites and at the time of shunting should be flushed out to decrease the risk of myocardial and renal toxicity. The bone can then be stabilized and the definitive vascular repair performed under more optimal conditions (Barros D'Sa 1992). The optimal choice of bony stabilization is considered below.

Definitive fracture management

The use of early locked intramedullary nailing has come to dominate the approach to the management of open femoral fractures and has largely eclipsed other methods of treatment over the past decade (Bucholz and Jones 1991). A number of reasons account for this gradual change. A series of retrospective studies appeared through the 1980s supporting the view that early fixation of long-bone fractures reduced the pulmonary complications that were responsible for much of the associated morbidity and mortality (Goris et al 1982, Riska and Myllynen 1982, Johnson et al 1985). These were followed by an influential study by Bone et al (1989) which randomized patients with femoral fractures into early- and delayed-fixation groups. They showed that the group undergoing early intramedullary fixation had lower mortality, had fewer respiratory complications and spent less time in intensive care units. Although other methods of treatment may still have an occasional role, they all have marked drawbacks in comparison to the locking nail for the management of open femoral diaphyseal fractures. The fracture stability, wound access and potential for early mobilization provided by intramedullary nailing has proved uniquely suited to the management of open femoral fractures. By comparison, the alternative methods of traction, cast-bracing, plating and external fixation all have significant drawbacks in the management of these injuries.

Traction and cast-bracing

Traction confines the patient to bed, and even modern methods are cumbersome (Browner et al 1981). Duration of hospital stay has been shown to be significantly longer in studies comparing traction followed by cast-bracing to intramedullary nailing (Thomas and Meggitt 1981, Pierre et al 1982). Delayed union and malunion are common sequelae and limb shortening is also not unusual (Nichols 1963, Dencker 1965, Carr and Wingo 1973, Schweigel and Gropper 1974). Loss of knee flexion is extremely common (Buxton 1981, Gates et al 1985). In a study comparing roller traction to interlocking nailing, Johnson et al (1984) reported a 66% incidence of malalignment and shortening in the traction group compared to 4% in the group treated with an interlocking nail. Since open femoral fractures are generally unstable injuries in patients with multiple injuries, traction, even with early cast-bracing, is probably the least satisfactory method of management.

Plating

Plating of open fractures has been recommended in the past but is rarely practised now. The operation is technically demanding, and the reported complication rates have been high. Rüedi and Lüscher (1979) reported on 131 comminuted femoral fractures treated by plating, of which 28 were open. The deep infection rate in the open fractures was 7% (2/28). In the series overall, there was a 7% incidence of implant failure and 7% of the patients required an additional bone-grafting procedure to achieve union. They recommended bone grafting in all patients at the index procedure.

Magerl et al (1979) reported on 67 femoral fractures of which nine were open injuries. Full weight-bearing was prohibited for three months. Twelve of the fractures (18%) required additional surgery to deal with complications or achieve union. Implant failure complicated 10% of cases. They encountered no deep infections in the open fractures. Of the nine open fractures, five were ultimately rated as having an excellent result and four a good result.

Other authors have reported much less favourable results of femoral plating. Loomer et al (1980) reported on 46 femoral diaphyseal fractures treated by plating. Seven were open. They recorded a 24% overall incidence of orthopaedic complications. Deep infection occurred in 7%, implant failure in 13% and non-union in 2%. Infection rates for plating of open femoral fractures are difficult to estimate since reported numbers in the literature are small, but in closed femoral plating deep infection rates are usually 7–8% (Jensen and Johansen 1977).

It seems reasonable to assume, therefore, that infection rates associated with plating of contaminated open femoral fractures will be even higher. In addition to these drawbacks, weight-bearing has to be restricted for prolonged periods postoperatively. More recently, in an effort to reduce the problems associated with plating, the AO group has introduced the low contact dynamic compression plate (LC-DCP) and the concept of 'biological plating'. Both are aimed at reducing the interference with the diaphyseal blood supply associated with more traditional methods of plating. Favourable results using the technique of biological plating have been reported in the treatment of subtrochanteric femoral fractures (Kinast et al 1989), but a report specifically detailing results for open femoral shaft fractures has yet to appear.

At present, the weight of evidence indicates that plating of open diaphyseal femoral fractures is a technically difficult procedure entailing the need for bone grafting in most cases and ultimately associated with a high rate of implant failure and other complications. A recommendation to use standard dynamic compression plating or newer plating techniques for these injuries must therefore await reports of these methods being used with acceptable results in a large number of patients.

External fixation

External fixation has been recommended for the treatment of open femoral fractures and has certainly been commonly used. Despite this, there is surprisingly poor documentation of the results of treatment with the method. It does have some theoretically useful attributes in the treatment of these injuries in the management of open femoral fractures. A modern uniaxial frame can be very rapidly applied, and this may be a particular advantage in the multiply traumatized patient with more than one long-bone fracture (Dabezies et al 1984, Murphy et al 1988). The relative ease and short time taken to apply may be a definite advantage in the early treatment of type IIIc open fractures where speed may be vital in the effort to save the limb.

Many varieties of frame types have been tried in the past. Some authors have used fixators with transfixation pins emerging on the medial aspect of the thigh (Coppola and Anzel 1983), but these take longer to apply and are associated with unacceptable rates of non-union (20%) and pin track infection (57%). The recent trend has been towards a simple uniaxial frame of which the Orthofix is probably most widely used. The complex circular frames of the Ilizarov type have very little part to play in the acute management of these injuries and are best reserved for the patients presenting with late problems such as long-standing deep infection and multiplanar deformity.

With the availability of strong uniaxial frames (Dabezies et al 1984, DeBastiani et al 1984) there is no indication now to use more complex configurations, since there is no evidence to suggest they have any advantage. An accurate assessment of results and complications treating open femoral fractures by external fixation is made difficult by the limited literature on the topic. Most series are small and consist of mixed open and closed fractures (Seligson and Kristiansen 1978, Gottschalk et al 1985). Most series have also reported experience with the Hoffman and Wagner frames.

Seligson and Kristiansen reported four cases of open femoral fracture treated with the Wagner device, noting no deep infection and no non-union. These authors gave no details regarding the need for bone grafting or the rate of malunion. Gottschalk et al (1985) reported three cases of open femoral fracture treated with either a Wagner or ASIF tubular external fixator. All fractures healed uneventfully but knee stiffness was a problem. Habboushe (1984) reported on 85 open femoral fractures treated with a simple uniaxial fixator comprising a methylmethacrylate plastic tube securing Schanz pins into bone. There was a 9% incidence of pin track infection and 14% of patients were described as having 'impaired function'. No other details were given.

Dabezies et al (1984) reported on the use of the Wagner device to treat a series of 20 complex femoral fractures of which 13 were open. Pin track infections complicated 20% and knee joint stiffness was noted in 9 patients. There were no deep infections.

Using either the AO double-bar frame or the Wagner device, Alonso et al (1989) reported union in eight grade II and five grade III open fractures. Infection was not a problem, but most of the patients developed some degree of knee stiffness. DeBastiani et al (1984) reported union in eight of nine cases of open femoral fractures treated with the dynamic axial fixator. There were apparently no deep infections but no details were given regarding other complications or functional outcome.

The small numbers of patients in these and other reports make firm conclusions difficult to draw. While the results are acceptable in terms of union and infection rates, external fixation of the femur carries a number of liabilities. Although uniaxial external fixators are not technically demanding to apply, achieving and maintaining an acceptable reduction against large deforming forces is a problem and malunion is a common complication, particularly in unstable open fractures. Pin track infection is a hazard associated with external fixation of any bone but this applies in particular to the femur where the pins must traverse vastus lateralis. Although rarely leading to deep infection, pin track sepsis is difficult to eradicate and very troublesome for the patient. Pin loosening is frequently associated with infection and may necessitate repositioning.

These problems often necessitate changing the mode of treatment. This is not without its hazards. A high rate of deep infection has been noted following conversion to intramedullary nailing (Dabezies et al 1984, Alonso et al 1989). Finally, the problem of knee stiffness is extremely common and can certainly compromise the functional result. In a study comparing the Wagner external fixator to use of the Grosse–Kempf interlocking nail for femoral fractures, the nail was associated with lower complication rates and proved superior in terms of functional results (Murphy et al 1988).

In summary, external fixation should be considered in the management of any open femoral fracture with an associated vascular injury. Some authors still recommend it as the method of choice in grade IIIb open femoral fractures (Brumback et al 1989, Sanders et al 1993), on the basis that it minimizes the deep infection rate. There is little basis for this assumption in the published literature, and the available evidence suggests that intramedullary nailing of grade IIIb fractures has a deep infection rate comparable with or lower than treatment with external fixation (Grosse et al 1993).

Intramedullary nailing

Following the introduction of locked intramedullary nailing, consistently excellent results have been reported for the management of closed femoral fractures. Initial experience with the method for complex femoral fractures suggested that it could also be used with success for open femoral fractures (Kempf et al 1985, Wiss et al 1986, Johnson and Greenberg 1987). The perceived risk of deep infection led some authors to recommend delayed nailing, with acceptable results (Chapman et al 1982). Over the past few years, a succession of reports have suggested that early reamed nailing of open femoral fractures could be used safely (Lhowe and Hansen 1988, Brumback et al 1989, O'Brien

et al 1991, Grosse et al 1993). These series have accumulated larger numbers and examined the outcome in more detail than earlier reports of other methods of treatment.

Lhowe and Hansen (1988) reported on 42 patients treated with nailing. There were 15 grade I injuries, 19 grade II and eight grade III injuries. Complications included an infection rate of 5%, with a 7% malunion rate and loss of fixation in 10%. In a larger series, Brumback et al (1989) reported on 89 open femoral fractures in 86 patients treated with locked nailing. In this series, there were 27 grade I fractures, 16 grade II and 46 grade III fractures. No fracture went on to a delayed or non-union. There were no deep infections in grade I, II or IIIa injuries but 3 of 27 (11%) grade IIIb fractures became infected. O'Brien et al (1991) reported the results of 63 fractures in 60 patients. There were 22 grade I, 26 grade II and 15 grade III fractures. Infection complicated 4.7% with no predilection for any grade of severity. Malunion and non-union occurred in 3% and 4.7%, respectively. In a combined series from the Edinburgh and the Strasbourg groups, 115 open femoral shaft fractures were treated with the Grosse–Kempf nail. Deep infection complicated three (2.6%) cases. Non-union affected four (3.4%) fractures. The malunion rate was not given. The mean range of knee motion at the time of final follow-up was 130°.

These series together comprise 297 open femoral fractures with deep infection complicating 11 cases, an overall rate of 3.7% (Table 6.1). Despite the view commonly expressed that reamed intramedullary nailing is unsuitable for

Table 6.1 Incidence of deep infection associated with locked intramedullary nailing of open femoral fractures

Series	No.	Type			Total
		I	II	III	
Lhowe and Hansen (1988)	42	0/15	2/19	0/8	2 (5%)
Brumback et al (1989)	89	0/27	0/16	3/46	3 (3.3%)
O'Brien et al (1991)	63	1/22	1/26	1/15	3 (4.7%)
Grosse et al (1993)	115		not given		3 (2.9%)
Total	309				11 (3.5%)

grade IIIb open femoral fractures, the available evidence suggests that the method can be used even in these severe injuries with the expectation of a favourable outcome. The occurrence of infection associated with intramedullary nailing is often considered a catastrophic complication but the reported experience suggests that this is not the case (Macausland and Eaton 1963). Deep infection following intramedullary nailing can usually be eradicated by the adoption of a suitable protocol for its management (Court-Brown et al 1992). In the case of infection complicating open femoral fractures after nailing, this usually involves re-exploration of the fracture site with debridement of all infected bone and soft tissue. Abandoning the nail is unnecessary, although it is usually exchanged for a larger one. This exchange facilitates access to the fracture site if a particularly radical debridement is deemed necessary. In addition, the original nail is replaced with one of larger diameter. By this manoeuvre, further reaming is carried out, which aids removal of potentially infected material from the canal.

The use of intramedullary nailing has also minimized the need for bone grafting for non-union. There were no non-unions in the series reported by Brumback (1989), and in the series reported by Grosse et al (1993) only three patients required bone grafting. This is in marked contrast to the use of plates or external fixators where the need for bone grafting has been much higher. Malunion rates with intramedullary nailing have varied from 2% to 7% (Lhowe and Hansen 1988, Brumback et al 1989, 1991). This problem can often be attributed to faulty technique or failure to use both locking screws at the time of the original surgery. Use of only one screw has been clearly identified as contributory to malunion and fixation failure and it therefore seems sensible to lock nails both proximally and distally in virtually all cases except those transverse fractures close to the isthmus (Brumback et al 1988a). In addition, the concept of 'dynamization' of the nail by removing one of the locking screws, though widely practised, has never been convincingly shown to enhance healing in either femoral or tibial fractures (Brumback et al 1988b, Court-Brown et al 1990b). It has been implicated in loss of fixation and development of malunion and the authors therefore do not recommend its use.

Table 6.2 Loss of knee flexion related to method of treatment

Series	Method	Patients with <90° flexion (%)
Lhowe and Hansen (1988)	IM nail	0
Murphy et al (1988)	IM nail	2
Murphy et al (1988)	External fixation	42
Dabezies et al (1984)	External fixation	45

Some reference has already been made to functional outcome in relation to the method chosen. The return of knee flexion is a commonly reported assessment of function in the assessment of patients at the time of follow-up. A comparison of a number of reports demonstrates that when external fixation is used, up to 50% of patients may be expected to have <90° of knee flexion. This compares very poorly with intramedullary nailing where it is exceptional for <90° to be obtained (Table 6.2). In addition, stiffness of the knee or hip joint has generally only been a problem when there was concomitant injuries to those joints.

There is still some controversy regarding the ideal timing of nailing for the more severe grades of open injury. There is general agreement that in situations where intramedullary nailing is to be used, the debridement and nailing should be carried out within eight hours of the original injury, although this guideline is based on what intuitively seems to be safe practice rather than on hard scientific data. Some authors have recommended initial immobilization with external fixation and subsequent conversion to intramedullary nailing in type IIIb fractures (Sanders et al 1993) although there are no studies to indicate the results with this approach for femoral fractures. In fact, the available evidence suggests that delaying the nailing procedure actually increases the infection rate (Kovacs et al 1973).

Studies in converting tibial fractures from external to an intramedullary nail have shown there is a serious risk of deep infection in cases where the external fixation has been complicated by pin track problems (McGraw and Lim 1988). More recent reports suggest that if conversion is planned, then it should be performed within the first 2–3 weeks of the injury and the fixator should be removed several days before the nailing procedure (Blachut et al 1990). We do not use this approach and have used immediate nailing of even type IIIb fractures with very satisfactory results and a low complication rate (Grosse et al 1993).

The use of intramedullary nailing for open femoral fractures as a result of gunshot injury has also been a source of debate. They have generally been considered to be a unique problem and the traditional approach has been treatment with traction (Ryan et al 1981) or external fixation. Even exponents of intramedullary nailing have recommended external fixation in this situation. However Wiss et al (1991) have recently reported excellent results using a protocol of minimal debridement and antibiotics with delayed intramedullary nailing performed at 10–14 days following gunshot injuries. There were no deep infections in a series of 56 cases and only two delayed unions. More recently, Nowotarski and Brumback (1994) have reported on immediate nailing of gunshot injuries with initial debridement and delayed wound closure in 46 femoral fractures. There was one delayed union and one deep infection.

Reamed or unreamed nails

Some concern has been expressed about the practice of reaming long bones in the presence of an open fracture. The damage caused to the endosteal circulation by reaming has been recognized for a long time (Rhinelander 1974). This is considered by some to potentially increase the risk of deep infection and non-union. There has been some more recent experimental work comparing the use of reamed and unreamed nails in a rabbit fracture model (Schemitsch et al 1994). The findings indicated a reduction in fracture blood flow early on in the reamed bones but no differences were observed in blood flow or callus strength at 12 weeks. This debate about unreamed nails may continue but the weight of clinical evidence presently supports the view that reamed locking nails can be used for open femoral fractures with a very low rate of bone grafting, non-union and deep infection.

Perhaps more importantly in relation to femoral fractures has been the association between reaming and the development of fat embolism syndrome. There has been concern that the reaming process may precipitate or exacerbate any tendency to develop fat embolus syndrome, based on experimental animal studies (Whitenack and Hausberger 1971, Manning et al 1983). In a study carried out at the author's unit, the presence of cardiac embolic material appearing during reamed intramedullary nailing was monitored using transoesophageal echocardiography (Pell et al 1993). The preliminary results indicated a rather variable relationship between the quantity of embolic material and reaming but larger volumes of material were observed in patients who had delayed nailing. Insertion of the nail was also associated with an increase in the volume of material seen. Similar observations have been made in experimental studies (Wozasek et al 1994). These findings may have particular relevance in the patient with an open femoral fracture who is likely to have other injuries, in particular rib fractures and underlying lung contusions.

Although there has been some re-evaluation of the use of reamed nails in these patients, the available evidence still favours the view that both morbidity and mortality in these patients is minimized by early nailing. The practice of venting the intramedullary canal to reduce pressures has been suggested and there has also been interest in altering reamer design in an effort to reduce systemic embolism. Clinical data are not yet available to determine the effect that may result from such modifications to the surgical procedure.

Open metaphyseal fractures

Open fractures of the proximal or distal end of the femur are even rarer than open fractures of the shaft, and consequently little has been written about them. No large series has been reported to the author's knowledge on open fractures of the peritrochanteric region, and clearly these are very rare injuries. There are a variety of classification systems for morphology of proximal femoral fractures but the most useful is that devised at the Hennepin County Medical Centre. This divides these fractures into high (type I) and low (type II) subgroups. A type I fracture is high and the fracture line extends into

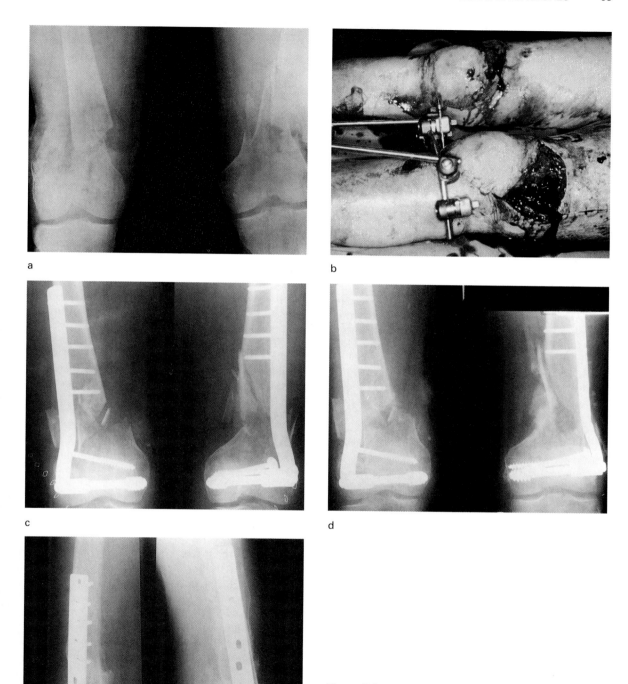

Figure 6.1

(a) Bilateral grade IIIa open distal femoral fractures in a 63-year-old female following a fall from a second floor window. (b) The wounds following debridement. (c) The wounds following internal fixation with dynamic condylar screw. (d) and (e) Early bone union occurring at 10 weeks.

the lesser trochanter region. For these fractures a standard interlocking nail is unsuitable and the choice rests between a second-generation locking nail or a sliding hip-screw device. The latter is usually preferable if the fracture comminution has destroyed the piriform fossa, making correct insertion of a nail difficult. In low (type II) fractures, the lesser trochanter is intact and a standard locking nail may be used.

Wiss and Brien (1992) reported on management of 95 subtrochanteric fractures of which 26 were open. Results were similar to open diaphyseal fractures, with no deep infections and one non-union. Intertrochanteric fractures are most commonly the result of low-energy injuries in elderly patients and are seldom open. However, it seems prudent to recommend that following debridement of the associated wound, internal fixation should be performed to stabilize the fracture. The implant of choice has been the sliding hip screw. Intramedullary devices such as the gamma nail are now being frequently used but there is as yet no clear evidence from published studies that they are superior (Halder 1992, Leung et al 1992). In situations where a femoral neck fracture occurs in association with a diaphyseal fracture, so-called 'second-generation locking nails' are now available where the neck fracture may be stabilized with proximal locking screws which are directed up the neck into the femoral head (Kyle et al 1994).

Open metaphyseal fractures of the distal femur are also an infrequent occurrence, although they are more common than open proximal femoral metaphyseal fractures. In an analysis of the epidemiology of distal femoral fractures, Kolmert and Wulff (1982) reported 137 fractures of which 10 (7%) were open. The Gustilo classification is generally used to describe the injury. The AO classification of the fracture morphology is also now being commonly used. Type A fractures are extra-articular metaphyseal injuries; type B are partial articular fractures; and type C are comminuted intra-articular fractures with no portion of the articular fracture in continuity with the diaphysis proximally. Mixed results have been reported in the literature from both non-operative and operative methods of management. For closed fractures of the metaphysis, it seems clear that best results are achieved by stable rigid internal fixation that allows early knee motion (Healy and Brooker 1983). Similarly,

the non-operative treatment of fractures with an intra-articular extension has been associated with poor functional results.

The presence of an open wound in association with either a metaphyseal or intra-articular fracture of the distal femur complicates the situation. Once again, the rarity of open fractures in this region means that recommendations regarding management are based on theoretical considerations and experience with management of closed fractures in this region. The use of interlocking nails augmented with screws may allow quite distal fractures to be treated with this method (Butler et al 1991) and this is the author's preference where it is technically feasible, particularly if there is an associated diaphyseal fracture.

In situations where this is not possible, other modes of fixation need to be considered. External fixation, if used, often needs to bridge the knee joint to adequately stabilize the fracture. This can only be a temporary measure and the subsequent conversion to an alternative fixation method may be hazardous if there has been pin track infection. Rigid internal fixation with either a blade plate or dynamic condylar screw if properly performed (Figure 6.1) has been associated with good results for closed fractures but there are very few data on the method with open fractures. Green and Trafton (1991) reported on 18 open distal femoral fractures and noted that three (17%) developed deep infection. They advised against using immediate internal fixation in type III open wounds.

Supracondylar nailing devices are now available which may be a very useful alternative to other methods in this situation. These nails are inserted via a distal entry point through the knee joint. Lucas et al (1993) have described the use of an intramedullary supracondylar nail to fix distal femoral fractures including those with intra-articular extensions. They reported on 34 fractures treated with the device. This included open fractures although the results for these were not given separately. There was one late infection and the mean arc of knee motion was 100°. To date, published experience with this and other similar devices is limited and a final assessment of the role of supracondylar nails awaits further clinical data.

The author's preference for these injuries is immediate internal fixation following debridement, using either a blade plate or a dynamic condylar screw (Figure 6.1a–e). The latter device is somewhat simpler to insert, although precise technique is still required for correct placement. If the fracture is very low, however, the screws inserted just proximal to the dynamic condylar screw will not engage the distal fragment. In this situation the condylar mass will be free to rotate around the condylar screw which offers minimal resistance to this tendency. Under these circumstances a blade plate is preferable, as it is impossible for the condylar fragments to rotate around the blade. Delayed secondary closure without the need for flap cover is usually feasible and bone-grafting may be performed as a secondary procedure if required.

In summary, immediate debridement followed by reamed intramedullary nailing is now the treatment of choice for open femoral fractures. External fixation has a limited role in their management and should be confined to situations where speed is the main consideration. Newer concepts of fixation such as biological plating and unreamed nailing await sound clinical evidence that they have any role to play. For metaphyseal fractures, immediate internal fixation with either a plate or an intramedullary nail if technically feasible seems to give the best results.

References

Alonso J, Geissler W, Hughes JL (1989) External fixation of femoral fractures. Indications and limitations, *Clin Orthop* **241**: 83–8.

Barros D'Sa AAB (1992) Editorial. Complex vascular and orthopaedic injuries, *J Bone Joint Surg* **74B**: 176–8.

Blachut PA, Meek RWN, O'Brien PJ (1990) External fixation and delayed intramedullary nailing, *J Bone Joint Surg* **72A**: 729–35.

Bone LB, Johnson KD, Weigelt J, Scheinberg R (1989) Early versus delayed stabilisation of femoral fractures. A prospective randomized study, *J Bone Joint Surg* **71A**: 336–41.

Browner BD, Kenzora JE, Edwards CC (1981) The use of modified Neufeld traction in the management of femoral fractures in polytrauma, *J Trauma* **21**: 779–87.

Brumback RJ, Jones AL (1994) Interobserver agreement in the classification of open fractures of the tibia, *J Bone Joint Surg* **76A**: 1162–5.

Brumback RJ, Reilly JP, Poka A, Lakatos RP, Bathon GH, Burgess AR (1988a) Intramedullary nailing of femoral shaft fractures. Part I. Decision making errors with interlocking fixation, *J Bone Joint Surg* **70A**: 1441–52.

Brumback RJ, Uwagie-Ero S, Lakatos RP, Poka A, Bathon GH, Burgess A (1988b) Intramedullary nailing of femoral shaft fractures. Part II. Fracture healing with static interlocking fixation, *J Bone Joint Surg* **70A**: 1453–62.

Brumback RJ, Ellison S, Poka A, Lakotos R, Bathon GH, Burgess AR (1989) Intramedullary nailing of open fractures of the femoral shaft, *J Bone Joint Surg* **71A**: 1324–31.

Bucholz RW, Jones A (1991) Current concepts review. Fractures of the shaft of the femur, *J Bone Joint Surg* **73A**: 1561–6.

Butler MS, Brumback RJ, Scott Ellison T, Poka A, Howard Bathon G, Burgess, A (1991) Interlocking intramedullary nailing for ipsilateral fractures of the femoral shaft and distal part of the femur, *J Bone Joint Surg* **73A**: 1492–502.

Buxton RA (1981) The use of Perkins traction in the treatment of fractures of the femoral shaft, *J Bone Joint Surg* **63B**: 362–6.

Carr CR, Wingo CH (1973) Fractures of the femoral diaphysis. A retrospective study of the results and costs of treatment by intramedullary nailing and traction and a spica cast, *J Bone Joint Surg* **55A**: 690–700.

Caudle RJ, Stern PJ (1987) Severe open fractures of the tibia, *J Bone Joint Surg* **69A**: 801–7.

Chapman MW, Pugh GA, Wood J, Day LJ, Bovill EG (1982) Closed intramedullary nailing of femoral shaft fractures, *Orthop Trans* **6**: 326.

Colton CL (1991) Editorial. Telling the bones, *J Bone Joint Surg* **73B**: 362–3.

Coppola AJ, Anzel SH (1983) Use of the Hoffmann external fixator in the treatment of femoral fractures, *Clin Orthop* **180**: 78–82.

Court-Brown CM, Wheelwright EF, Christie J, McQueen MM (1990a) External fixation for type III open tibial fractures, *J Bone Joint Surg* **72B**: 801–4.

Court-Brown CM, Christie J, McQueen MM (1990b) Closed intramedullary nailing, *J Bone Joint Surg* **72B**: 601–11.

Court-Brown CM, McQueen MM, Quaba AA, Christie J (1991) Locked intramedullary nailing of open tibial fractures, *J Bone Joint Surg* **73B**: 959–64.

Court-Brown CM, Keating JF, McQueen MM (1992) Infection after intramedullary nailing of the tibia. Incidence and protocol for management, *J Bone Joint Surg* **74B**: 770–4.

Dabezies EJ, D'Ambrosia R, Shoji H, Norris R, Murphy G (1984) Fractures of the femoral shaft treated by external fixation with the Wagner device, *J Bone Joint Surg* **66A**: 360–4.

DeBastiani G, Aldegheri R, Brivio LR (1984) The treatment of fractures with a dynamic axial fixator, *J Bone Joint Surg* **65B**: 538–45.

Dellinger EP, Caplan ES, Weaver LD, Wertz MJ, Grypma M, Droppert B, Anderson PA (1988a) Risk of infection after open fracture of the arm or the leg, *Arch Surg* **123**: 1320–7.

Dellinger EP, Caplan ES, Weaver LD, Wertz MJ, Droppert B, Hoyt N, Brumback R, Burgess A, Poka A, Benirschke SK, Lennard ES, Lou MA (1988b) Duration of preventive antibiotic administration for open extremity fractures, *Arch Surg* **123**: 333–9.

Dencker H (1965) Shaft fractures of the femur. A comparative study of the results of various methods of treatment in 1003 cases, *Acta Chir Scand* **130**: 173–84.

Gates DJ, Alms M, Cruz MM (1985) Hinged cast and roller traction for fractured femur. A system of treatment for the Third World, *J Bone Joint Surg* **67B**: 750–6.

Goris RJA, Gimbrére JSF, van Niekerk JLM, Schoots FJ, Booy LHD (1982) Early osteosynthesis and prophylactic mechanical ventilation in the multitrauma patient, *J Trauma* **22**: 895–903.

Gottschalk FAB, Graham AJ, Morein G (1985) The management of severely comminuted fractures of the femoral shaft, using the external fixator, *Injury* **16**: 377–81.

Green A, Trafton PG (1991) Early complications in the management of open femur fractures: a retrospective study, *J Orthop Trauma* **5**: 51–6.

Grosse A, Christie J, Taglang G, Court-Brown C, McQueen M (1993) Open adult femoral shaft fracture treated by early intramedullary nailing, *J Bone Joint Surg* **75B**: 562–5.

Gustilo RB, Anderson JT (1976) Prevention of infection in the treatment of one thousand and twenty-five open fractures of long bones: retrospective and prospective analysis. *J Bone Joint Surg* **58A**: 453–8.

Gustilo RB, Mendoza RM, Williams DN (1984) Problems in the management of type III (severe) open fractures: a new classification of type III open fractures, *J Trauma* **24**: 742–6.

Gustilo RB, Gruninger RP, Davis T (1987) Classification of type III (severe) open fractures relative to treatment and results, *Orthopedics* **10**: 1781–8.

Gustilo RB, Merkow RL, Templeman D (1990) Current concepts review. The management of open fractures, *J Bone Joint Surg* **72A**: 299–304.

Habboushe MP (1984) Al-Rasheed Military Hospital. External fixation system for compound missile wounds of bone, *Injury* **15**: 388–9.

Halder SC (1992) The Gamma nail for peritrochanteric fractures, *J Bone Joint Surg* **74B**: 340–4.

Healy WL, Brooker AF (1983) Distal femoral fractures. Comparison of open and closed methods, *Clin Orthop* **174**: 167–71.

Jensen JS, Johansen J, Mörch A (1977) Middle third femoral fractures treated with medullary nailing or AO compression plates, *Injury* **8**: 174–81.

Johnson KD, Greenberg M (1987) Comminuted femoral shaft fractures, *Orthop Clin N Am* **18**: 133–47.

Johnson KD, Johnston DWC, Parker B (1984) Comminuted femoral shaft fractures: treatment by roller action, cerclage wires and an intramedullary nail, or an intramedullary nail, *J Bone Joint Surg* **66A**: 1222–35.

Johnson KD, Cadambi A, Seibert GB (1985) Incidence of adult respiratory distress syndrome in patients with multiple musculoskeletal injuries: effect of early operative stabilisation of fractures, *J Trauma* **25**: 375–84.

Kempf I, Grosse A, Beck G (1985) Closed locked intramedullary nailing. Its application to comminuted fractures of the femur, *J Bone Joint Surg* **67A**: 709–19.

Kinast C, Bolhofner BR, Mast JW, Ganz R (1989) Subtrochanteric fractures of the femur, *Clin Orth Rel Res* **238**: 122–30.

Kolmert L, Wulff K (1982) Epidemiology and treatment of distal femoral fractures in adults, *Acta Orthop Scand* **53**: 957–62.

Kovacs AJ, Richard LB, Miller J (1973) Infection complicating intramedullary nailing of the femur, *Clin Orthop Rel Res* **96**: 266–70.

Kyle RF, Cabanela ME, Russell TA et al (1994) Fractures of the proximal part of the femur, *J Bone Joint Surg* **76A**: 924–50.

Lange RH, Bach AW, Hansen ST, Johansen KH (1985) Open tibial fractures with associated vascular injuries. Prognosis for limb salvage, *J Trauma* **25**: 203–8.

Leung KS, So WS, Shen WY, Hui PW (1992) Gamma nails and dynamic hip screws for peritrochanteric fractures, *J Bone Joint Surg* **74B**: 345–51.

Lhowe DW, Hansen ST (1988) Immediate nailing of open fractures of the femoral shaft, *J Bone Joint Surg* **70A**: 812–20.

Loomer RL, Meek R, De Sommer F (1980) Plating of femoral shaft fractures: the Vancouver experience, *J Trauma* **20**: 1038–42.

Lucas SE, Seligson D, Henry SL (1993) Intramedullary supracondylar nailing of femoral fractures, *Clin Orthop Rel Res* **296**: 200–6.

Macausland WR, Eaton RG (1963) The management of sepsis following intramedullary fixation for fractures of the femur, *J Bone Joint Surg* **45A**: 1643–53.

McGraw JM, Lim EVA (1988) Treatment of open tibial shaft fractures. External fixation and secondary intramedullary nailing, *J Bone Joint Surg* **70A**: 900–11.

Magerl F, Wyss A, Brunner C, Binder W (1979) Plate osteosynthesis of femoral shaft fractures in adults. A follow-up study, *Clin Orthop* **138**: 62–73.

Manning JB, Bach AW, Herman CM, Carrico CJ (1983) Fat release after femur nailing in the dog, *J Trauma* **23**: 322–6.

Müller ME, Nazarian S, Koch P, Schatzker J (1990) *The Comprehensive Classification of Fractures of Long Bones* (Springer-Verlag: New York) 128–31.

Murphy CP, D'Ambrosia RD, Dabezies EJ, Acker JH, Shoji H, Chuinard RG (1988) Complex femur fractures: treatment with the Wagner external fixation device or the Grosse-Kempf interlocking nail, *J Trauma* **28**: 1553–61.

Nichols PJR (1963) Rehabilitation after fractures of the shaft of the femur, *J Bone Joint Surg* **45B**: 96–102.

Nowotarski PJ, Brumback RJ (1994) Immediate interlocking nailing of gunshot femoral fractures, *Orthop Trans* **18(1)**: 5–6.

O'Brien PJ, Meek RN, Powell JN, Blachut PA (1991) Primary intramedullary nailing of open femoral shaft fractures, *J Trauma* **31**: 113–16.

Pell A, Christie J, Keating JF, Sutherland G (1993) The detection of fat embolism by transoesophageal echocardiography during reamed intramedullary nailing. A study of 24 patients with femoral and tibial fractures, *J Bone Joint Surg* **75B**: 921–5.

Perren S (1991) Concept of biological plating using the limited contact dynamic compression plate. Scientific background, design and application, *Injury* **22** (Suppl): 1–41.

Pierre RK St, Fleming SS, Fleming LL (1982) Fractures of the femoral shaft: a prospective study of closed intramedullary nailing, modified open intramedullary nailing and cast-bracing, *South Med J* **75**(7): 827–35.

Rhinelander FW (1974) Tibial blood supply in relation to fracture healing, *Clin Orthop* **105**: 34–81.

Riska EB, Myllynen P (1982) Fat embolism in patients with multiple injuries, *J Trauma* **22**: 891–4.

Rittmann WW, Schibli M, Matter P, Allgower M (1979) Open fractures. Long term results in 200 consecutive cases, *Clin Orthop* **138**: 132–40.

Rüedi T, Lüscher JN (1979) Results after internal fixation of comminuted fractures of the femoral shaft with DC plates, *Clin Orthop* **138**: 74–8.

Ryan JR, Hensel RT, Salciccioli GG, Pedersen HE (1981) Fractures of the femur secondary to low velocity gunshot wounds, *J Trauma* **21**: 160–2.

Sanders R, Swiontkowski M, Nunley J, Spiegel P (1993) The management of fractures with soft tissue disruptions, *J Bone Joint Surg* **75A**: 778–89.

Schemitsch E, Kowalski M, Swiontkowski M, Senft D (1994) Effects of reamed versus unreamed locked intramedullary nailing on bone blood flow in a fractured sheep tibia model, *Orthop Trans* **18**: 6–7.

Schlickewei W, Kuner EH, Mullaji AB, Götze B (1992) Upper and lower limb fractures with concomitant arterial injury, *J Bone Joint Surg* **74B**: 181–8.

Schweigel JF, Gropper PT (1974) A comparison of ambulatory versus non-ambulatory care of femoral shaft fractures, *J Trauma* **14**: 474–81.

Seligson D, Kristiansen TK (1978) Use of the Wagner apparatus in complicated fractures of the distal femur, *J Trauma* **18**: 795–9.

Thomas TL, Meggit BF (1981) A comparative study of methods for treating fractures of the distal half of the femur, *J Bone Joint Surg* **63B**: 3–6.

Whitenack S, Hausberger F (1971) Intravascularisation of fat from the bone marrow cavity, *Am J Pathol* **65**: 335–45.

Winquist RA, Hansen ST (1980) Comminuted fractures of the femoral shaft treated by intramedullary nailing, *Orthop Clin N Am* **11**: 633–48.

Wiss DA, Fleming CH, Matta JM, Clark D (1986) Comminuted and rotationally unstable fractures of the femur treated with an interlocking nail, *Clin Orthop* **212**: 35–47.

Wiss DA, Brien WW, Becker V (1991) Interlocking nailing for the treatment of femoral fractures due to gunshot wounds, *J Bone Joint Surg* **73A**: 598–606.

Wozasek GE, Simon P, Redl H, Schlag O (1994) Fat embolism during intramedullary nailing. *Orthop Trans* **18**: 4.

7
Open tibial fractures

C.M. Court-Brown

The epidemiological data contained in Chapter 3 show that the tibia has a greater incidence of open fractures than that of any other bone, except those of the fingers. Not only are open fractures of the tibia common, but their treatment is contentious. The fact that external skeletal fixation and intramedullary nailing have both been adopted by orthopaedic surgeons in recent years has merely served to fuel the debate as to how these difficult fractures should be treated. Orthopaedic surgeons tend to have a preoccupation with fixation methods and often attribute the quality of their results to the use of a particular implant or device. Thus in the last 20 years, improved results in the management of open fractures of the tibia have been attributed to the use of dynamic compression plates, rigid external fixation, dynamic external fixation, small pin external fixation and both reamed and unreamed intramedullary nails. In reality, the use of different metallic implants or explants has probably had little effect on the incidence of infection or non-union following open fracture, these outcome criteria depending mainly on the nature of the injury and the quality of the treatment of the soft-tissue injury associated with the fracture. It is likely that the prognosis of an open tibial fracture is governed mainly by the adequacy of the initial debridement and the skill with which the soft tissues are treated by the plastic surgeons. This is not to denigrate the role of the orthopaedic surgeon and the choice of implant. There is no doubt that outcome criteria such as the incidence of malunion, the requirement for open bone grafting, joint mobilization and return of the patient to full function and to work are affected by the choice of treatment method. As with closed fractures the surgeon can choose between four basic treatment methods, these being non-operative management using a cast or brace, dynamic compression plating, external

skeletal fixation using one of many different designs of external fixator, or intramedullary nailing. In recent years, there has been a marked trend away from cast or brace treatment of open tibial fractures, particularly when they are Gustilo type II or III in severity. This is understandable as there has been a realization that immobilization is important for the healing of both soft tissue and bone. In addition, immobilization of open fractures undoubtedly lessens further injury to the soft-tissue envelope as well as relieving pain and facilitating inspection and treatment of the open wound. Until relatively recently, immobilization of open fractures could only be achieved by the use of casts or splints made of plaster of Paris or other similar material. However, internal and external fixation techniques have been in widespread use for the last 50 years or so and many surgeons now use both techniques as primary treatment for open tibial fractures.

Blood supply of the tibial diaphysis

The rationale for the use of different fixation methods is often attributed to the effect that they have on the diaphyseal blood supply at bone union. It is certainly true that alteration of the blood supply to the tibial diaphysis and associated changes in medullary and periosteal osteogenesis following tibial diaphyseal fracture are of paramount importance not only when considering the need for stabilization of open fractures, but also when analysing the role of different fracture fixation methods. The vascular supply of the normal tibial diaphysis is well known following studies by Brookes (1971) and Rhinelander (1972). These researchers showed that the direction of normal blood flow through the diaphyseal cortex is centrifugal, travelling from the medulla to the periosteum. The direction of flow is influenced by the pressure gradient from the medullary canal to the periosteum. Under normal circumstances, the periosteal circulation supplies the outer third of the bone cortex and the relative importance of the medullary blood supply in the intact tibia is not in doubt, although in occlusive vascular disease and osteoarthritis the flow can be reversed.

Following tibial diaphyseal fracture, the cortical vascular supply changes and a new external supply develops. This has been named the extraosseous blood supply of healing bone. Unlike the periosteal blood supply this is not conveyed through fascial attachments but reaches bone wherever healing is in progress. Gothman (1961) showed that the source of the extraosseous blood supply was the injured soft tissues adjacent to the fracture. It develops immediately after injury and supplies the early periosteal callus. It conveys much of the blood to healing bone and as Rhinelander (1974) indicated that the tibial nutrient artery was often damaged in even slightly displaced fractures it is obvious that the extraosseous blood supply has a dominant role after fracture.

The vascular supply to the bone has been examined after both undisplaced and displaced closed fractures. Since open fractures are rarely undisplaced it is logical to examine the vasculature of displaced closed fractures when considering open fractures. Rhinelander et al (1968) clearly showed that stabilization was essential for displaced closed fractures to heal. They showed that stabilization increased both the osseous blood supply and the amount of medullary callus when compared with cast-managed patients. They also considered that stabilization was more important than accurate reduction as long as an adequate blood supply was present.

Use of rigid bone plates

Early work by Rahn et al (1971) suggested that the use of bone plates promoted primary bone union or direct cortical healing without callus formation. These experiments were done in animals using an osteotomy made with a very thin saw and held under direct compression with a plate. They were carried out under ideal conditions without significant soft-tissue stripping and it is unlikely that they duplicated the circumstances found in an open tibial fracture.

Rahn et al (1971) stated that the important factor was direct osteonal crossing of the cortical defect but in fact Rhinelander (1972) showed that the technique actually served to promote medullary osteogenesis with minimal periosteal callus being formed. Further vascular studies showed that the application of a bone plate deleteriously affects the vascularization of that segment of cortex under the plate as a normal circulatory flow is blocked. The other significant vascular problem associated with plating is that excessive soft-tissue stripping to allow the application of a plate may compromise fracture vascularity and lead to non-union.

External skeletal fixation

External fixation has some of the same effects on bone vascularization as plating by the nature of the stability conferred on the fracture. Unlike with plating or nailing, the stiffness of an external fixation device can be altered and some surgeons use this property in the management of open fractures, applying a stiff configuration at the beginning of treatment and then reducing the stiffness to facilitate callus formation once the soft tissues have healed. The effect of a stiff external fixation device on the healing of osteotomized rabbit tibiae was examined by Court-Brown (1985). This experiment compared the blood flow and histology in osteotomized rabbit tibiae, one tibia being fixed by a stiff unilateral frame, with the osteotomy in the contralateral tibia being immobilized by plaster cast. Striking differences were seen in the histological analysis of both osteotomies. This showed that with rigid external fixation medullary osteogenesis was markedly enhanced, with the periosteal callus formation being increased by plaster management. However, while rigid external fixation was associated with decreased callus formation, there was little doubt that there was acceleration of the endochondral ossification of the periosteal callus that was formed. The overall effect was that bone union was facilitated by external fixation compared with cast management.

Intramedullary nailing

Rhinelander (1974) detailed the effects of introducing a single large intramedullary nail into the tibial diaphysis. He used the Küntscher technique, employing reaming to ensure a secure fit in the medullary canal. The combination of reaming and nailing obliterated the medullary blood supply. He demonstrated gradual return of the medullary vasculature, but concluded that cortical regeneration of the nutrient arterial supply was so slow in reaching the osteotomy that delayed osseous union was inevitable. Further experimentation using a four-fluted nail showed faster regeneration of the intramedullary blood supply. Rhinelander showed that at four weeks, the nutrient artery had regenerated, but he still emphasized the relative slowness of revascularization via the medullary supply. More recently, Klein et al (1990) have examined the difference between reamed and unreamed nails with reference to interference with the cortical circulation of the canine tibia. They demonstrated that both techniques disturbed the cortical circulation but on average the diaphyseal vascular supply was reduced by 31% with unreamed nails and 70% with reamed nails. Schemitsch et al (1994) have confirmed the findings of Klein and his co-workers. They used a spiral fracture model in sheep tibia and demonstrated that after unreamed nailing cortical revascularization had occurred by six weeks. If reamed nails were used, the revascularization was not complete until 12 weeks. The consistency of these findings since certainly suggests that reaming has a deleterious effect on the cortical vasculature but there is little evidence from clinical trials that it greatly matters. Indeed a recent publication by Reichert et al (1995) has suggested that reaming may be advantageous in causing increased periosteal vascularity. Certainly in closed fractures the results from Court-Brown et al (1990a) do not indicate a vascularization problem.

A review of the literature regarding bone vascularity and fracture fixation suggests a number of overall conclusions with reference to open tibial fractures:

1. Stabilization promotes bone union.
2. The incidence of infection is likely to be less in stabilized open fractures as revascularization is facilitated.
3. Plated fractures heal mainly by medullary osteogenesis. The absence of periosteal callus may account for the high incidence of refracture that is seen with this technique.
4. Nailed fractures heal by periosteal new bone formation. Clinical trials fail to confirm the importance of the damage to the medullary blood supply by reaming.
5. Externally fixed fractures allow for an altered biomechanical environment promoting either medullary or periosteal ossification depending on stiffness of the particular frame used by the surgeon.

External casting for open tibial fractures

Until relatively recently, the standard method of treating all tibial fractures whether open or closed was by the application of a cast or brace. Theoretically, this method should lead to poor results especially in the management of more serious open fractures and indeed this is probably the case. However, the trend towards operative fixation of open fractures has also been accompanied by other changes of surgical practice, such as the use of antibiotics, improved soft-tissue management and more sophisticated bone-reconstruction techniques. Another reason why comparison of cast-treated open fractures with internally or externally fixed fractures is impossible, is that most of the literature dealing with external casting or traction is at least 25 years old and was written before the advent of modern classification systems and outcome measurements. It is likely that the older literature dealing with cast management overstates the usefulness of the technique. In addition, there is virtually no literature dealing exclusively with open fractures, and it is usually impossible to distil the facts about the open fractures from the mixed data supplied about the treatment of the whole tibial fracture group. Two reports illustrate the difficulty of comparing the older literature with current literature. Brown and Urban (1969) and Burkhalter and Protzman (1975) analysed

Table 7.1   Treatment of tibial fractures with long-leg casts

Author	Number of fractures	Open fractures (%)	Time to union (weeks)	Malunion (%)	Joint stiffness (%)
Nicoll (1964)	674	22.5	15.9	8.6	25.0
Slatis and Rokkinen (1967)	198	33.3	19.8	?	?
Karahaju et al (1979)	80	23.7	?	11.2*	27.5*
Steen Jensen et al (1977)	102	?	?	21.0*	7.0*
Van der Linden and Larsen (1979)	50	12.0	17.0	50.0	24.0
Haines et al (1984)	91	36.3	16.3	25.3	33.0
Kay et al (1986)	79	22.8	19.1	9.1	?
Kyro et al (1991)	165	21.0	13.7	30.0*	42.0*

*Value is a minimum figure. The true value is probably higher. ? data not available.

Table 7.2   Treatment of tibial fractures with patellar-tendon-bearing casts

Author	Number of fractures	Open fractures (%)	Time to union (weeks)	Malunion (%)	Joint stiffness (%)
Mollan and Bradley (1978)	106	38.3	10.0	?	?
Austin (1981)	132	11.4	16.7	39.0	?
Bostmann and Hanninen (1982)	114	16.0	15.3	40.0	?
Hooper et al (1991)	33	21.0	18.3	27.3	15.0

? data not available.

Table 7.3   Treatment of tibial fractures with functional braces

Author	Number of fractures	Open fractures (%)	Time to union (weeks)	Malunion (%)	Joint stiffness (%)
Sarmiento (1970)	135	24.4	15.5	?	?
Sarmiento et al (1989)	780	31.0	18.7	13.7	?
Suman (1982)	82	36.6	14.7	?	9.7
Digby et al (1983)	82	20.7	17.4	9.0*	45.0
Den Outer et al (1990)	94	11.7	?	40.0	?
Pun et al (1991)	97	7.2	17.1	23.7*	28.9*
Alho et al (1992)	35	31.4	17.0	8.6*	26.0*

*Value is a minimum figure. The true value is probably higher. ? data not available.

their results of the use of long-leg casts in the management of tibial fractures. These authors dealt with many of the late problems following the Vietnam War. They presumably saw their patients at a late stage, initial management having been carried out earlier. Brown and Urban (1969) reviewed 63 tibial fractures treated by long-leg casts and documented a mean time to union of 19 weeks despite the presence of 'massive loss of skin and muscle' in many wounds. Fifty-seven patients had 'no disability' although many showed only 'good to normal'

knee movement. There was a considerable incidence of malunion and infection was not thought to be a problem despite 15 fractures discharging for at least 27 weeks. Burkhalter and Protzman (1975) documented an infection rate of 3% despite treating 159 open fractures with exposed bone without the use of flaps. Comparison with modern papers is difficult and the most likely explanation of the apparent difference in standards is that the surgeons had different criteria for the definition of successful results. The use of casts in the management of tibial fractures is analysed in Tables 7.1 and 7.2. The incidence of open fractures varies between 12% and 38.3%, but it is impossible to break down the overall results into those for closed and open fractures.

A number of authors have used casting techniques for less severe fractures, reserving fixation methods for severe problems. It is therefore obvious that little can be gleaned from much of the literature regarding the usefulness of cast management in open fractures. However, Nicoll (1964) and Karahaju et al (1979) both commented on the association between wound size and soft-tissue damage and eventual joint stiffness. Steen-Jensen et al (1977), in a study comparing bone plating with the use of long-leg casts, showed a 34% incidence of skin necrosis or infection in open fractures treated with a cast. They also found a 21% incidence of non-union in the open fracture group.

The results of the use of the patella tendon bearing cast popularized by Sarmiento (1967) are shown in Table 7.2. Bostmann and Hanninen (1982) had a 15% infection rate in open fractures using such a cast. They detailed the overall complications for conservative management of tibial fractures as 18% with 22% for screw fixation, 28% for plate fixation and 12% for intramedullary nailing. The use of functional bracing is detailed in Table 7.3. These braces theoretically allow for movement of knee, ankle and subtalar joints. However, comparison of Tables 7.1–7.3 shows that, despite the theoretical freedom provided by the brace, the results in terms of joint mobility are poor and there is little evidence that joint stiffness is improved by the use of functional braces. Sarmiento et al (1989) published their results on the use of functional bracing with 780 tibial fractures. However, they used a number of exclusion criteria and treated Gustilo type III open fractures with external fixation, although they often applied a functional brace after the soft tissues had united. Their open fractures took on average 4.3 weeks longer than their closed fractures to unite and they felt that functional bracing was appropriate for closed and Gustilo type I fractures, but not for type III fractures. Den Outer et al (1990) and Alho et al (1992) both undertook retrospective studies comparing the use of functional braces with other methods of treating tibial diaphyseal fractures. Den Outer et al (1990)

used functional braces for closed and type I open fractures only and concluded that functional bracing was the preferred method of management for these fractures. Alho et al (1992) took the view that intramedullary nailing was a better technique. Analysis of the literature dealing with cast management of open tibial fractures does not help to specify the role of this technique in different types of open fractures. It seems that Gustilo type II and III open fractures are not well treated by cast management. The difficulty of treating the wound and the relatively high incidence of infection suggests that internal or external fixation is better. As regards type I open tibial fractures, these probably have a similar prognosis to closed fractures and the surgeon should use whichever technique he or she is familiar with. However, the incidence of malunion and joint stiffness noted in Tables 7.1–7.3 indicates that cast or brace management of these fractures is not without its problems.

Plating of open tibial fractures

The introduction of the dynamic compression plate (Figure 7.1) stimulated considerable interest in the plating of open tibial fractures. A study of the literature relevant to this technique in the 1970s and early 1980s suggests that the use of the technique was not always accompanied by surgical excellence and possibly because of this, the technique is no longer widely used. Tibial plating is the most difficult of all the operative techniques commonly used to stabilize open tibial fractures. The soft-tissue dissection must be undertaken very carefully to avoid excessive stripping of the periosteum, fascia and muscle, thereby increasing the incidence of non-union. In addition, skin closure over a plate in a traumatized limb can often be difficult and a high incidence of skin necrosis or superficial infection is reported for tibial plating of open fractures (Steen-Jensen et al 1977, Van der Linden and Larsson 1979, Rommens and Schmidt-Neuerberg 1987).

It should be remembered that many of the commonly used reconstructive plastic surgery techniques had not been devised in the late 1970s and there was certainly less awareness of the problems of apparently superficial skin necrosis. It is therefore not surprising that some

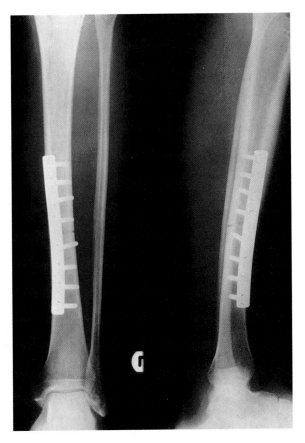

Figure 7.1

The use of a dynamic compression plate to stabilize a tibial diaphyseal fracture.

authors had a relatively high infection rate (Table 7.4) following tibial plating of open fractures. However, the incidence of infection in plated open tibial fractures is complicated by the terminology used in dealing with the problem. The terms 'superficial infection', 'osteitis' and 'deep infection' are all in widespread use. There seems little doubt that all these terms are synonyms for bone infection and it is possible that the incidence of bone infection is actually greater than the reports suggest.

In recent years, with increased interest in external fixation and intramedullary nailing, there has been less interest in tibial plating and the report by Bach and Hansen (1989) represents one of the very few dealing with the tibial plating of open fractures using modern techniques.

The early work of Ruedi et al (1976) produced very good results. They analysed 95 open fractures, of which 83 were grade I or II according to Allgöwer's criteria (see Chapter 2). Their results are detailed in Table 7.4. It would appear that their poor results were mainly seen in grade III open fractures where they had two amputations. Rittman et al (1979) examined 200 consecutive fractures of which 131 were in the lower leg. They had ten infections (7.6%) of which nine occurred in type II or III open fractures. The severity of infection in these particular fractures is highlighted by the fact that the average time to union following surgery to treat the infection was 33.2 months.

Van der Linden and Larsson (1979) carried out a prospective study comparing plate fixation with non-operative management of tibial fractures. Only six fractures were open in each

Table 7.4 The use of plates in the management of tibial fractures

Author	Number of fractures	Fracture type*	Infection (%)	Fixation failure (%)	Malunion (%)	Refracture (%)	Joint stiffness (%)
Ruedi et al (1976)	95	O (GI–III)	11.6	6.3	?	1.0	?
Steen Jensen et al (1977)	44	O (GI–III)	11.3	0	2.8	4.8	6.8
Van der Linden and Larsson (1979)	50	C,O	4	2	0	0	16
Rommens and Schmidt-Neuerberg (1987)	113	O (GI–III)	12.1	0	6	3	?
Clifford et al (1988)	97	O (GI–III)	10.3	7.2	3.1	0	11.4
Bach and Hansen (1989)	26	O (GII–III)	19.2	11.5	3.8	3.8	?
Den Outer et al (1990)	76	C,O (GI)	2.6	5.3	7.0	3.9	?

*C denotes closed fractures, O denotes open fractures and GI–III signifies the Gustilo fracture types that were treated. ? data not available.

group, but they documented a greater incidence of complications in the plating group with more superficial infections, skin necrosis and osteomyelitis. The difference in complications between the two groups was significant.

Rommens and Schmidt-Neuerberg (1987) analysed ten years' experience of operatively managed tibial fractures, 217 cases being treated by plating of which 113 were open fractures. The results are shown in Table 7.4. However, as with other series, most open fractures were Gustilo type I or type II in severity and only seven type III fractures were plated. The authors comment that 80% of the open fractures healed within four months, 15 patients required secondary surgery for non-union and 11 patients developed osteitis. All of these patients had either type II or type III fractures for which the primary operation time exceeded two hours. Control of infection was clearly difficult as multiple surgical procedures were required.

Clifford et al (1988) analysed 97 open fractures of the tibial shaft of which 60 were either type II or type III in severity. The overall infection rate was 10.3%, but detailed analysis showed that the infection rate of the type I wounds was 5.4% with 7.8% for the type II wounds and 44.4% for the type III wounds. They commented on the importance of patient selection and meticulous surgical technique but felt that plating was a reasonable treatment for the type I or type II open fractures.

Bach and Hansen (1989) carried out a prospective randomized trial of plate fixation and external fixation in severe open tibial fractures. All 59 patients had Gustilo type II or III fractures. Twenty-six patients were plated. There were three cases of fixation failure and nine patients (34.5%) had superficial infection with five of them (19.2%) developing chronic osteomyelitis. The complication rate of plating considerably exceeded that of external fixation and the authors felt that plating was an inappropriate technique for Gustilo type II and III open fractures.

The stated potential problems of plating open tibial fractures are that the plate itself obstructs the normal centrifugal blood flow and that the rigid nature of the plate so minimizes callus formation that there is a high incidence of non-union and refracture. In addition, the need to strip soft tissues from the bone to facilitate plate placement contributes to non-union. These factors have encouraged surgeons to develop new plates and techniques to attempt to circumvent these problems. The use of the low contact dynamic compression (LCDC) plate is said to minimize interference with cortical blood flow.

Animal experiments (Monney et al 1991) have suggested that conventional dynamic compression plates produce a greater disturbance of the cortical blood supply and early clinical results using the LCDC plate suggest good biocompatibility, but further research is necessary to demonstrate its superiority over the conventional dynamic compression plate.

Another innovation in plating is the use of 'biological' plating techniques. The early philosophy of the AO group was that rigid fixation was mandatory, but the later success of non-rigid fixation systems has encouraged them to develop plating techniques that permit greater callus formation (Perren et al 1991). Such techniques include the use of biocompatible plates such as the low contact dynamic compression plate (Figure 7.2) and restricting the number

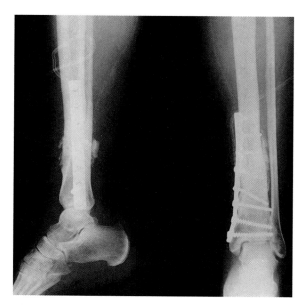

Figure 7.2

A low contact dynamic compression (LCDC) plate used to treat a refracture of a tibial diaphyseal fracture which occurred in a skiing accident. Theoretically, the sculpted surface of the plate facilitates vascular ingrowth although it must be stressed that there is little clinical evidence of the benefit of this type of plate.

of screws placed in the diaphysis. Again, much more work is needed to analyse these changes.

The need for extensive soft-tissue stripping has been addressed by the use of subcutaneous plating. This technique involves the careful contouring of long plates to the exact shape of the tibia. These are inserted subcutaneously into the leg on the subcutaneous border of the tibia and the position of the plate is checked by fluoroscopy. Screws are then inserted percutaneously under fluoroscopic control with minimal soft-tissue damage. This technique is reported to be successful in occasional cases (Sanders, personal communication 1993) but it clearly requires considerable skill and may not be generally applicable.

External skeletal fixation

The use of external skeletal fixation utilizing metallic transosseous screws or pins seems to have started with the work of Cucel and Rigaud (1850). However, it was Albin Lambotte (1913) who documented the advantages and complications of external fixation. He utilized the technique in the management of open fractures as did Parkhill (1898) and Hey-Groves (1921) in Great Britain. External skeletal fixation continued to be used in both Europe and North America until 1950 when, despite excellent results in the literature, a report from the American Academy of Orthopaedic Surgeons (Johnson and Stovald, 1950) criticized the technique and its use waned considerably in North America.

In Europe, however, external fixation continued to be popular, with the Hoffmann multiplanar fixator being studied in considerable detail. Lindahl (1962) published the first biomechanical evaluation of the Hoffmann device and Burney and Bourgois (1965) and Vidal (1970) and Adrey (1970) all examined the clinical usefulness of this fixator. There was a difference of opinion as to the type of frame that should be applied. Burney and his co-workers have consistently favoured the simple, non-rigid Hoffmann configurations which allow callus formation, whereas Vidal and Adrey proposed that a rigid fixation using a quadrilateral frame was superior.

The work of these researchers rekindled interest in North America and the 1970s and 1980s

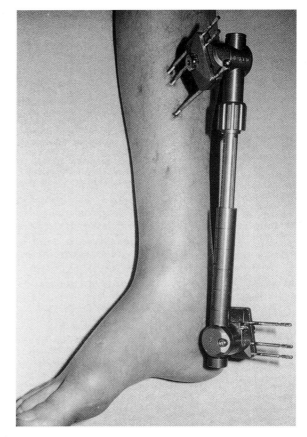

Figure 7.3

A unilateral external fixator used to treat a tibial pilon fracture by the principle of ligamentotaxis. Pins have been placed in the tibial diaphysis and the calcaneus.

heralded an explosion of interest in external skeletal fixation, particularly with reference to open fractures of the tibial diaphysis. The evolution of external fixation has followed a number of paths. A number of surgeons advocated the use of simple unilateral fixators as shown in Figure 7.3 (Edge and Denham 1981, Sukhtian and Hughes 1979, Evans et al 1981, De Bastiani et al 1984) on the grounds that these simple frames maximized soft-tissue access while permitting satisfactory bone fixation. Other surgeons promoted the use of multiplanar fixators as

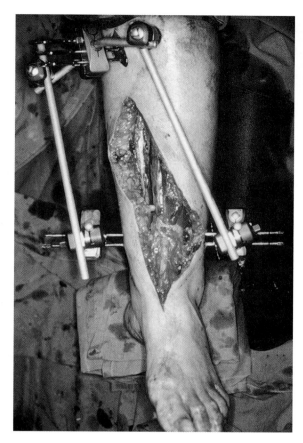

Figure 7.4

A Hoffmann external fixator used in a biplanar configuration. The advantage of this type of device is that a large number of different frame configurations can be constructed.

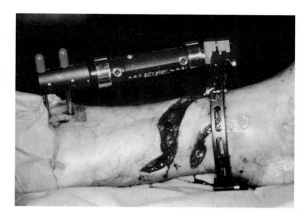

Figure 7.5

An Orthofix hybrid fixator used to treat an open tibial pilon fracture. Small wires have been used to transfix the distal fragments, with conventional half-pins being employed in the diaphysis.

demonstrated in Figure 7.4 (Vidal 1970, Adrey 1970) and circular devices which greatly restricted soft-tissue access, this being a considerable problem in the management of open tibial fractures (Oganesyan 1982, Fischer 1983).

Recent interest in external fixation has focused around the dynamization of the fracture to allow for fracture motion and thereby increasing callus formation. This facility has been advocated mainly by proponents of the Orthofix fixator (De Bastiani 1984, Melendez and Colon 1989, Keating et al 1991). This type of fixator is usually applied in a static mode with dynamization being allowed after a short period. Kenwright and his co-workers (1991) have assessed the usefulness of a pneumatic pump in the application of controlled axial fracture displacement.

Recently, there has been a resurgence of interest in circular external fixators, although the modern circular frames have utilized multiple small wires rather than larger more traditional half-pins or transfixion pins. This interest in small wire fixation has followed the work of Ilizarov (1992). Initially, this type of device was used for the late reconstruction of deformity, but recently its use in open fractures has been advocated. In the last few years surgeons have been interested in hybrid external fixation devices (Figure 7.5) for the management of metaphyseal or intra-articular fractures. These fixators consist of a circular or semi-circular frame utilizing small wires or half-pins which are used to stabilize the metaphysis. Any intra-articular fracture is usually treated by limited internal fixation and the metaphysis is secured to the diaphysis by a conventional single bar fixator utilizing half-pins. Early work with these devices suggests that they may be superior to conventional plating techniques in the stabilization of open metaphyseal and intra-articular fractures.

Table 7.5 Use of unilateral external fixators

Author	Fixator type	Number of fractures	Fracture type*	Pin sepsis (%)	Malunion (%)	Duration of fixation (weeks)	Infection (%)
Edge and Denham (1981)	Portsmouth	38	C,O	42	60	22	51
De Bastiani et al (1984)	Orthofix	131	C,O	0.6	?	?	0.3
Court-Brown and Hughes (1985)	Hughes	48	C,O (GI–III)	25.5	38.6	?	4.2
Evans et al (1988)	Shearer	30	C,O (GI–III)	2.8	10	16.5	?
Melendez and Colon (1989)	Orthofix	45	O,G (I–III)	17	4.4	?	22
Keating et al (1991)	Orthofix	100	C,O (GI–III)	30	24	12	1
Kenwright et al (1991)	Oxford Static	40	C,O (GI–III)	19.2	?	>12	0
Kenwright et al (1991)	Oxford Dynamic	40	C,O (GI–III)	12	?	>12	0
Krettek et al (1991)	Monofixator	44	O (GI–III)	11	13	?	5

*C denotes closed fractures, O denotes open fractures and GI–III signifies the Gustilo fracture types that were treated. ? data not available.

The most recent development in external fixation has been a pinless fixator (Babst et al 1992). This device has been developed by the AO group and is based on the principle of the bone clamp. Babst et al state that it provides good temporary bone fixation and is particularly useful if the surgeon is contemplating secondary intramedullary nailing, but there are few clinical results available at this time.

At present, there are three major groups of external fixators which merit further discussion. These are unilateral frames, most of which now permit axial movement at the fracture site, multiplanar frames which can be built into a number of different configurations and circular or hybrid fixators utilizing small wires or half-pins.

Unilateral external fixation

The results of a number of studies detailing the use of unilateral external fixation (Figure 7.3) in the management of tibial diaphyseal fractures are shown in Table 7.5. Most studies deal with both open and closed fractures and therefore the stated union times are merely an average of time to union for different severities of fracture. In addition, the incidence of non-union is also a poor outcome measure as some authors adopt an aggressive bone-grafting policy thereby lowering the incidence of non-union. Time to union and the incidence of non-union are therefore not included in Table 7.5. There is some evidence that static unilateral external fixation

tends to delay union. Court-Brown and Hughes (1985) found that the average time to union for their closed and Gustilo type I open fractures was 29.2 weeks and noted that this was considerably in excess of the average time to union for other fracture treatment measures. Similar results were obtained by Evans et al (1988) who also found an average time to union of 29 weeks in closed fractures treated by closed techniques with a static Shearer fixator. Kenwright et al (1991) found that the static form of the unilateral Oxford fixator appeared to delay union when compared with the dynamized form.

Unilateral external fixators which permit micromovement of the fracture site appear to have better results. De Bastiani et al (1984) had remarkable healing times for tibial fractures using the Orthofix fixator. Their closed tibial fractures united in an average of 15 weeks and the open fractures in 23 weeks. Melendez and Colon (1989) used the Orthofix device in the treatment of 45 open tibial fractures. The mean healing time was 22.6 weeks with a range of 9.5 to 35.5 weeks. Keating et al (1991) had a mean time to union of 15.2 weeks for closed tibial fractures with 20.5 weeks for open fractures.

In the only prospective randomized trial examining the effects of dynamization using a unilateral frame, Kenwright et al (1991) showed that micromovement with a pneumatic pump significantly reduced the union time in closed and type I open tibial fractures which were not comminuted. In comminuted or more severe open fractures, the effect of dynamization was less pronounced.

Table 7.6 Use of multiplanar external fixators

Author	Fixator type	Number of fractures	Fracture type*	Pin sepsis (%)	Malunion (%)	Duration of fixation (weeks)	Infection (%)
Benum and Svenningsen (1982)	Hoffmann	50	C,O (GI–III)	50.0	50.0	24.0	2.0
Chan et al (1984)	AO	17	O III	?	41.0	?	38.0
Behrens and Searls (1986)	AO	75	C,O	12.0	1.3	14.4	3.0
Edwards et al (1988)	Hoffmann	202	O (GIII)	29.0	9.0	12.0	15.0
Blick et al (1989)	Hoffmann	53	C,O (GI–III)	28.0	?	23.0	7.5
Holbrook et al (1989)	AO Hoffmann Orthofix	28	O (GI–III)	13.6	10.7	10.0	14.0
Whitelaw et al (1990)	Hoffmann ICCH	17	O (GI–III)	12.0	35.0	8.2	18.0
Court-Brown et al (1990b)	Hughes Hoffmann	57	G–III	35.0	47.0	10.9	17.6

*C denotes closed fractures, O denotes open fractures and GI–III signifies the Gustilo fracture types that were treated. ? data not available.

Table 7.5 indicates that the main complications of unilateral external fixation are pin track sepsis and malunion. There is no accepted definition of what constitutes pin track sepsis and the considerable differences seen in Table 7.5 are probably largely accounted for by a failure to standardize the definition of this problem. However, an incidence of between 20% and 42% is not uncommon.

Malunion is usually caused by the premature removal of the frame. Patients often tire of wearing an external frame for a prolonged period and wish its removal. If this is done prior to the formation of adequate callus, fracture malposition and subsequent malunion may result. Court-Brown and Hughes (1985) examined the incidence of tibial malunion with reference to a number of parameters. The parameters they examined were the alteration of pin angle, pin location and pin length as well as fixation locator. None of these parameters altered time to union or the incidence of malunion. They found that adequacy of fracture reduction and the duration of external fixation were the only factors to alter time to union, incidence of malunion and the requirement for bone grafting.

It is perhaps unfair to compare papers dealing with external fixation written a decade apart. The awareness of the importance of adequate debridement and flap cover has certainly increased since Edge and Denham (1981) documented their results. However, the results in Table 7.5 must give rise to some concern. It would appear that static unilateral fixation tends to prolong union when compared with other techniques, although the use of dynamized fixators improves the result. However, it is interesting to note that the results of Kenwright et al (1991) using a dynamic fixator, although better than their static fixation results, are equivalent to those using bracing (Digby et al 1982) and nailing (Court-Brown et al 1990a).

Multiplanar external fixation

External fixation differs from other fracture-fixation methods in two principal ways. Some external fixators can be applied in many different configurations ranging from simple unilateral frames to complex arrangements which impart considerable rigidity to the fracture. They can also be used to stabilize many different types of fracture whether they be intra-articular, metaphyseal or diaphyseal. The use of external fixation to stabilize metaphyseal or intra-articular fractures usually requires a multiplanar frame (Figure 7.4) and although many surgeons have employed unilateral frames for diaphyseal fractures (Table 7.5), others have advocated more rigid frames (Table 7.6).

Many workers have investigated the biomechanical properties of different fixators and their configuration (Chao et al 1989) and there is no doubt that fracture healing is altered by the stiffness of the frame. However, there is no clinical evidence that any one fixator or fixator configuration is superior to others and good results are obtained by adherence to good surgical practice (Behrens and Searls 1986, Court-Brown and Hughes 1985, Court-Brown et al 1990b). This indicates that the philosophy of Burney and his co-workers is probably correct and that the simplest frame to offer adequate fixation of the fracture should be used. Table 7.6 analyses the use of multiplanar fixation. As with the unilateral fixator (Table 7.5) a number of reports have included some closed fractures in their series, although these are usually relatively few in number. Benum and Svenningsen (1982) compared two different Hoffmann configurations, finding no difference in the results between bilateral uniplanar Hoffmann planes and the Vidal–Adrey double-frame mounting. They, like the other reports listed in Table 7.6, found a high incidence of pin track sepsis and malunion despite maintaining the frame for an average of 24 weeks.

Behrens and Searls (1986) analysed 75 fractures, of which most were open, using the AO frame. Most fractures were treated with a unilateral configuration but 17.3% of the group had a bilateral construct. They defined a safe surgical corridor for pin fixation and concluded that external fixation was a good method of managing open tibial fractures, but that a uniplanar device was usually adequate. Their low pin track sepsis rate was attributed to accuracy of pin placement, pin design, predrilling and good postoperative care.

A number of authors have examined the use of external fixation in the management of Gustilo type III open fractures. Chan et al (1984), mainly using the AO fixator, had a high complication rate, finding a 38% incidence of infection and a 41% incidence of malunion. They did not document their pin track sepsis rate, but it was clearly very high and they commented that pin loosening was present in virtually every case. They advocated perfect fracture alignment, fixation of the fracture with semi-rigid external fixation and early cancellous bone grafting. Edwards et al (1988) analysed 202 type III open fractures and noted a 7% amputation rate with an average union time of 39 weeks. They had

15% infection, as well as 9% malunion and 29% of the patients had pin track sepsis. They did not distinguish between Gustilo type IIIa and IIIb fractures, but both Blick et al (1989) and Court-Brown et al (1990b) did. Blick and his co-workers realized the importance of early and repeated aggressive debridement, early soft-tissue cover and early bone grafting. Their complications were relatively few although 28% of the patients had pin track problems. They defined their time to union as 39.8 weeks and 44.0 weeks for IIIa and IIIb fractures without bone loss, the time to union for IIIb fractures with bone loss being 57.8 weeks. The results of Court-Brown et al (1990) were not dissimilar. They used both the Hughes and the Hoffmann fixators to treat type III open fractures, finding no difference in the results between the two fixators despite their obvious biomechanical differences. Twenty type IIIa fractures united in 26.5 weeks, 14 IIIb fractures united in 47.4 weeks and 85.7% of the IIIc fractures were amputated.

Holbrook et al (1989) and Whitelaw et al (1990) both compared external fixation mainly using multiplanar devices, with Ender nails. Whitelaw's study was retrospective but concluded that there were significantly fewer complications with Ender nails in the treatment of Gustilo type I, II and IIIa fractures. The study of Holbrook et al (1989) was prospective. They showed that Ender nails were associated with a significantly lower malunion rate and less pain in the fracture site. They felt that Ender nailing was a safe alternative to external fixation in type II and III open fractures.

Circular fixators

In recent years there has been considerable interest in the principles of Ilizarov, and his circular frame has been used to treat complex deformities and to facilitate limb lengthening. There has been some work undertaken to study the usefulness of this device in open and closed tibial fractures. Tucker et al (1992) used the Ilizarov fixator in 41 consecutive open and closed tibial fractures and analysed 26 fractures which did not have bone loss. Six were closed, the remainder being Gustilo type I, II and III fractures. Their pin track sepsis was 10% and there was an 18.5% incidence of malunion. They had 21 excellent results by their criteria, although an excellent result did not require full joint movement. Schwartsman et al (1992) examined 18 tibial fractures of which 14 were open. They had no malunion but 'many' pin infections. The average time for wearing the device was 18 weeks, although the patients required a cast for an average of another six weeks.

The comparison of Tables 7.5 and 7.6 shows that no matter which external fixator is used, the principal problems are those of pin track sepsis and malunion. The use of a ring fixator also appears to be associated with similar problems. In view of the lack of evidence of multiplanar fixators being superior to unilateral devices there seems no need to use them unless the pattern and location of the fracture demands it. If the surgeon chooses to use external fixation to treat a diaphyseal fracture, a unilateral frame capable of dynamization should ideally be used. Multiplanar devices should be reserved for proximal and distal metaphyseal and intra-articular fractures which are more difficult to stabilize with a unilateral device. There can be no logical place for the use of a ring fixator utilizing multiple small wires for the treatment of open diaphyseal fractures. They merely serve to restrict soft-tissue access and apparently have no advantages over simpler frames. Their use should be restricted to the management of complex reconstructive procedures.

The importance of pin track sepsis is that it is unpleasant for the patient and the treatment utilizes a good deal of patient and nurse time. Poorly inserted pins which become infected and loose may give rise to bone infection, but in general pin track sepsis does not actually lead to osteomyelitis very often. Malunion, however, can provide more significant problems and if external fixation is to be employed, consideration should be given to utilizing the method until bone union is obtained to avoid subsequent malunion.

Open tibial metaphyseal and intra-articular fractures

Conventionally, open tibial plateau and pilon fractures have been treated using AO plates with initial accurate repositioning of the fracture fragments using interfragmentary screws and subsequent bone plating to rigidly fix the fracture. Open tibial plateau fractures are relatively rare, but when they occur are often severe. Surgeons have found that the tissue mobilization associated with the application of two proximal tibial plates can result in major soft-tissue defects and infection. The same is true for pilon fractures where the use of plates is technically demanding and the incidence of infection is high.

Surgeons have recently turned to the use of external fixation supplemented by minimal internal fixation for proximal and distal tibial metaphyseal and intra-articular fractures, particularly those of the tibial plafond. This type of external fixation can take three forms. The surgeon may employ 'ligamentotaxis' for very comminuted tibial pilon fractures (Figure 7.3). This involves placing the external fixation device between the mid-diaphyseal area and the calcaneum. If the external fixator is used to distract the fracture, partial or occasionally complete fracture reduction can be obtained. Secondly, the surgeon may choose to internally fix the pilon fracture with plates and screws in the conventional manner but supplement the internal fixation with external fixation between the mid-diaphysis and the calcaneus. Thirdly, the surgeon may elect to use minimal internal fixation to reposition the intra-articular bone fragments and then use a ring or half-ring hybrid fixator to stabilize the metaphyseal bone to the diaphysis. Similar techniques can be used for tibial plateau fractures (Figure 7.6).

Bone et al (1993) have reported on 20 patients with severely comminuted or open tibial pilon fractures treated with the multiplanar AO fixator. Some of their patients were treated with plates and screws and the external fixator was placed between the mid-tibia and the calcaneum to support the internal fixation. In other patients the fixator replaced the plate as supplementary fixation, with the surgeons using minimal internal fixation. All the patients, however, had calcaneal fixation.

Where possible, it is logical to attempt to reconstruct the intra-articular fracture using minimal internal fixation and then use external fixation employing either a ring fixator or half-pins to stabilize the metaphyseal component onto the diaphysis. This, combined with appropriate bone grafting, allows for fracture union with adequate ankle and subtalar mobility.

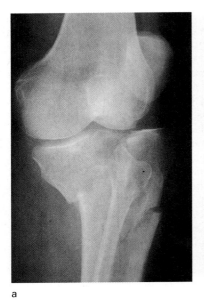
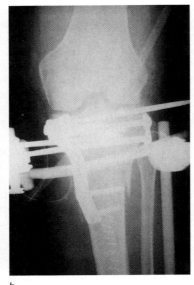
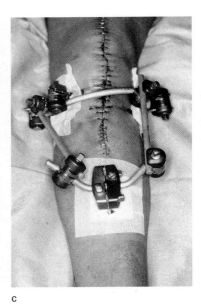

a   b   c

Figure 7.6

(a) A bicondylar tibial plateau fracture. (b) The joint surface has been reconstructed with interfragmentary screws and a medial plate. Rather than elevate the muscles from the lateral side and risk devascularization, an external fixator has been used to stabilize the fracture. (c) A semi-circular hybrid Hoffmann configuration has been used. Half-pins, rather than small wires, have been utilized.

Saleh and co-workers (1993) have taken another approach to preserving ankle movement and pilon fractures. They have used an Orthofix unilateral device, the distal pins being placed in the talus and calcaneum. A hinging unit has been incorporated in the construct and they suggest that ankle movement can be allowed with the correct application of the fixator. They also combine external fixation with internal fixation techniques.

Intramedullary nailing of open tibial fractures

The use of intramedullary nails to treat open tibial fractures was popularized in the 1960s and 1970s following the introduction of the Kuntscher–Herzog nail. Considerable success was achieved with this nail (Zucman and Maurer 1970, Merle d'Aubigne et al 1974) but the absence of locking screws in the original nails meant that only a relatively small number of tibial fractures could be adequately stabilized without the use of an ancillary cast. Many tibial fractures either occur at the junction of the middle and distal thirds of the bone or are spiral or comminuted; and a single nail could often not be used to stabilize these fractures. Lottes (1952) attempted to improve on the original Künstcher design by developing a flexible unreamed nail. However, he still needed to use postoperative casts because of the inherent instability of many tibial fractures.

The invention of interlocking intramedullary tibial nails by Klemm and Schellman (1972) and Kempf et al (1978) allowed surgeons to combine the advantages of closed tibial nailing with the avoidance of postoperative casts (Figure 7.7). Once interlocking nailing had been perfected, it was clear that the tibia was easier to nail than

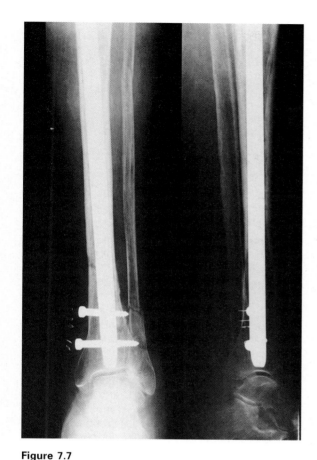

Figure 7.7

A Grosse–Kempf interlocking tibial nail.

(1974) reported a 6.6% incidence of infection in 256 open tibial fractures. Their incidence of non-union in the open fracture group was only 2.4%.

Lottes (1974) using his unreamed nail reported a 7.3% infection rate following nailing of open single tibial fractures and a 6.3% infection rate in open segmental fractures. He, like other workers, felt that the intramedullary tibial nailing was a good technique for open tibial fractures.

The introduction of the Klemm–Schellman and Grosse–Kempf nails permitted adequate stabilization of virtually all tibial diaphyseal fractures. Both these nails were designed to be used with prior reaming but interest in unreamed nails continued and improvements in metallurgy and nail design allowed for the introduction of unreamed interlocking intramedullary nails. Examples of this type of unreamed nail include the Russell Taylor nail (Whittle et al 1992) and the AO nail (Haas et al 1993, Oedekoven et al 1993, Renner et al 1993).

Reamed interlocking tibial nailing

Table 7.7 shows some of the clinical results obtained using reamed interlocking nailing mainly for closed and Gustilo type I open fractures, although some type II fractures were included. It is obvious that the complication rate for intramedullary nailing is less than that for external fixation, but it must be remembered that Tables 7.5 and 7.6 include Gustilo type III open fractures. However, Table 7.7 does show that there is a low infection rate and a low incidence of malunion, joint stiffness and compartment syndrome in closed and Gustilo type I and II open tibial fractures.

A number of surveys of the use of intramedullary nailing have involved selected patient groups. However, Court-Brown et al (1990a) adopted a policy of nailing all tibial fractures that required an anaesthetic in their treatment. In their 125 patients, 11 had Gustilo type I open fractures and they considered that their results illustrated in Table 7.7 vindicated their policy. They also found the functional results following intramedullary nailing to be better than those reported for other treatment methods.

the femur and the technique of interlocking tibial nailing rapidly became accepted.

The relative success of tibial nailing is demonstrated by reviewing the results of the surgeons who only had unlocked nails. Despite this disadvantage and the necessity of having to use postoperative casts Zucman and Maurer (1970) treated 136 open tibial fractures with an 8.1% infection rate. Their incidence of aseptic non-union was 0.7% and they had no malunions. However, only 15% of their open fractures were severe. Merle d'Aubigne et al

Table 7.7   Use of interlocking nails in the management of tibial diaphyseal fractures

Author	Fracture type*	Infection (%)	Non-union (%)	Malunion (%)	Joint stiffness (%)
Henley (1989)	C,O (GI,II)	0	0	4.2	?
Hooper et al (1991)	C,O (GI)	0	?	3.4	<17
Court-Brown et al (1990)	C,O (GI)	1.6	1.6	2.4	7.2
Court-Brown et al (1991)	O (GII,III)	8.8	†	5.8	47
Whittle et al (1992)	O (GI,II,III)	8	†	4	?
Tornetta et al (1994)	O (GIIIb)	6.6	†	0	?

*C denotes closed fractures, O denotes open fractures and GI–III signifies the Gustilo grade.
†Prophylactic bone grafting used and therefore a true non-union incidence is impossible to determine.
? data not available.

Hooper et al (1991) undertook a prospective randomized study of intramedullary nailing and cast management for closed and Gustilo type I tibial fractures. They examined a number of parameters and showed significant improvement in time to union, time off work, time in hospital, out-patient visits and the number of radiographs between the two groups. They also showed a decreased incidence of malunion and improved function following intramedullary nailing. They actually abandoned their prospective study and declared that intramedullary nailing was a far more effective method of treating these types of tibial fractures than non-operative management.

The use of reamed intramedullary nailing in the management of type III open tibial fractures (Figure 7.8) remains controversial (Gustilo et al 1990). Opponents of the technique suggest that its use further damages the vascular supply of a diaphysis that is already compromised as a result of the severity of the injury. This is said to increase the incidence of infection and non-union in these fractures. Although Bone and Johnson (1986) criticized the use of reamed intermedullary nailing in the management of type II and III open fractures, very few of their fractures were type III in severity and the majority were treated with unlocked tibial nails. Currently there is still relatively little literature dealing with the management of Gustilo type III open tibial fractures using intramedullary nailing. Comparison of two similar works is interesting. In one, Court-Brown et al (1991) detailed the use of the reamed Grosse–Kempf nail and in the second Whittle et al (1992) discussed the use of the unreamed Russell Taylor nail. Comparison of this latter work with the later work of Court-Brown et al (1992) is instructive as both deal with the intermedullary nailing of 34 type III open tibial fractures, although Whittle et al also looked at a further 16 type II fractures.

The selection policy for both groups was different. In Edinburgh (Court-Brown et al 1992), the majority of diaphyseal fractures are nailed and only very distal and very proximal tibial fractures were excluded. In Memphis (Whittle et al 1992), fractures of the distal quarter of the tibia were excluded from nailing and these were treated by external fixation. In both centres, early aggressive debridement was used and nailing was carried out early with a static lock being employed. Postoperatively, in Edinburgh, there was no restriction on mobility, although 36% of the patients were multiply injured and mobilization was therefore slow. In Memphis, the surgeons placed some restrictions on mobility; all patients were protected with a patella tendon bearing cast or orthosis. Those patients with an 8-mm nail were protected until callus was formed and those patients who had 50% of bone comminution remained non-weight-bearing until callus was seen. Dynamization was undertaken between 12 and 16 weeks after fracture if callus was not evident. Dynamization was not used in the Edinburgh series.

Union was not a problem in either series. In Memphis, bone grafting was performed as part of the trial protocol and all except two patients united. These patients were paraplegic and an active decision was made not to treat their non-unions. In Edinburgh, all fractures united, bone grafting being performed in cases where there was bone loss measuring >2 cm and 50% of the bone circumference. In other cases, exchange nailing was used.

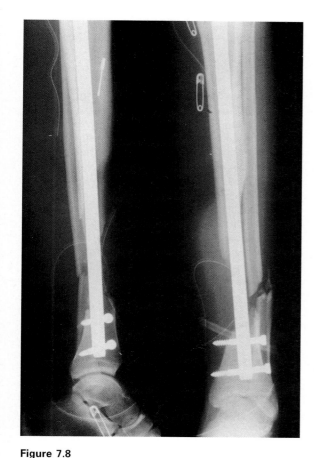

Figure 7.8

A Grosse–Kempf nail used to stabilize a Gustilo IIIb open tibial fracture.

In Edinburgh, there were no infections in 18 type IIIa fractures and a 16.6% infection rate in 16 Gustilo type IIIb fractures. In Memphis, there was a 4.5% infection rate in 22 type IIIa fractures and a 25% infection rate in 12 type IIIb fractures. Implant failure in Edinburgh consisted of one broken cross screw which did not interfere with the management of fracture, but in Memphis there was an incidence of 10% screw failure and 6% nail failure despite postoperative bracing of the fracture.

Comparison of the results of these two series illustrates their similarities and suggests that the incidence of non-union and infection between reamed and unreamed nails in type III open fractures is very similar. However, the increased incidence of implant failure associated with unreamed nails means that these patients require postoperative bracing, this interfering with mobilization. More work is required to assess the usefulness of reamed nailing in the management of type III open fractures, but this initial study suggests that the belief that the technique is associated with increased infection and non-union is fallacious. This view is confirmed by a further study from Vancouver (Keating et al 1994). In Vancouver, 100 open tibial fractures were randomly allocated between reamed and unreamed nails. The epidemiological characteristics of both groups were very similar. A comparison of the mean union times between the reamed and unreamed groups showed no difference in any of the Gustilo groups. In addition, there was no statistical difference in the incidence of infection and non-union between the groups.

Court-Brown et al (1991) pointed out the similarity of their results with those obtained for external fixation in type III open fractures and concluded that the incidence of infection and non-union was independent of the method of fracture management, although they suggested that the incidence of malunion, joint stiffness and the requirement for bone grafting was less with intramedullary nailing. This view has been confirmed in two recent studies from the United States (Tornetta et al 1994, Henley et al 1994). Tornetta et al randomized 29 patients with Gustilo IIIb fractures to either an unreamed nail group or an external fixator group. Both groups had the same initial management, soft-tissue procedures and early bone grafting. There were no differences in time to union or range of joint motion but the authors found the nailed fractures easier to manage especially in terms of soft-tissue procedures and bone grafting. Similar results were gained by Henley et al (1994) who reiterated many previous authors in stating that the degree of soft-tissue injury and not the implant determined the prognosis. They actually found that external fixation was associated with a higher incidence of malunion, wound problems and requirement for reoperation.

The recent introduction of the AO unreamed tibial nail has extended the debate between reamed and unreamed nailing. The nail is solid and inserted without the use of a guide wire.

Haas et al (1993) examined the use of the AO unreamed nail in Tscherne C2 and C3 closed fractures and Gustilo type II and III open fractures. They reported no infections, but had a 13.7% incidence of screw breakage and a 13.7% incidence of peroneal nerve palsy. Ten per cent of their patients required ancillary fixation to gain adequate rigidity. In addition, they reported that 42% of their patients required a fasciotomy although they did not state whether these were therapeutic or prophylactic.

The work of Oedekoven et al (1993) is also of interest. They treated 100 tibial fractures using either an AO or Russell Taylor unreamed nail, 44% of the fractures being open. They documented a delayed union rate of 11.6% with an incidence of non-union of 7%. Again they had no deep infections, but a 2.3% incidence of superficial infection. As with Haas et al (1993), they had a high incidence of compartment syndrome at 9%, with 11.6% incidence of malunion. Renner et al (1993) analysed 17 open and closed tibial fractures. They had no infections, but reported an 11.8% incidence of compartment syndrome, a 17.6% incidence of screw breakage and a 5.9% malunion rate. These reports all stress the fact that they have had no infection and Haas et al (1993) implied that this nullifies the effect of any other complication that they might have. The authors have not, however, fully defined their policies on debridement, antibiotic policy and early skin cover and it may well be these factors along with the undoubted surgical expertise of the authors which have resulted in a zero infection rate.

Sequential external fixation and intramedullary nailing

There has been a flurry of interest in this technique during the last five years (Figure 7.9). The perceived advantages of external fixation in controlling the fracture while soft-tissue cover is undertaken, combined with the definite advantages of the use of intramedullary nailing once soft-tissue cover has been successfully carried out, have encouraged surgeons to combine the two techniques and to treat the fracture primarily with an external fixation device and secondarily with an intramedullary nail. Table 7.8 summarizes the results of a number of papers dealing with this technique. It is interesting to note that there are two basic patterns of results. A number of authors have reported good results following the use of the sequential technique, but others such as Tornquist (1990) report a very poor result. Analysis of Table 7.8 to try to find a reason for the difference points only to the fact that a relatively short delay between the removal of the external fixation device and the insertion of the nail seems to be associated with a lower infection rate. This view is carried to its extreme when analysing Tornquist's work where there was an average delay of 218 days and a 66% infection rate. Wheelwright and Court-Brown (1990) advocated a short period of traction or cast management between removal of the fixation device and the introduction of an intramedullary nail. This allows for granulation of the pin tracks and they believed that nailing should be delayed until the pin tracks had granulated. This view is supported by other authors. When combined with the observation that the delay between procedures should be short, it suggests that if a surgeon is contemplating the use of this sequential procedure, he or she should insert the external fixation pins with maximum care to ensure a low rate of pin sepsis.

Flexible intramedullary nailing

The use of flexible intramedullary nails was popularized by the Rush family in the United States and the use of Rush pins in the management of tibial fractures has become popular with some surgeons. Rush (1955) detailed the techniques of using both single and double flexible nails in different types of tibial fractures. He recognized that there was an inherent problem with this technique in that it failed to control the rotation and spiral fractures or preserve length in comminuted fractures. Enders nails have recently superseded the use of Rush pins and the use of these nails has been documented by Wiss (1986). Wiss has suggested that contraindications to this technique are fractures that involve the proximal or distal tibia within 7.5 cm of the knee or ankle joint as well as fractures of extensive bicortical or circumferential comminution. He also suggested that their use in type III open

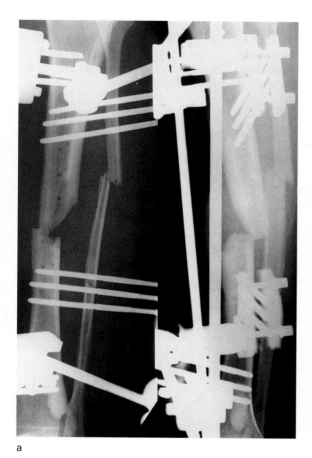
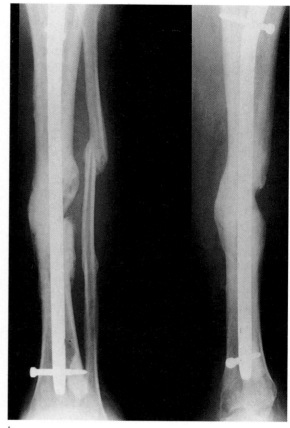

a   b

Figure 7.9

(a) A Gustilo IIIb open tibial fracture initially stabilized with a Hoffmann external fixator. (b) A Grosse–Kempf interlocking tibial nail was substituted successfully and the fracture united. The patient regained good function.

Table 7.8   Use of sequential external fixation and intramedullary nailing in tibial fractures

Author	Number of fractures	Duration of external fixation (days)	Time before nailing (days)	Pin track sepsis (%)	Infection rate (%)
McGraw and Lim (1988)	16	59.5	21	44	44
Maurer et al (1989)	24	52	65	29	25
Johnson et al (1990)	16	84	13	12.5	0
Blachut et al (1990)	41	17	9	5	5
Tornquist (1990)	6	72	218	100	66
Wheelwright and Court-Brown (1992)	21	57.4	11.7	33.3	4.8
Siebenrock et al (1993)	24	45	?	0	4

? data not available.

fractures was limited. This view has been supported by other authors. If surgeons wish to use flexible intramedullary nails for the management of open tibial fractures, they must be quite clear that they are dealing with an inherently stable fracture configuration, these being uncommon in more severe open fractures.

Suggested treatment

The overall prognosis of the open tibial fracture depends on the severity of the fracture and its associated soft-tissue damage. Good results are obtained by an adequate initial debridement and good subsequent soft-tissue surgery. It is clear that internal or external stabilization of the fracture should be performed and the surgeon must choose between the alternative treatment methods. Bone plating is the most difficult technique to use, although with care good results can be obtained in type I and II open fractures. Currently, their use in type III open diaphyseal fractures cannot be advised. External skeletal fixation is widely used for the management of all open tibial fractures and good results have been obtained. There is, however, no evidence that one fixation device or configuration is superior to another and it is advised that if external fixation is to be used, the simplest possible device commensurate with adequate stabilization of the fracture be used. For diaphyseal fractures this will frequently be a uniplanar device, but for metaphyseal and interarticular fractures, a ring or half-ring fixator may well be employed. This may be combined with minimal internal fixation or in very severely comminuted metaphyseal or interarticular fractures the technique of ligamentotaxis may be used. There seems no place for the use of complex small wire-ring fixators in the primary management of open tibial diaphyseal fractures where soft-tissue access is essential.

The debate between reamed and unreamed intramedullary nailing of open tibial fractures will continue. Early results suggest little difference between the two techniques in the management of type III open fractures. There seems little doubt that intramedullary nailing is associated with a lower rate of malunion, joint stiffness and bone grafts than external fixators. Currently, the author employs intramedullary nailing for open tibial diaphyseal fractures regardless of their severity and external skeletal fixation with or without minimal internal fixation for open fractures of the tibial metaphysis.

References

Adrey J (1970) Le Fixateur externe d'Hoffmann couplé en cadre. Étudie bioméchanique dans les fractures des jambe (Editions Gead: Paris).

Alho A, Benterud JG, Hogevold HE, Ekeland A, Stromsoe K (1992) Comparison of functional bracing and locked intramedullary nailing in the treatment of displaced tibial shaft fractures, Clin Orthop 277: 243–50.

Austin RT (1981) The Sarmiento tibial plaster: a prospective study of 145 fractures, Injury 13: 10–22.

Babst R, Regazzoni P, Renner N, Rosso R, Heberer M (1992) Stable temporary traction substitute with the pinless fixation, Injury 23: Suppl 3.

Bach AW, Hansen ST (1989) Plates versus external fixation in severe open tibial fractures: a randomised trial, Clin Orthop 241: 89–94.

Behrens F, Searls K (1986) External fixation of the tibia. Basic concepts and prospective evaluation, J Bone Joint Surg (Am) 68B: 246–54.

Benum P, Svenningsen S (1982) Tibial fractures treated with Hoffmann's external fixation, Acta Orthop Scand 53: 471–6.

Blachut PA, Meek RN, O'Brien PJ (1990) External fixation and delayed intramedullary nailing of open fractures of the tibia shaft. A sequential protocol, J Bone Joint Surg (Am) 72A: 729–35.

Blick SS, Brumback RJ, Lakatos R, Poka A, Burgess AR (1989) Early prophylactic bone grafting of high-energy tibial fractures, Clin Orthop 240: 21–41.

Bone LB, Johnson KD (1986) Treatment of tibial fractures by reaming and intramedullary nailing, J Bone Joint Surg (Am) 68A: 877–87.

Bone L, Stegemann P, McNamara K, Seibel R (1993) External fixation of severely comminuted and open tibial pilon fractures, Clin Orthop 292: 101–7.

Bostmann O, Hanninen A (1982) Tibial shaft fractures

caused by indirect violence, *Acta Orthop Scand* **53**: 981–90.

Brookes M (1971) *The Blood Supply of Bone* (Butterworths: London).

Brown PW, Urban JG (1969) Early weight-bearing treatment of open fractures of the tibia, *J Bone Joint Surg (Am)* **51A**: 59–75.

Burkhalter WE, Protzman R (1975) The tibial shaft fracture, *J Trauma* **15**: 785–94.

Burney FL (1975) Elastic external fixation of tibial fractures: study of 1421 cases. In: Brooker AF, Edwards CC, eds, *External Fixation: The Current State of the Art* (Williams and Watkins: Baltimore) 55–74.

Burney FL, Bourgois R (1965) Étude bioméchanique de l'osteotaxis. In: *La Fixation externe en chirurgie* (Imp Medicale et Scientifique: Brussels).

Chan KM, Leung YK, Cheng JCY, Leung PC (1984) The management of type III open tibial fractures, *Injury* **16**: 157–65.

Chao EYS, Aro HT, Lewellan DG, Kelly PJ (1989) The effect of rigidity on fracture healing in external fixation, *Clin Orthop* **241**: 24–35.

Clifford RP, Beauchamp CG, Kellar JF, Webb JK, Tile M (1988) Plate fixation of open fractures of the tibia, *J Bone Joint Surg (Br)* **70B**: 644–8.

Court-Brown CM (1985) The effect of external skeletal fixation on bone healing and bone blood supply. An experimental study, *Clin Orthop* **201**: 278–9.

Court-Brown CM, Hughes SPF (1985) Hughes external fixation in treatment of tibial fractures, *J R Soc Med* **78**: 830–7.

Court-Brown CM, Christie J, McQueen MM (1990a) Closed intramedullary tibial nailing. Its use in closed and type I open fractures, *J Bone Joint Surg (Br)* **72B**: 605–11.

Court-Brown CM, Wheelwright EF, Christie J, McQueen MM (1990b) External fixation for type III open tibial fractures, *J Bone Joint Surg (Br)* **72B**: 801–4.

Court-Brown CM, McQueen MM, Quaba AA, Christie J (1991) Locked intramedullary nailing of open tibial fractures, *J Bone Joint Surg (Br)* **73B**: 959–64.

Court-Brown CM, McQueen MM, Quaba AA, Christie J (1992) *Reamed Intramedullary Nailing of Grade III Open Tibial Fractures* (AAOS: Washington).

Cucel LR, Rigaud R (1850) Des vis metalliques enfonces dans les tissues des os, pour le traitement de certaines fractures, *Rev Med Chir Paris* **8**: 115.

De Bastiani G, Aldegheri R, Brivio LR (1984) The treatment of fractures with a dynamic axial fixation, *J Bone Joint Surg (Br)* **66B**: 538–45.

Den Outer AJ, Meeuwis JD, Hermans J, Zwaveling A (1990) Conservative versus operative treatment of displaced noncomminuted tibial shaft fracture, *Clin Orthop* **252**: 231–7.

Digby JM, Holloway GMN, Webb JK (1983) A study of function after tibial cast bracing, *Injury* **14**: 432–9.

Edge AJ, Denham RA (1981) External fixation for complicated tibial fractures, *J Bone Joint Surg (Br)* **63B**: 92–7.

Edwards CC, Simmons SC, Browner BD, Weigel MC (1988) Severe open tibial fractures. Results treating 202 injuries with external fixation, *Clin Orthop* **230**: 98–115.

Evans G, McLaren M, Shearer JR (1988) External fixation of fractures of the tibia. Clinical experience of a new device, *Injury* **19**: 73–6.

Gothman L (1961) Vascular reactions in experimental fractures, *Acta Clin Scand* Suppl 284.

Gustilo RB, Merkow RC, Templeman RB (1990) Current concepts review. The management of open fractures, *J Bone Joint Surg (Am)* **72A**: 299–304.

Haas N, Krettek C, Schandelmaier P, Frigg R, Tscherne H (1993) A new solid unreamed tibial nail for shaft fractures with severe soft tissue injury, *Injury* **24**: 49–54.

Henley MB (1989) Intramedullary devices for tibial fracture stabilisation, *Clin Orthop* **240**: 87–96.

Henley MB, Chapman JR, Agel J, Swionkowski MF, Benirschke MD, Mayo KA (1994) *Comparison of Unreamed Tibial Nails and External Fixateurs in the Treatment of Grade II and III Open Tibial Shaft Fractures* (Orthopaedic Trauma Association: Los Angeles).

Hey-Groves EW (1921) *On Modern Methods of Treating Fractures*, 2nd edn (John Wright and Sons: Bristol).

Holbrook JL, Swiontkowski MF, Sanders R (1989) Treatment of open fractures of the tibial shaft: Ender nailing versus external fixation. *J Bone Joint Surg (Am)* **71A**: 1231–8.

Hooper GJ, Keddell RG, Penny ID (1991) Conservative management or closed nailing for tibial shaft fractures, *J Bone Joint Surg (Br)* **73B**: 83–5.

Ilizarov GA (1992) Ilizarov method, *Clin Orthop* **280**: 2–169.

Johnson EE, Simpson LA, Helfet DL (1990) Delayed intramedullary nailing after failed external fixation of the tibia, *Clin Orthop* **253**: 251–7.

Johnson HE, Stovald SL (1950) External fixation of fractures, *J Bone Joint Surg (Am)* **32A**: 466–7.

Karahaju EO, Alho A, Nieminen J (1979) The results of operative and non-operative management of tibial fractures, *Injury* **7**: 49–52.

Kay L, Hansen BA, Raaschou HO (1976) Fracture of the tibial shaft conservatively treated, *Injury* **17**: 5–11.

Keating JF, Gardner E, Leach J, McPherson S, Abrami G (1991) Management of tibial fractures with the Orthofix external fixator, *J R Coll Surg Edin* **36**: 272–7.

Keating JF, O'Brien PJ, Blachut PA, Meek RN, Broekhuize H (1994) *Interlocking Intramedullary Nailing of Open Fractures of the Tibia—a Prospective Randomised Comparison of Reamed and Unreamed Nails* (Canadian Orthopaedic Association, Winnipeg).

Kempf I, Grosse A, Laffourge D (1978) L'apport du verrouillage dans l'enclouge centromedullaire des os longs, *Rev Chir Orthop* **64**: 635.

Kenwright J, Richardson JB, Cunningham JC, White SH, Goodship AE, Adams MA, Magnussen PA, Newman JH (1991) Axial movement and tibial fractures, *J Bone Joint Surg (Br)* **73B**: 654–9.

Klein MPM, Rahn BA, Frigg R, Kessler S, Perren SM (1990) Reaming versus non-reaming in medullary nailing: interference with cortical circulation of the canine tibia, *Arch Orthop Trauma Surg* **109**: 314–16.

Klemm K, Schellmann WD (1972) Dynamische und statische Verriegelung des Marknagels, *Monatsschr Unfallheilkunde* **75**: 568.

Krettek C, Haas N, Tscherne H (1991) The role of supplemental leg-screw fixation for open fractures of the tibial shaft treated with external fixation, *J Bone Joint Surg (Am)* **73A**: 893–7.

Kyro A, Tunturi I, Soukka A (1991) Conservative management of tibial shaft fractures, *Ann Chir Gynaecol* **80**: 294–300.

Lambotte A (1913) *Chirurgie operatoire des fractures* (Masson et Cie: Paris).

Lindahl O (1962) Rigidity of immobilisation of transverse fractures, *Acta Orthop Scand* **32**: 237–46.

Lottes JO (1952) Intramedullary fixation for fractures of the shaft of the tibia, *South Med J* **45**: 407–14.

Lottes JO (1974) Medullary nailing of the tibia with the triflange nail, *Clin Orthop* **105**: 253–66.

Maurer DJ, Merkow RL, Gustilo RB (1989) Infections after intramedullary nailing of severe open tibial fractures initially treated with external fixation, *J Bone Joint Surg (Am)* **71A**: 835–8.

McGraw JM, Lim EVA (1988) Treatment of open tibial shaft fractures. External fixation and secondary intramedullary nailing, *J Bone Joint Surg (Am)* **70A**: 900–11.

Melendez EM, Colon C (1989) Treatment of open tibial fractures with the Orthofix fixation, *Clin Orthop* **241**: 224–30.

Merle d'Aubigne R, Maurer P, Zucman P, Masse Y (1974) Blind intramedullary nailing for tibial fractures, *Clin Orthop* **105**: 267–75.

Mollan RAB, Bradley B (1978) Fractures of the tibial shaft treated in a patellar-tendon-bearing cast, *Injury* **10**: 124–7.

Monney G, Cordey J, Rahn B (1991) Studies concerning the blood supply after plating with the DCP and LC-DCP, *Injury* **22**: Suppl 1.

Nicoll EA (1964) Fractures of the tibial shaft. A survey of 705 cases, *J Bone Joint Surg (Br)* **46B**: 373–87.

Oedekoven G, Claudi B, Frigg R (1993) Treatment of open and closed tibial fractures with unreamed interlocking tibial nails, *Orthop Traumatol* **2**: 115–28.

Parkhill C (1898) Further observations regarding the use of the bone clamp in ununited fractures, fractures with malunion and recent fractures with a tendency to displacement, *Ann Surg* **27**: 553–70.

Perren SM, Allgower M, Brunner H, Burch HB (1991) The concept of biological plating using the limited contact–dynamic compression plate (LC-DCP), *Injury* **22**: Suppl 1.

Pun WK, Chow SP, Fang D, Ip FK, Leong JCY, Ng C (1991) A study of function and residual joint stiffness after functional bracing of tibial shaft fractures, *Clin Orthop* **267**: 157–63.

Rahn BA, Gallinaro P, Baltensperger A, Perren SM (1971) Primary bone healing. An experimental study in the rabbit, *J Bone Joint Surg (Am)* **53A**: 783–6.

Reichert ILH, McCarthy ID, Hughes SPF (1995) The acute vascular response to intramedullary reaming, *J Bone Joint Surg (Br)* **77B:** 490–3.

Renner N, Regazzoni P, Babst R, Rosso R (1993) Initial experiences with the unreamed tibial nail, *Helv Chir Acta* **59**: 665–8.

Rhinelander FW (1968) The normal microcirculation of diaphyseal cortex and its response to fracture, *J Bone Joint Surg (Am)* **50A**: 784–800.

Rhinelander FW (1972) Circulation in bone. In: Bourne R, ed, *The Biochemistry and Physiology of Bone* (Academic Press: New York).

Rhinelander FW (1974) Tibial blood supply in relation to fracture healing, *Clin Orthop* **105**: 34–81.

Rittman WW, Schibli M, Matter P, Allgöwer M (1979) Open fractures. Long term results in 200 consecutive fractures, *Clin Orthop* **138**: 132–40.

Rommens P, Schmidt-Neuerberg KP (1987) Ten years experience with the operative management of tibial shaft fractures, *J Trauma* **27**: 917–27.

Ruedi T, Webb JK, Allgöwer M (1976) Experience with the dynamic compression plate (DCP) in 418 recent fractures of the tibial shaft, *Injury* **7**: 252–7.

Rush LV (1955) *Atlas of Rush Pin Techniques* (Bervion: Meridian, Miss).

Saleh M, Shanahan MDG, Fern ED (1993) Intra-articular fractures of the distal tibia: surgical management by limited internal fixation and articulated distraction, *Injury* **24**: 37–40.

Sarmiento A (1967) A functional below-the-knee cast for tibial fractures, *J Bone Joint Surg (Am)* **49A**: 855–75.

Sarmiento A (1970) A functional below-the-knee brace for tibial fractures, *J Bone Joint Surg (Am)* **52A**: 295–311.

Sarmiento A, Gersten LM, Sobol PA, Shankwiler JA, Vangsness CT (1989) Tibial shaft fractures treated with functional braces, *J Bone Joint Surg (Br)* **71B**: 602–9.

Schemitsch EH, Kowalski MJ, Swiontkowski MF, Senft D (1994) Cortical bone blood flow in reamed and unreamed locked intramedullary nailing: a fractured tibial model in sheep, *J Orthop Trauma* **8**: 373–82.

Schwartsman V, Martin SN, Ronquist RA, Schwartsman R (1992) Tibial fractures. The Ilizarov alternative, *Clin Orthop* **278**: 207–16.

Siebenrock KA, Schillig B, Jakob RP (1993) Treatment of complex tibial shaft fractures: arguments for early secondary intramedullary nailing, *Clin Orthop* **290**: 269–74.

Slatis P, Rokkanen P (1967) Conservative treatment of tibial shaft fractures, *Acta Chir Scand* **134**: 41–7.

Steen Jensen J, Wang Hansen F, Johansen J (1977) Tibial shaft fractures, *Acta Orthop Scand* **48**: 204–12.

Suman RK (1982) Ortholast brace for the treatment of tibial shaft fractures, *Injury* **13**: 133–8.

Tornetta P, Bergman M, Watnik N, Berkowitz G, Steuer J (1994) Treatment of grade IIIb open tibial fractures. A prospective, randomised comparison of external fixation and non-reamed locked nailing, *J Bone Joint Surg (Br)* **76B**: 13–19.

Tornquist H (1990) Tibia non-unions treated by interlocking nailing: increased risk of infection after previous external fixation, *J Orthop Trauma* **4**: 109–14.

Tucker HL, Kendra JC, Kinnebrew TE (1992) Management of unstable open and closed tibial fractures using the Ilizarov method, *Clin Orthop* **280**: 125–35.

Van der Linden W, Larsson K (1979) Plate fixation versus conservative treatment of tibial shaft fractures, *J Bone Joint Surg (Am)* **61A**: 873–8.

Vidal J, Rabischong P, Boneel F (1970) Etude biomechanique du fixateur d'Hoffman dans les fractures de jambe, *Soc Chir Montpelier* Seance 20 Jan: 43–52.

Wheelwright EF, Court-Brown CM (1992) Primary external fixation and secondary intramedullary nailing in the treatment of tibial fractures, *Injury* **23**: 373–6.

Whitelaw GP, Wetzler M, Nelson A, Segal D, Fletcher J, Hadley N, Sawka M (1990) Ender rods versus external fixation in the treatment of open tibial fractures, *Clin Orthop* **253**: 258–69.

Whittle AP, Russell TA, Taylor JC, Lavelle DG (1992) Treatment of open fractures of the tibial shaft with the use of interlocking nailing without reaming, *J Bone Joint Surg (Am)* **74A**: 1162–71.

Wiss DA (1986) Flexible medullary nailing of acute tibial shaft fractures, *Clin Orthop* **212**: 122–32.

Zucman J, Maurer P (1970) Primary medullary nailing of the tibia for fractures of the shaft in adults, *Injury* **2**: 84–92.

8
Open fractures of the humerus

M.M. McQueen

Open fractures of the humerus occur with relative infrequency and consequently have received little attention in the orthopaedic literature. The results of a Medline search for open humeral fractures in the last five years reveal one article whilst the same search for open tibial fractures reveals 71 articles. Perhaps partly because of this the management of the open humeral fracture remains an unsolved problem and whereas most are associated with little soft-tissue injury, it is important to realize that the severe open injuries can lead to significantly more serious disability than their equivalent in the lower limb.

Epidemiology

Over the five-year period from 1988 to 1992 inclusive, 14 open humeral diaphyseal fractures, 13 open intra-articular distal humeral fractures and five open fractures of the proximal humerus presented to the Edinburgh Orthopaedic Trauma Unit. This Unit has a catchment area of 750 000. Smaller units such as an average District General Hospital serving a population of 250 000 will therefore only treat approximately two open humeral fractures per year. Assuming an average of four orthopaedic consultants, each would only have experience of one open humeral fracture every two years.

During the five-year period, there were a total of 249 humeral diaphyseal fractures treated. The incidence of open fractures in this group is therefore 5.6%.

Of the 14 patients with open diaphyseal fractures, there were eight men and six women with an average age of 47 years ranging from 16 to 83 years. Five patients had a simple fall and

these five were all over 50 years of age with an average age of 73 years. All were Gustilo type I injuries and all were spiral fractures. Four of the five were AO type A or simple spiral fractures (Figure 8.1) whilst the youngest patient had an AO type B fracture. It is likely that the major

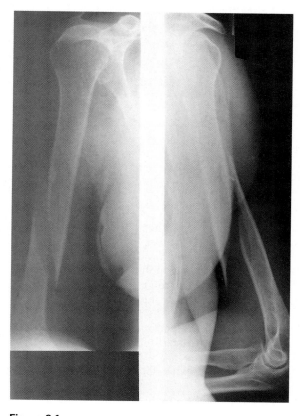

Figure 8.1

AO Type A1.2 humeral diaphyseal fracture.

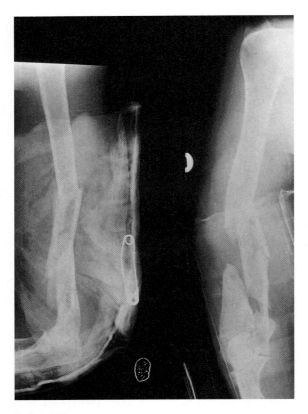

Figure 8.2

AO Type C humeral diaphyseal fracture.

Table 8.1 Complications of open humeral diaphyseal fractures

Complication	n	%
Non/delayed union	3/10	30
Nerve injury		
radial	1/14	7
median/ulnar	1/14	7
Fixation failure	3/10	30
Joint stiffness	1/10	10

AO type B fractures, three of which were short oblique or transverse, whilst two had type C or severely comminuted fractures (Figure 8.2).

Overall the morbidity was high. Four patients (29%) died shortly after injury. Of the remaining ten, eight patients (80%) experienced complications (Table 8.1).

It is difficult to extract the true incidence and prevalence of open humeral diaphyseal fractures from other series since they are usually selected groups of patients. Rojczyk (1984) reported on the localization of 678 open fractures of which 43 (6.3%) were in the humerus but not specifically diaphyseal. Bleeker and his co-authors (1991) studied 239 consecutive non-pathological fractures in a 16-year period, of which ten (4%) were open. North American authors report generally higher incidences ranging from 8% to 36% (Bell et al 1985, Brumback et al 1986, Hall and Pankovich 1987) but these series have a high proportion of patients with high-energy injury with multiple associated injuries. The other striking difference between North America and Europe in the aetiology of open humeral fractures is the high number of gunshot wounds in North America (Hall and Pankovich 1987).

In the five-year period, there were 224 intra-articular fractures of the distal humerus: 13 of these were open, giving an incidence of 5.8%. There were eight women and five men with an average age of 43 years ranging from 21 to 83 years. Ten of the 13 occurred as a result of high-energy injuries. These patients were a younger group, with an average age of 38 years ranging from 21 to 58 years. The fracture configurations of this group were all severe with intra-articular comminution (AO type C) (Figure 8.3). The

underlying cause of these fractures was osteoporosis and the open wound was an 'inside-out' injury from the spike on the fracture end.

Nine patients had high-energy injuries, seven of which were road traffic accidents. Six of these patients had multiple injuries. The average age of this group was 36 years. The soft-tissue injuries were more serious with five Gustilo type I wounds, two Gustilo type II wounds, one type IIIa and one type IIIb. There were no type IIIc injuries in this series and no patient required amputation.

In general, the fracture configurations were more severe than in the osteoporotic low-energy group with three AO type A fractures either short oblique or transverse in shape. Four patients had

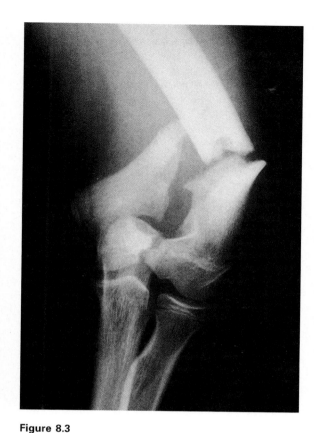

Figure 8.3

AO Type C distal humeral fracture.

remaining three low-velocity injuries were in older patients with an average age of 61 years and generally a more benign fracture pattern.

The epidemiology of open intra-articular distal humeral fractures is poorly documented in the available literature. Holdsworth and Mossad (1990) reported on 62 patients with distal humeral fractures treated by internal fixation over a six-year period, of which 13 were open (21%). The series reported by Jupiter and his colleagues (1985) and by Zagorski and his co-authors (1986) have incidences of open fractures of 41% and 33%, respectively. All of these series, however, are selected patients and it is likely that the true incidence is considerably lower.

Management

Soft tissues

In the management of any open fracture, the handling of the soft tissues is of prime importance. It is upon the soft tissues that the bone depends for its blood supply, without which the immune system cannot mobilize its defences against infection and without which bone is unable to unite. Once the bone is stabilized either by fixation or bone union, it is also the soft tissues upon which the limb depends in order to regain its maximum possible function.

Initial assessment of the soft tissues in an open fracture of the humerus must take into account the nature, extent and site of the open wound. Although rare, there are occasions when the open wound in the humerus is so severe that amputation may be considered. Generally, in the upper limb, this will be in the presence of severe neurological and vascular injury such that a useful extremity cannot be obtained by reconstructive procedures or when the patient's continued survival is threatened. It must be remembered that amputation in the severe open humeral fracture is much more disabling than in a lower limb fracture, but fortunately is required much less frequently.

More commonly, an open wound overlies a humeral fracture without significant threat to life or limb. The general principles of management of any open fracture apply to the humerus with a thorough and meticulous debridement being carried out under aseptic conditions, with excision of all dead and contaminated soft and bony tissues. The fracture ends must always be visualized regardless of the size of the initial wound which usually requires surgical extension. When the wound is deemed to be excised fully, then copious irrigation should be used. Effective antibiotic therapy is also important in the prevention of infection after open fractures (Patzakis and Wilkins 1989, Gustilo et al 1990).

There is no indication for primary closure of open wounds of the humerus as even in small wounds this will result in skin tension if adequate debridement has been carried out. Many wounds in the humerus can be closed either by secondary suture or split-skin graft 48 hours after debridement. Because of the good soft tissue envelope around the humerus, it is rare to require flap cover except in the most severe cases. The principles of wound debridement discussed in more detail in Chapter 5 apply as closely to the humerus as to the lower limb.

Radial nerve palsy

In closed humeral fractures, it is generally recommended that radial nerve palsy be treated expectantly as usually the nerve is in continuity and spontaneous recovery is common (Mast et al 1975, Pollock et al 1981, Stern et al 1984, Bostman et al 1986). In open humeral fractures, however, it is less likely that the radial nerve is in continuity. Foster and his colleagues (1993) reported on their experience of ten years of exploration of the radial nerve at debridement of an open humeral shaft fracture. During this time, there were 14 patients with open humeral shaft fractures complicated by radial nerve palsy, nine of whom (64%) had either a transected or interposed nerve at surgery. Repair or removal of the nerve from between the fracture ends resulted in good motor recovery in seven patients. The state of the nerve was not significantly influenced by the extent of the open wound. Levin and his co-authors (1990) found that four of eight severe open humeral fractures had radial nerve injury and three of these were transected. Repair resulted in one excellent, one good and one fair functional result. Along with others (Omer 1982, Shah and Batti 1983), they recommend early exploration and primary repair of nerve injury after open humeral fracture.

Median and ulnar nerve palsy occur much more frequently in open humeral shaft fractures than in closed fractures, especially after missile wounds (Mast et al 1975, Levin et al 1990). The ulnar nerve is at particular risk in open fractures of the distal end of the humerus because of its intimate relationship to bone at this level. In a review of reported incidences of complications of bicondylar distal humeral fractures Helfet and Schmeling (1993) quote a 7–15% incidence of ulnar nerve palsy but do not differentiate between closed and open fractures. The same principles of early exploration and repair apply to injuries to the median and ulnar nerve in open humeral injuries as to radial nerve injury.

Skeletal stabilization

It is now accepted practice that skeletal stabilization be carried out in open fractures of long bones, especially in the lower limb (Chapman 1979, Tscherne 1984, Gustilo et al 1990, Court-Brown et al 1991, Sanders et al 1993, Grosse et al 1993). A stable skeleton ensures optimum conditions for soft-tissue healing and functional recovery as well as allowing easy access to the soft tissues for any plastic surgery required to achieve skin cover. The open fracture of the humerus usually causes fewer problems than its equivalent in the tibia mainly because of the excellent soft-tissue envelope and blood supply of the humerus, but nevertheless advantage is still to be gained by achieving skeletal stability. This can be achieved in several ways.

Methods of internal fixation include intramedullary nailing with and without reaming and plate fixation, both of which remain controversial as a method of management of open long-bone fractures, especially in the tibia (Patzakis and Wilkins 1989, Gustilo et al 1990, Court-Brown et al 1991). The stated reason for avoiding internal fixation in open fractures is usually the risk of infection (Chapman and Mahoney 1979, Gustilo et al 1990, Sanders et al 1993) although these same authors agree that the most important factor reducing infection rates is a meticulous and aggressive debridement. The humeral diaphysis is relatively more protected from infection than the tibia because of its good blood supply and thus concerns about infection are minimal provided the open wound is adequately treated.

External fixation is used but probably less so than in the lower limb while some authors still advocate conservative management for the less severe open fractures.

In open fractures of the metaphysis of the humerus, the injury is usually intra-articular. The same indications for skeletal stabilization apply as in the diaphysis and added to this is the importance of achieving rigid stabilization of intra-articular fractures to allow early motion. Metaphyseal fractures have a good blood supply, thus largely protecting the injury from infection provided the soft tissues are appropriately handled.

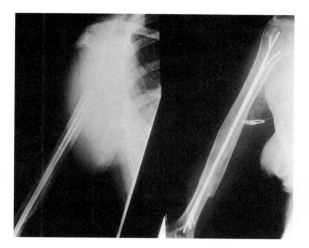

Figure 8.4

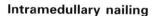
Multiple pin fixation of an open diaphyseal fracture of the humerus.

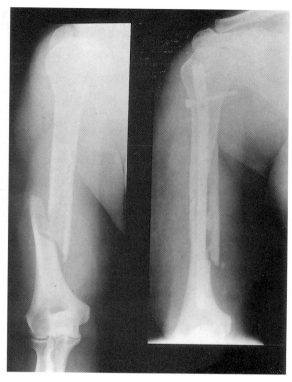

Figure 8.5

Antegrade interlocking humeral nailing.

Intramedullary nailing

The use of intramedullary nailing is only appropriate for diaphyseal and not metaphyseal fractures in the humerus. There are several different techniques including unreamed, unlocked nailing using multiple pins (Figure 8.4) and reamed or unreamed interlocking nailing (Figure 8.5). Their use is controversial and as yet no clear advantage has emerged with any specific nailing technique.

Selection of approach

Intramedullary nailing of the humerus may be carried out in an antegrade manner with an entry portal at the shoulder or retrograde from the elbow.

Antegrade nailing is performed with the patient supine and draping, allowing access to the shoulder. An incision is made anterolaterally on the shoulder over the area of the greater tuberosity of about 4 cm in length. Blunt dissection is performed through deltoid and the incision deepened on to bone. A bone awl is then used to make the entry portal in bone. Care must be taken not to extend the wound too far distally as this may damage the axillary nerve. If a flexible nail is to be used, the portal of entry can be made distal to the greater tuberosity but it must be appreciated that this puts the axillary nerve at added risk.

Retrograde nailing of the humerus is performed with the patient either in the lateral position or prone. The arm is prepared and draped from shoulder to forearm and placed on a radiolucent board with the elbow flexed to 90° and the forearm hanging vertically (Figure 8.6). An incision is made posteriorly, one finger's breadth above the olecranon extending 5 cm proximally. The underlying triceps is split in the same direction and an entry portal made with a burr in the centre of the humerus just proximal to the extra-articular fat of the olecranon fossa.

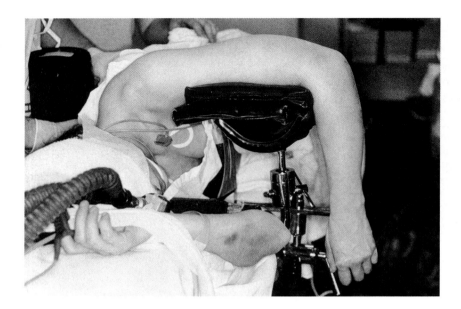

Figure 8.6

The lateral position for retro-grade humeral nailing.

This should be oval in shape and is usually about 4 cm long by 2.5 cm wide for a single reamed nail but may be smaller if multiple flexible nails are used.

Type of nail

Although several types of intramedullary nail are available there are two basic methods of fixation: multiple flexible rods or a single interlocking nail inserted with or without reaming.

Multiple flexible nailing can be carried out using Rush pins or Enders nails or by the Hackethal stacked nailing technique (Hackethal 1961). The advantage of these techniques is the flexibility of the implant which makes their inser-tion easier, particularly when used in a retrograde fashion. Except for tightly stacked nails, they do not provide rotational stability although this has not proven to be a problem clinically. In commin-uted fractures these implants do not prevent shortening of the humerus which may be more problematical. The most troublesome complica-tion is nail back out which has been reported in

a significant number of patients (Stern et al 1984, Brumback et al 1986) and was the main cause of complications in Hall and Pankovich's series (1987). Durbin and his colleagues (1983) had no instances of nail back out with tightly stacked Steinman pins inserted using Hackethal's technique.

In contrast, the interlocking intramedullary rod allows more rigid fixation and has a lower incidence of rotational malalignment or shorten-ing and therefore may be more applicable to open injuries of the humerus, which are more likely to be high-energy comminuted fractures. Migration of the nail has been reported, despite proximal and distal locking in osteoporotic patients (Robinson et al 1992, Rommens et al 1995). The rigid nature of the nail makes inser-tion more difficult and great care must be taken to avoid causing iatrogenic fracture, especially with retrograde insertion.

Interlocking nails may be inserted with or without reaming of the humerus. The debate about reaming has centred around the manage-ment of tibial fractures with proponents arguing that reaming is beneficial because it stimulates periosteal osteogenesis and the reaming products act as an internal bone graft (Danckewardt-Lilliestrom 1969). Reaming also has the advantage of allowing the insertion of a larger and therefore stronger nail which is less important in the humerus. Opponents of reaming believe that reaming damages the medullary blood vessels and can lead to bone ischaemia and thereby infection, especially in severe open fractures, although this has not been substantiated clinically.

Outcome

In principle, intramedullary nailing with interlocking nails should have as successful an outcome with open fractures of the humerus as it has proven to have in the lower limb (Court-Brown et al 1991). Because of the specific problems of the humerus, this has not as yet been achieved.

Union rates for open humeral fractures treated with intramedullary nails are difficult to extract from the available literature. Brumback and his colleagues (1986) report a 6% delayed union rate in 56 fractures of which 11 were open but the authors do not specify the union rate for the open fractures alone. One of 28 open fractures in Hall and Pankovich's series (1987) failed to heal. This was one of six Gustilo type III open fractures (Gustilo and Anderson 1976). A higher rate of delayed union is reported by Stern et al (1984) with four of their 12 open fractures taking over 17 weeks to unite, although this definition of delayed union in an open fracture is debatable. No open fractures were considered to have proceeded to non-union in this study.

All of these studies reported the results of unlocked, unreamed nails. Using interlocking nails with reaming, Rommens and his colleagues (1995) had two patients with delayed union in 39 closed and open fractures. Robinson et al (1992) reported seven of 30 (23%) patients with delayed union using a reamed Seidel nail in a mixed group of different fracture types.

Reports of the results of locked nailing with mixed open and closed fractures demonstrate very low infection rates (Riemer et al 1991, Ingman and Waters 1994). Rommens and his colleagues (1995) encountered no infections in their series which included four type II open

injuries, but type III injuries were excluded. Similarly, low infection rates were reported for unreamed unlocked nailing in mixed groups of open and closed fractures ranging from 0% to 5% (Stern et al 1984, Brumback et al 1986, Hall and Pankovich 1987). Stern and his colleagues noted that 17% of open fractures became infected compared to 2% of open fractures. In none of these series were infection rates reported for individual open fracture types.

The choice of approach for nailing can have a significant effect on outcome. The major disadvantage of the antegrade approach is violation of the rotator cuff. High incidences of shoulder problems have been reported ranging from 24% to 69% (Stern et al 1984, Foster et al 1985, Brumback et al 1986, Riemer et al 1991, Robinson et al 1992) with particular problems with slow rehabilitation in the elderly patient (Hall and Pankovich 1987). Although shoulder stiffness and pain is particularly associated with prominence of the nail, it also occurs in a significant number of patients without nail prominence (Robinson et al 1992). This may be because of the formation of a defect in the rotator cuff which can propagate to a tear, especially in the older patient.

The retrograde approach has the advantage of avoiding damage to the rotator cuff. Limitation of elbow movement has been reported (Durbin et al 1983, Ingman and Waters 1994, Rommens et al 1995) and may be due to fibrosis in the triceps, ossification at the entry portal (Rommens et al 1995) or a protruding nail causing impingement. The insertion of a non-elastic straight nail can also cause iatrogenic fracture, particularly with small distal fragments (Ingman and Waters 1994).

Although closed nailing could theoretically cause radial nerve damage this does not seem to have occurred in significant numbers (Durbin et al 1983, Stern et al 1984, Robinson et al 1992, Crolla et al 1993, Rommens et al 1995). Adequate debridement in open fractures should ensure that the radial nerve is not trapped between the bone ends and therefore not at risk of reamer damage.

Plating

Open reduction and internal fixation with plates and screws may be used in open fractures of the

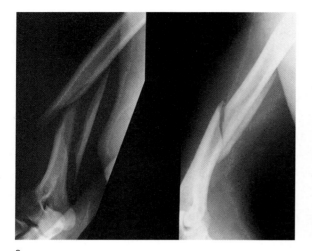

a

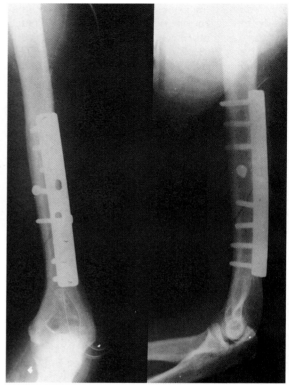

b

Figure 8.7

Open humeral diaphyseal fracture treated by plating.

diaphysis (Figure 8.7) or metaphysis (Figure 8.8) of the humerus.

Approach

To a certain extent, the choice of approach for the open humeral fracture will depend on the site of the open wound which should be incorporated if possible. Extension of the open wound to allow adequate debridement should take into consideration the chosen approach.

The anterolateral approach of Henry (1973) is the most appropriate choice for fractures of the proximal and middle thirds of the diaphysis without radial nerve palsy. With the patient supine and the arm abducted a longitudinal incision is made, centred over the fracture site. Biceps is retracted medially and brachialis is split longitudinally to expose the fracture.

The posterior approach is used for fractures of the diaphysis, requiring exploration of the radial nerve or fractures of the distal third of the diaphysis or of the distal end of the humerus. The patient is placed in the prone or lateral decubitus position with the arm resting on a support and the elbow flexed and free. For diaphyseal fractures, a longitudinal skin incision followed by a longitudinal split in triceps exposes the bone although care must be taken to protect the radial nerve.

For metaphyseal fractures, especially those which are intra-articular, adequate exposure cannot be achieved without an olecranon osteotomy. The initial skin incision is extended distally with radial deviation round the tip of the olecranon. The ulnar nerve is identified and protected and a straight or V-shaped intra-articular osteotomy (Jupiter et al 1985) made with a saw and completed with an osteotome after

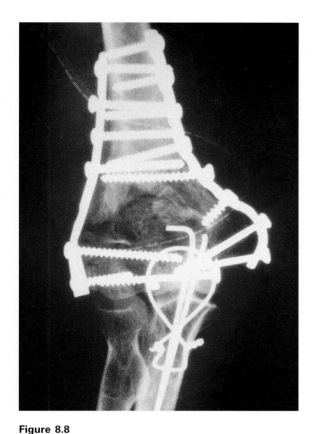

Figure 8.8

Plating of an open fracture of the distal humerus.

predrilling for subsequent fixation. This gives excellent exposure for reconstruction of the joint surface.

Outcome

Although earlier reports of open reduction and internal fixation of humeral shaft fractures reported high complication rates (Bohler 1965, Klenerman 1966, Christensen 1967) this has not been substantiated by more recent studies and has never been proven by a prospective random-ized study comparing treatment methods. Older studies used older techniques and a multiplicity of implants and attempted to compare these with non-operative methods (Klenerman 1966,

Christensen 1967) which were generally chosen for less complex fractures. Modern authors report relatively high success rates with open reduction and plating and several quote open fractures as an indication for the use of this technique (Bell et al 1985, Van der Griend et al 1986, Heim et al 1993). Previous objections to plating mainly centred on high rates of non-union, infection or radial nerve injury. Dabezies et al (1992) and Van der Griend et al (1986) report no non-union in 13 and 11 open fractures of the humerus, respectively, stabilized by plates. Others report low non-union rates of around 2% (Bell et al 1985, Heim et al 1993) in mixed groups of open and closed fractures.

Theoretically, the extra disturbance of the soft tissues, stripping of the periosteum and subse-quent drop in blood flow to bone following open reduction and plating could predispose to non-union and it is important to employ a meticulous technique. In very severe open fractures with bone loss, where the periosteum is destroyed already, these concerns are less important and plating can allow simultaneous segmental graft-ing (Calkins et al 1987).

There remains controversy also about the use of plate fixation in open humeral fractures because of concern about infection in more severe fractures. Bell and his colleagues (1985) had no infections in 13 open fractures treated by plating although the majority of their patients were Gustilo type I open injuries. Van der Griend et al (1986) matched this experience with no deep infection in 13 patients with open fractures treated by plating, although they did not give any indication of the severity of the soft-tissue damage. Of 127 fractures treated by plating, Heim and his co-authors (1993) report a 3.1% infection rate. None of these infections occurred in the nine open fractures which were again mainly type I. On the basis of one deep infection of seven open fractures occurring in a type IIIb open fracture (Gustilo et al 1984) treated by a plate, Rogers and his colleagues (1984) recom-mended external fixation for severe open fractures. There is no evidence to support this recommendation, and it is likely that the quality of the debridement and the handling of the soft tissues has a much greater influence on infection rates than the type of fixation employed.

There has been concern that damage to the radial nerve may occur during plating. Reported incidences of radial nerve palsy first appearing after surgery are low (Bell et al 1985, Foster et al 1985, Van der Griend et al 1986, Heim et al 1993) and all of these authors report early resolution of the palsy.

Open reduction and internal fixation with plates is the method of choice for open fractures of the distal humerus, especially those which are intra-articular since this allows anatomical restoration and early movement of the joint (Jupiter et al 1985, Zagorski et al 1986, Helfet and Schmeling 1993). Complications of infection or non-union are poorly reported in open fractures of the distal humerus. Jupiter et al (1985) had four open fractures of 34 of which one deep infection occurred in the only type III injury. There is general agreement that the outcome of these severe injuries is determined by the experience of the surgeon and the adequacy of debridement and fixation (Jupiter et al 1985, Collins and Temple 1989, Holdsworth and Mossad 1990).

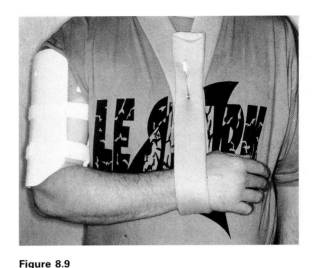

Figure 8.9

Bracing of a humeral shaft fracture.

Non-operative management

Although closed fractures of the humeral shaft are often treated non-operatively there remains debate about the use of this technique in open fractures, although even proponents of non-operative management agree that massive soft-tissue injury or bone loss are contraindications to primary non-operative management (Zagorski et al 1988).

The most common methods used are hanging casts or prefabricated braces (Figure 8.9) both of which are intended to use a combination of soft-tissue compression and the effect of gravity to maintain reduction. It must be emphasized, however, that the use of these non-operative fixation devices does not remove the need to perform a thorough and aggressive debridement.

Technique

In the early years of humeral fracture bracing, the brace was applied after acute pain and swelling had subsided with the fracture initially being immobilized in plaster. Current practice has resulted in the brace being applied earlier

and even as primary treatment (Sarmiento et al 1977, Zagorski et al 1988). After a few days, the patient is allowed to perform pendulum exercises, passive shoulder movement and active elbow exercises which may cause some angulatory deformities to correct (Zagorski et al 1988, Sarmiento et al 1990). Regular radiological and clinical review is required to assess the fracture position although the humerus is tolerant of a moderate amount of deformity (Klenerman 1966, Zagorski et al 1988, Sarmiento et al 1990). Functional bracing commonly allows some varus deformity (Zagorski et al 1988, Sarmiento et al 1990) but in neither of these series was this a functional or cosmetic problem.

Outcome

Union times for brace-treated open fractures appear similar to those of fractures treated operatively. Zagorski and his colleagues (1988) reported an average union time of 13.6 weeks for 43 open fractures treated by debridement and bracing. They do not detail the types of open fracture but all soft tissue wounds were left to heal by secondary intention, and thus by implication were likely to be type I. One of the 43 patients (2.3%) had a non-union. Sarmiento et al (1990) had one non-union in 11 open fractures treated with braces. One of these, a type IIIc open fracture, was treated with an external fixator for six weeks prior to bracing, implying that braces were not used primarily for severe open fractures. In an earlier report, Sarmiento and his colleagues (1977) had no non-unions in 13 open fractures treated with braces.

Infection rates with open fractures treated with bracing were also reported as low (Zagorski et al 1988, Sarmiento et al 1990) but severe open fractures again were excluded.

Joint stiffness can be a significant problem after non-operative management of humeral shaft fractures. Ciernik and his co-authors (1991) reported compromise of shoulder and elbow movement with treatment by hanging cast. Klenerman (1966) reported nine of 30 patients (30%) examined after U-slab and sling treatment with restriction of elbow and shoulder movement or both.

Although theoretically functional bracing should avoid most of these problems, significant loss of motion in the shoulder and elbow are reported. Sarmiento et al (1990) report 45% of patients with limitation of shoulder external rotation, 26% with some limitation of elbow flexion and 24% with limitation of elbow extension in a group of 65 patients with either open or closed fractures of the distal third of the humeral diaphysis.

One other disadvantage of bracing is the requirement for close supervision by physiotherapists. Close supervision is also required to ensure that correct hygiene is performed, as otherwise problems may arise with severe skin maceration (Zagorski et al 1988). Other possible soft-tissue problems reported are oedema distal to the brace and inferior shoulder subluxation (Zagorski et al 1988).

Functional bracing or plaster management is not recommended for severe open humeral shaft fractures. Minor open injuries may be treated by splinting provided an adequate debridement is performed and there is close clinical and physiotherapy supervision during the rehabilitation periods.

Non-operative management is not recommended for open articular fractures of the distal humerus.

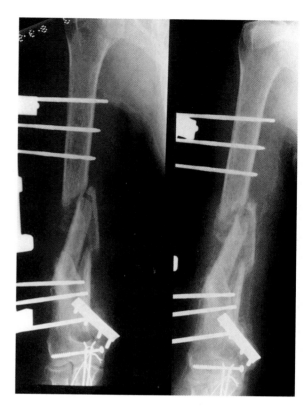

Figure 8.10

External fixation for a severe open humeral fracture. Note the associated distal humeral injury.

External fixation

The relative indications for the use of external fixation in the open fracture of the humeral diaphysis include severe open fractures with associated vascular damage or associated burns (Choong and Griffiths 1988) or severe open segmental fractures where internal fixation would be technically difficult (Levin et al 1990). These situations are rare and therefore external fixation is not commonly used in open humeral fractures. Indications for external fixation in open intra-articular fractures of the distal humerus are very limited and only occur when bone loss is sufficiently severe as to preclude internal fixation or where soft-tissue injury leads to loss of elbow stability.

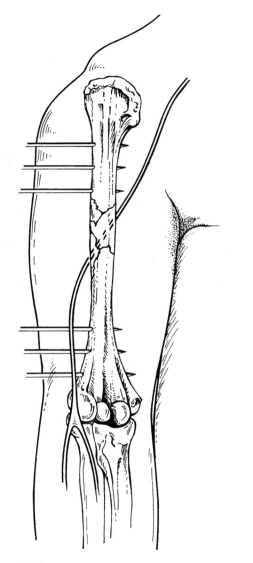

Figure 8.11

Ideal pin placement for external fixation of the humerus avoiding the radial nerve.

ity of the neurovascular structures to bone. Because of this, pin placement should always be carried out using an open technique to avoid inadvertent damage to important structures.

Half-pins inserted laterally with a single bar are usually adequate to stabilize the humerus (Figure 8.10). Pins should not be inserted at the surgical neck or at the junction of the middle and lower thirds of the shaft to avoid damage to the axillary and radial nerves respectively (Figure 8.11). Alternatively, for distal fractures, pins may be placed posteriorly through the triceps aponeurosis. If possible, intermuscular planes should be used to minimize transfixion of muscle groups and avoid shoulder or elbow stiffness.

Outcome

There have been limited reports of the outcome of open fractures treated by external fixation. Delayed union or non-union is a common problem (Choong and Griffiths 1988, Smith and Cooney 1990, Kim et al 1994) and some authors recommend conversion to plating and bone grafting at an early stage after soft-tissue healing is complete (Choong and Griffiths 1988). Sepsis rates are poorly reported with the use of external fixation but are likely to be related to the severity of the soft-tissue injury and the adequacy of debridement rather than to the external fixation.

Joint stiffness is a predictable problem with the use of external fixation in a bone with such a good soft-tissue envelope as the humerus. Smith and Cooney (1990) report a 22% incidence of significant impairment of shoulder motion after external fixation of severe open fractures. Other potential problems include poor patient compliance, shoulder subluxation and radial nerve injury (Choong and Griffiths 1988, Putnam and Walsh 1993).

Technique

More difficulty is encountered in applying an external fixator to the humerus than to the tibia. This is because of the absence of a subcutaneous border in the humerus and the relative proxim-

References

Bell MJ, Beauchamp CG, Kellam JK, McMurtry RY (1985) The results of plating humeral shaft fractures in patients with multiple injuries, *J Bone Joint Surg* **67B**: 293–6.

Bohler L (1965) Conservative treatment of fresh closed fractures of the shaft of the humerus, *J Trauma* **5**: 464–8.

Bleeker WA, Nijsten MWN, Yen Duis H-J (1991) Treatment of humeral shaft fractures related to associated injuries, *Acta Orthop Scand* **62**: 148–53.

Bostman O, Bakalim G, Vainionpaa S, Wilppula E, Patiala H, Rokkanen P (1986) Radial palsy in shaft fracture of the humerus, *Acta Orthop Scand* **57**: 316–19.

Brumback RJ, Bosse MJ, Poka A, Burgess AR (1986) Intramedullary stabilisation of humeral shaft fractures in patients with multiple trauma, *J Bone Joint Surg* **68A**: 960–70.

Calkins MS, Burkhalter W, Reyes F (1987) Traumatic segmental bone defects in the upper extremity. Treatment with exposed grafts of corticocancellous bone, *J Bone Joint Surg* **69A**: 19–27.

Chapman MW, Mahoney M (1979) The role of early internal fixation in the management of open fractures, *Clin Orthop* **138**: 120–30.

Choong PFM, Griffiths JD (1988) External fixation of complex open humeral fractures, *Aust NZ J Surg* **58**: 137–42.

Christensen S (1967) Humeral shaft fractures, operative and conservative treatment, *Acta Chir Scand* **133**: 455–60.

Ciernik IF, Meier L, Hollinger A (1991) Humeral mobility after treatment with hanging cast, *J Trauma* **31**: 230–3.

Collins DN, Temple SD (1989) Open joint injuries. Classification and treatment, *Clin Orthop* **242**: 48–56.

Court-Brown CM, McQueen MM, Quaba AA, Christie J (1991) Reamed intramedullary nailing: its use in type II and III open tibial fractures, *J Bone Joint Surg* **73B**: 959–64.

Crolla RM, de Vries LS, Clevers GJ (1993) Locked intramedullary nailing of humeral fractures, *Injury* **24**: 403–6.

Dabezies EJ, Banta CJ, Murphy CP, d'Ambrose RD (1992) Plate fixation of the humeral shaft for acute fractures, with and without radial nerve injuries, *J Orthop Trauma* **6**: 10–13.

Danckewardt-Lilliestrom G (1969) Reaming of the medullary cavity and its effect on diaphyseal bone, *Acta Orthop Scand Suppl* **128**.

Durbin RA, Gottesman MJ, Saunders KC (1983) Hackethal stacked nailing of humeral shaft fractures, *Clin Orthop* **179**: 168–74.

Foster RJ, Dixon GL, Bach AW, Appleyard RW, Green TM (1985) Internal fixation of fractures and non-unions of the humeral shaft, *J Bone Joint Surg* **66A**: 857–64.

Foster RJ, Swiontkowski MF, Bach AW, Sack JT (1993) Radial nerve palsy caused by open humeral shaft fractures, *J Hand Surg* **18A**: 12–124.

Grosse A, Christie J, Taglang G, Court-Brown C, McQueen MM (1993) Open adult femoral shaft fracture treated by early intramedullary nailing, *J Bone Joint Surg* **75B**: 562–5.

Gustilo RB, Anderson JT (1976) Prevention of infection in the treatment of one thousand and twenty-five open fractures of long bones, *J Bone Joint Surg* **58A**: 453–8.

Gustilo RB, Mendoza RM, Williams DN (1984) Problems in the management of type III (severe) open fractures: a new classification of type III open fractures, *J Trauma* **24**: 742–6.

Gustilo RB, Merkow RL, Templeman D (1990) Current Concepts Review. The management of open fractures, *J Bone Joint Surg* **72A**: 299–304.

Hackethal KH (1961) *Die Bundel-Nagelung* (Springer-Verlag: Berlin).

Hall RF, Pankovich AM (1987) Ender nailing of acute fractures of the humerus, *J Bone Joint Surg* **69A**: 558–67.

Heim D, Herkert F, Hess P, Regazzoni P (1993) Surgical treatment of humeral shaft fractures—the Basel experience, *J Trauma* **35**: 226–32.

Helfet DL, Schmeling GJ (1993) Bicondylar intra-articular fractures of the distal humerus in adults, *Clin Orthop* **292**: 26–36.

Henry AR (1973) *Extensile Exposure*, 2nd edn. (Churchill Livingstone: Edinburgh).

Holdsworth BJ, Mossad MM (1990) Fractures of the adult distal humerus, *J Bone Joint Surg* **72B**: 362–5.

Ingman AM, Waters DA (1994) Locked intramedullary nailing of humeral shaft fractures, *J Bone Joint Surg* **76B**: 23–9.

Jupiter JB, Neff V, Holzach P, Allgower M (1985) Intercondylar fractures of the humerus. An operative approach, *J Bone Joint Surg* **67A**: 226–39.

Kim NH, Hahn SB, Park HW, Yang IH (1994) The Orthofix external fixator for fractures of long bones, *Int Orthop* **18**: 42–6.

Klenerman L (1966) Fractures of the shaft of the humerus, *J Bone Joint Surg* **48B**: 105–11.

Levin LS, Goldner RD, Urbaniak JR, Hurley JA, Hardaker WT (1990) Management of severe musculo-skeletal injuries of the upper extremity, *J Orthop Trauma* **4**: 432–40.

Mast JW, Spiegel PG, Harvey JP, Harrison C (1975) Fractures of the humeral shaft. A retrospective study of 240 adult fractures, *Clin Orthop* **112**: 254–63.

Omer GE (1982) Results of untreated peripheral nerve injuries, *Clin Orthop* **163**: 15–19.

Patzakis MJ, Wilkins J (1989) Factors influencing infection rate in open fracture wounds, *Clin Orthop* **243**: 36–40.

Pollock FH, Drake D, Bovill EG, Day L, Trafton PG (1981) Treatment of radial neuropathy associated with fractures of the humerus, *J Bone Joint Surg* **59A**: 596–601.

Putnam MD, Walsh TM (1993) External fixation for open fractures of the upper extremity, *Hand Clinics* **4**: 613–23.

Riemer BL, Butterfield SL, D'Ambrosia R, Kellam J (1991) Seidel intramedullary nailing of humeral diaphyseal fractures: a preliminary report, *Orthopaedics* **14**: 239–46.

Robinson CM, Bell KM, Court-Brown CM, McQueen MM (1992) Locked nailing of humeral shaft fractures. Experience in Edinburgh over a two year period, *J Bone Joint Surg* **74B**: 558–62.

Rogers JF, Bennett JB, Tullos HS (1984) Management of concomitant ipsilateral fractures of the humerus and forearm, *J Bone Joint Surg* **66A**: 552–6.

Rojczyk M (1984) Results of treatment of open fractures, aspects of antibiotic therapy. In: Tscherne H, Gotzen L, eds, *Fractures with Soft Tissue Injuries*, pp. 33–8 (Springer-Verlag: Berlin).

Rommens PM, Verbruggen J, Broos PL (1995) Retrograde locked nailing of humeral shaft fractures, *J Bone Joint Surg* **77B**: 84–9.

Sanders R, Swiontkowski M, Hurley J, Spiegel P (1993) The management of fractures with soft tissue disruptions, *J Bone Joint Surg* **75A**: 778–89.

Sarmiento A, Kinman PB, Galvin EG, Schmitt RH, Phillips JG (1977) Functional bracing of fractures of the shaft of the humerus, *J Bone Joint Surg* **59A**: 596–601.

Sarmiento A, Horowitch A, Aboulafia A, Vangsness CT (1990) Functional bracing for comminuted extra-articular fractures of the distal third of the humerus, *J Bone Joint Surg* **72B**: 283–7.

Shah JJ, Bhatti NA (1983) Radial nerve paralysis associated with fractures of the humerus, *Clin Orthop* **172**: 171–7.

Smith DK, Cooney WP (1990) External fixation of high-energy upper extremity injuries, *J Orthop Trauma* **4**: 7–18.

Stern PJ, Mattingly DA, Pomeroy DC, Zenni EJ, Kreig JK (1984) Intramedullary fixation of humeral shaft fractures, *J Bone Joint Surg* **66A**: 639–46.

Tscherne H (1984) In: Tscherne H, Gotzen L, eds, *Fractures with Soft Tissue Injuries*, pp. 10–32 (Springer-Verlag: Berlin).

Van der Griend R, Tomasin J, Ward EF (1986) Open reduction and internal fixation of humeral shaft fractures, *J Bone Joint Surg* **68A**: 430–3.

Zagorski JB, Jennings J, Burkhalter WE, Uribe JW (1986) Comminuted intra-articular fractures of the distal humeral condyles, *Clin Orthop* **202**: 197–204.

Zagorski JB, Latta L, Zych GA, Finnieston AR (1988) Diaphyseal fractures of the humerus. Treatment with prefabricated braces, *J Bone Joint Surg* **70A**: 607–10.

9
Open fractures of the forearm

M.M. McQueen

Open fractures of the forearm occur with varying degrees of frequency along the lengths of the radius and ulna involving both metaphyseal and diaphyseal bones. Because of the importance of the soft tissues in this area, especially for hand function, an open fracture of any severity with ensuing complications is potentially a very disabling condition.

Epidemiology

During the five-year period from January 1988 to December 1992, 98 open fractures of the radius and ulna were admitted to the Edinburgh Orthopaedic Trauma Unit. Twelve of these (12%) were in the proximal ends of the radius and ulna, 31 (32%) in the diaphyses and 55 (56%) involved the distal ends of the radius and ulna. During this period, there was a total of 1392 fractures of the proximal radius and ulna giving an incidence of 0.9% of open fractures. The diaphyseal fractures were open in 8.5% of patients and the distal radius and ulna were open in 2% of patients.

Of the 12 patients with proximal fractures, eight were male and four female with an average age of 41 years ranging from 16 to 80 years. Seven patients had been involved in road traffic accidents and two were assaulted. One patient was injured in a simple fall, one in a fall from a height and one due to sport. Overall, eight (66%) injuries were high energy in nature.

All the fractures involved the olecranon alone, none having radial head involvement. All but one were intra-articular with the majority being AO class B1.1, i.e. olecranon unifocal and intra-articular (Figure 9.1), although six were at the

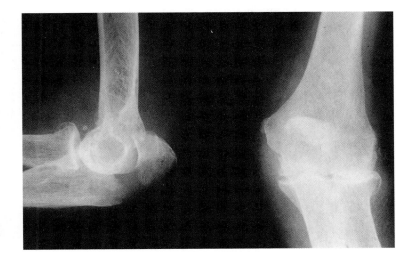

Figure 9.1

An AO type B1.1 olecranon fracture.

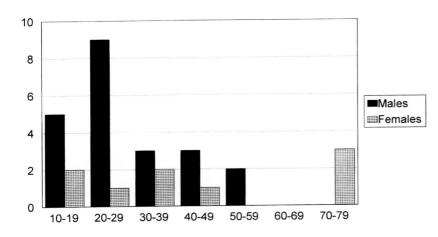

Figure 9.2

Age/sex distribution of open forearm diaphyseal fractures. Note the bimodal distribution.

complex end of this spectrum with more than one fracture line in the olecranon.

Three patients had Gustilo type I (Gustilo and Anderson 1976) injuries, six Gustilo type II and three Gustilo type IIIa (Gustilo et al 1984). All the wounds were either closed secondarily or left to granulate. None was sufficiently severe to require plastic surgery.

Open fractures of the proximal forearm usually involve the olecranon; open radial head fractures are extremely rare. They tend to be high-energy injuries in a relatively young age group with moderately severe soft-tissue injuries and complex intra-articular fractures of the olecranon.

There were 31 patients with open fractures of the diaphyses of the radius and ulna. During the same time period, a total of 366 diaphyseal fractures were treated giving an incidence of 8.5% of open fractures at this site. The majority (71%) were males and the average age was young at 33 years. The age/sex distribution is bimodal (Figure 9.2) with a large peak of young males and a small peak of older women. Twenty-one of the 31 patients (68%) had had high-energy injuries either as a result of road traffic accidents, crushing injuries or high-velocity sporting injuries. Twelve of the 31 fractures were AO class A or a simple configuration. Thirteen were AO type B with wedge fragments (Figure 9.3) and the remainder were segmental or severely comminuted fractures classified as AO type C (Figure

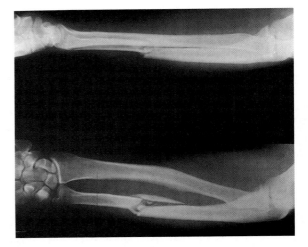

Figure 9.3

AO type B forearm diaphyseal fracture.

9.4). Overall, 61% of the fractures had varying severities of comminution. The simple fractures occurred in a younger age group with an average age of 24 years compared to 36 years for the more complex fractures. Both high- and low-velocity injury caused AO type A and B fractures although all the type C fractures were caused by high-energy injuries.

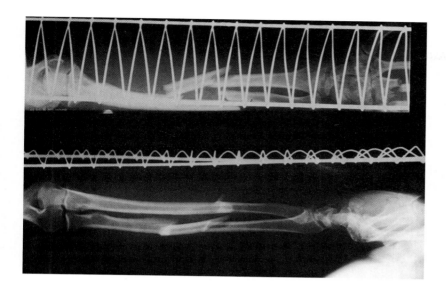

Figure 9.4

AO type C forearm diaphyseal fracture.

Eighteen of the 31 fractures involved both bones of the forearm with nine being isolated ulnar fractures and four isolated radial fractures. None was a Monteggia or Galeazzi fracture.

Overall, the soft-tissue injuries were more severe than those proximally or distally. Almost half (48%) of the injuries were Gustilo type I and 23% were type II. Nine injuries (29%) were type III with three type IIIa and six type IIIb injuries. Three injuries required either local or free flap cover and six required split-skin grafting. None of the type I or II injuries required plastic surgery, which is an indication of the relatively good soft-tissue cover on the forearm bones.

Open fractures of the diaphyses of the forearm bones are epidemiologically similar to other long bone fractures, with a bimodal distribution but a preponderance of young males, a high incidence of high-energy complex injuries, and a significant number of severe soft-tissue injuries. However, the overall incidence is less than for the tibia, presumably because of the good soft tissue envelope in the forearm.

The commonest open fracture of the forearm involves the distal ends of the radius and ulna, being 56% of all open forearm fractures. There were 55 patients with this injury over a five-year period which was 2% of all the distal radial

fractures treated during this time. Unlike fractures in the rest of the forearm, the majority of cases were female (65%) and the average age was older at 62 years. Their mode of injury is shown in Table 9.1. The most common cause was a simple fall (56%) with most of the remainder being high-energy injuries. This is in contrast with the mode of injury of the total population of distal radial fractures where 80% are caused by simple falls.

The fracture configurations also show some differences from the total population of distal radial fractures. In the total population, there are roughly equal proportions of AO type A or extra-articular fractures (Figure 9.5) and AO type C or complete articular fractures (Figure 9.6) while in the open fractures, 57% are AO type C and 38%

Table 9.1 Mode of injury of open distal forearm fractures

Fall	31
Fall from height	9
Road traffic accident driver	3
Road traffic accident pedestrian	9
Other	3

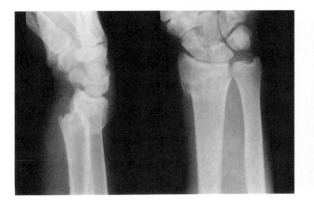

Figure 9.5

An extra-articular fracture of the distal radius.

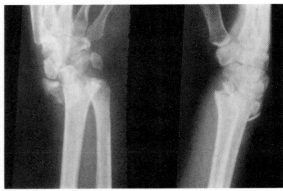

Figure 9.6

An AO type C or complete articular fracture of the distal radius.

are AO type A. The most obvious difference between open and closed fractures is the preponderance of severe comminution extending into the diaphysis in the open fractures. Twenty-three of the 55 open fractures (42%) were either AO type A3.3 (Figure 9.7) or type C3.3 compared to 0.1% of closed fractures.

Most of the soft-tissue injuries were Gustilo type I (76%) with 22% being type II injuries and only one type III injury which was a type IIIa. The majority of the type I injuries were open through an associated fracture of the distal ulna or diaphyseal comminution.

There were two main groups of patients with open distal radial fractures. There were 21 patients less than 60 years of age, 16 (76%) of whom had sustained high-energy injury. Eighteen (86%) had AO type C fractures all but two of which were complex articular fractures. Ten (48%) had diaphyseal comminution. Twelve of the 21 (57%) had either multiple system injuries or multiple orthopaedic injuries.

Of the group over 60 years of age, 27 (79%) had sustained low-energy injury. Twelve (35%) had AO type C injuries while 13 (38%) had diaphyseal comminution. Only eight (24%) had associated injuries.

Little has been published on the subject of epidemiology of open forearm fractures. Rojczyk (1984) reported that 12.6% of open fractures

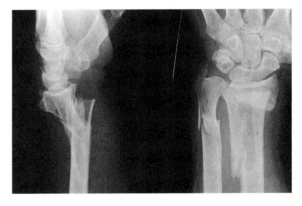

Figure 9.7

An open distal radial fracture with diaphyseal comminution.

treated at the Hanover Medical School occurred in the forearm, a figure very similar to the experience in Edinburgh (Chapter 3). Open forearm diaphyseal fractures are reported by Moed et al (1986) to occur in a young population with high-energy injuries. They also reported a relatively high incidence (22%) of type III soft-tissue injury.

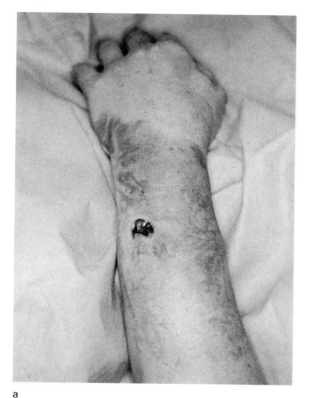

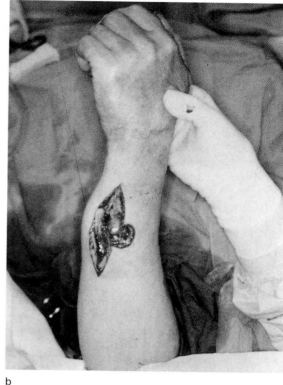

a

b

Figure 9.8

(a) An open fracture of the ulnar shaft. (b) The same fracture after excision.

Management

Management of the soft tissues

The management of the soft-tissue injury in open fractures is the key to a successful outcome. Aggressive and thorough debridement removing all necrotic or contaminated tissue whether soft or bony is essential to ensure a clean non-infected wound without which further management will not be successful. The ideal outcome of an open fracture of the forearm is a non-infected healed fracture with normal hand, wrist and elbow function. With adequate handling of the soft tissues, the first two aims should be consistently achieved. The third is

partly dependent on the severity of the initial soft-tissue injury since the soft tissues of the forearm are crucial to a normally functioning hand and forearm. In the most severe injuries with severe neurological and vascular impairment, significant soft-tissue loss and a threat to life, amputation may have to be considered in open forearm fractures. In this context Slauterbeck et al (1994) have shown that the mangled extremity severity score (MESS), which depends on the severity of the soft-tissue injury, limb ischaemia, degree of shock and age, is an accurate predictor of the upper extremities best treated by amputation. Considering the unique functional importance of the upper limb and the financial and psychological sequelae of its loss, it is fortunate that such severe injuries are rare. More commonly the open wound is not life or limb threatening and vigorous immediate treatment is indicated.

Aggressive debridement of the open wound should be performed immediately, excising all dead and contaminated soft or bony tissue. Debridement is not complete unless the bone ends are visualized by delivering them through the wound. This will usually involve extension of the open wound to allow adequate access. Figure 9.8a shows an open fracture of the ulnar shaft with the proximal end of the ulna protruding. Figure 9.8b demonstrates the wound extension necessary to achieve an adequate debridement. Copious irrigation and antibiotic therapy are important adjuncts to an aggressive debridement (Gustilo et al 1990).

The wound should be left open after debridement although surgical extensions may be closed provided this does not apply tension to the skin edges. The wound extensions in the patients in Figure 9.8b were left open because swelling precluded closure of the extensions without tension. A 'second look' procedure should be performed 24–48 hours after initial debridement and further debridement undertaken if necessary. If the wound is clean at this stage, then cover may be achieved by whatever means are necessary ranging from secondary closure to a free flap.

Injury to nerves or tendons is not uncommonly associated with open forearm fractures. Moed and his colleagues (1986) reported nine of 50 patients (18%) with open forearm diaphyseal fractures and nerve, tendon or arterial injury. The more severe soft-tissue injuries such as the 18 type III open diaphyseal fractures in Jones' series (1991) have a higher incidence of nerve or tendon injury (44%). In a series of open forearm fractures with bone loss, Grace and Eversmann (1980a) reported a 61% incidence of nerve injury. The majority of the patients required either repair of the nerve or tendon grafting. Smith and Cooney (1990) reported vascular injury in 45% and neurological injury in 34% of their group of 32 open fractures most of which were Gustilo type III. Repair of the soft tissues is generally carried out where possible; secondary tendon transfers or nerve grafts should be performed if necessary after stable soft-tissue healing is achieved.

Management of the bone injury

Proximal metaphyseal fractures of the radius and ulna

As can be seen from the epidemiology of open forearm fractures, open fractures of the proximal ulna are uncommon and those of the proximal radius extremely rare. Open fractures of the ulna are amenable to several different treatment techniques including tension band wiring, plating, screw fixation or excision of the fragment with repair of the extensor apparatus.

Tension band wiring

This technique was first described by Weber and Vasey (1963). The fracture is reduced and two longitudinal parallel Kirschner wires are inserted. A figure-of-eight wire is then passed round the K wires under the triceps tendon and through a hole in the proximal ulnar shaft. The bent ends of the K wires are then punched through the triceps tendon to engage the wire. The wire is then tightened to apply compression across the fracture site (Figure 9.9).

The aim of tension band wiring of an olecranon fracture is to reduce the joint surface anatomically and to fix the reduction rigidly so

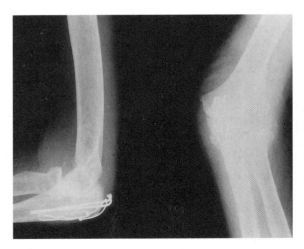

Figure 9.9

Tension band wiring of an olecranon fracture.

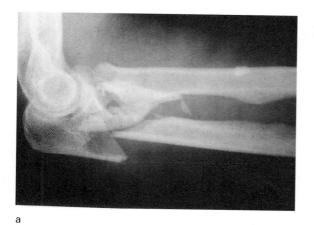

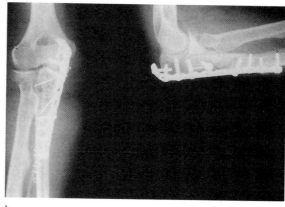

a   b

Figure 9.10

(a) A complex proximal ulnar fracture; note the associated radial head fracture. (b) The same fracture with interfragmentary fixation and a contoured plate.

that early movement and rehabilitation may be started. Most authors publish a high proportion of good results with union rates ranging from 85% to 98% (Horne and Tanzer 1981, Gartsman et al 1981, Holdsworth and Mossad 1984, Hume and Wiss 1992, Teasdall et al 1993) even in the most complex of fractures. Equally, these authors agree that a functional range of movement is regained, albeit with fairly frequent slight extension losses, and there is generally excellent recovery of rotation provided there was not an associated radial head fracture.

Holdsworth and Mossad (1984) measured elbow flexor and extensor strength after tension band wiring and found 85% with good or excellent functional scores although the older patients fared less well. Gartsman and his colleagues (1981) reported 27% loss of elbow extension for patients treated by internal fixation.

The major drawback of tension band wiring is the frequency with which the implants cause significant problems. K-wire backout, skin problems from poorly buried wire knots or pain requiring removal of the device have been reported with considerable frequency (Horne and Tanzer 1981, Holdsworth and Mossad 1984, Macko and Szabo 1985, Jensen and Olsen 1986, Hume and Wiss 1992).

Plating

Plate fixation is generally used for the more complex olecranon fracture (Figure 9.10a) and requires a sufficiently large proximal fragment to allow the insertion of two or preferably three screws. The plate must be contoured to fit the olecranon proximally (Figure 9.10b). Experimentally, Fyfe et al (1985) showed that comminuted osteotomies were held most rigidly by a contoured 1/3 tubular plate while transverse osteotomies fared best with tension band wiring. For oblique osteotomies, there was no difference between tension band wiring and plating. Hume and Wiss (1992) randomly compared two groups of patients with displaced olecranon fractures treated with tension band wiring or plate fixation. They found better clinical results in terms of pain and range of movement in the plated group along with a significant reduction in symptomatic metal prominence. The only drawback was a slightly longer operating time for the plated fractures. A potential drawback in treating open fractures by plating, however, is the increased bulk of a plate on a subcutaneous bone thereby increasing the difficulties of secondary wound closure. This is, however, not a contraindication to plate fixation, especially with good plastic surgery facilities.

Excision of the fragment and triceps repair

There is general agreement that the non-articular small fragment or AO type A1.1 fracture is successfully treated by excision of the fragment and triceps repair (Horne and Tanzer 1981). There is more debate, however, about the treatment of articular fractures of the olecranon by this method although there is also agreement that those with associated injury and possibly elbow instability should not be treated with excision.

Gartsman and his colleagues (1981) reviewed 107 patients who had been treated either by open reduction and various methods of fixation or primary excision. They found similar outcomes functionally and radiologically for each group. There was a higher rate of complications in the fixation group but these were treated mostly with intramedullary screws without tension band wiring.

It would seem that at the present state of knowledge open fractures of the olecranon may be treated after a thorough wound excision by one of three methods. Excision of the fragment and triceps repair may be used for the extra-articular proximal fractures. The simpler more proximal articular fractures may be treated by tension band wiring with attention to detail to reduce the complications related to the implant (Jensen and Olsen 1986). More complex or distal articular fractures are best held by plates and screws, although this may require more complex soft-tissue cover.

Diaphyseal fractures of the radius and ulna

Open fractures of the shaft of the forearm bones are usually treated operatively either by internal or external fixation although it is possible to manage the less severe open isolated ulnar shaft fractures non-operatively. Nevertheless, it is important to achieve bone stability in order to protect the integrity of the remaining soft tissues, to facilitate soft-tissue healing, to reduce the rate of infection (Gustilo et al 1990) and to ensure that rehabilitation is started as expeditiously as possible. Keeping in mind that the main aims of treatment are achieving fracture union with minimal restriction of movement in the forearm, elbow

and wrist and restoration of full pain-free function to the upper extremity, fixation of the forearm bones can be achieved by plating, intramedullary fixation or external fixation.

Plating

At present, plating is the most commonly used and best proven method of internal fixation of forearm diaphyseal fractures. To a certain extent, the approach to open forearm diaphyseal fractures is dictated by the site of the open wound. Wound extensions will be required in all but the most severe soft-tissue injuries and should incorporate the open wound where possible. The radius and ulna should be approached through separate incisions since a single incision may predispose the patient to develop cross-union (Breit 1983).

Radius
The radius may be approached through a volar or dorsal incision depending on the site of the open wound.

The volar approach is that of Henry. The skin incision is from a point just proximal and lateral to the biceps tendon and extends into the forearm along the medial border of brachioradialis as far as the radial styloid if necessary. All, or part, of this incision may be used depending on the circumstances. The deep fascia is incised in the line of the skin incision protecting the radial vessels. Brachioradialis is retracted laterally and flexor carpi radialis medially and, with the hand pronated, the periosteum is incised lateral to the origin of flexor pollicis longus. The radius may then be exposed subperiosteally. Proximally the supinator muscle should be stripped subperiosteally from the radius as must pronator quadratus distally.

Should the dorsal surface of the radius be the site of the open wound then the dorsal approach of Thompson may be used. The skin excision extends from the centre of the dorsum of the wrist to a point anterior to the lateral epicondyle of the humerus. The interval between extensor digitorum and extensor carpi radialis brevis is developed and these muscles retracted towards the ulnar and radial sides respectively. As much of extensor digitorum and the supinator muscle as required is stripped subperiosteally off the radius, taking care not to damage the deep branch of the radial nerve in the substance of supinator.

The ulna is exposed by a longitudinal incision along its subcutaneous border. This is deepened to bone in the interval between the flexor and extensor muscles.

Outcome of plating

The advent of compression plating revolutionized the management of forearm diaphyseal fractures. Prior to this, non- or delayed union rates ranged from 6% to 40% (Hicks 1961, Caden 1961) while the functional results had a high incidence of unsatisfactory ratings (Knight and Purvis 1949, Hughston 1957, Caden 1961). In contrast, the majority of modern reports on compression plating of forearm fractures demonstrate a high proportion of good to excellent results ranging from 66% to 92% (Anderson et al 1975, Grace and Eversmann 1980b, Hadden et al 1984, Moore et al 1985, Moed et al 1986, Chapman et al 1989, Jones 1991). Most of these assessments are based on fracture union and range of motion, particularly forearm rotation, and it is clear from many authors that in open fractures the severity of the initial soft-tissue injury is the major determinant of the final outcome.

Fracture union is always considered as an outcome criterion. Anderson and his co-authors (1975) set the standard for rates of fracture union in compression plating of forearm fractures, reporting an overall union rate of 97.9% for the radius and 96.3% for the ulna in a large series of fractures. There was no difference between single bone or both bone fractures for union. Bone grafting was carried out primarily in 135 fractures but did not diminish the rate of non-union. They reported 38 open fractures and 292 closed fractures in which the union rates were 97.4% and 97.2%, respectively. Anderson and his colleagues attributed the non-unions to infection or poor technique. The average time to union was just over seven weeks for both the radius and the ulna. Similar high rates of union in forearm diaphyseal fractures treated with plating have been reported by others in mixed series of open and closed fractures (Grace and Eversmann 1980b, Chapman et al 1989) and in series of open fractures (Moed et al 1986, Jones 1991, Duncan et al 1992) despite the fact that Jones' series was exclusively type III open fractures.

There are no clear criteria for the use of early bone grafting in open forearm fractures except in cases with bone loss when grafting should be performed when there is good soft-tissue coverage (Elstrom et al 1978, Calkins et al 1987). The general recommendation is to use early bone grafting either at the time of wound closure or after soft-tissue healing in severely comminuted fractures (Anderson et al 1975, Moed et al 1986, Chapman et al 1989, Jones 1991, Langkamer and Ackroyd 1991) although added to this Chapman and his colleagues bone grafted all open fractures. Although this protocol does not show any decrease in union rates with grafting (Anderson et al 1975, Chapman et al 1989) it must be appreciated that the bone-grafted fractures are more severe configurations and ought to take longer to unite.

The risk of infection in open fracture has been cited as a reason for either not using internal fixation or delaying plating for ten days to reduce the risk of sepsis (Anderson et al 1975, Elstrom et al 1978, Grace and Eversmann 1980b). Those authors who felt internal fixation to be contraindicated were usually considering the management of open lower limb injuries whilst the advocates of delayed plating report relatively small numbers of open fractures in their series without detailing the severity of the soft-tissue injury. In more recent series, with large numbers of open fractures treated by immediate plating, infection rates are low (Moed et al 1986, Chapman 1989). Jones' (1991) series of exclusively type III open forearm fractures had a low deep infection rate of 5% with immediate plating in all cases although Duncan et al (1992) found increased infection rates in type IIIb and IIIc open forearm fractures treated by plating. They acknowledge that the infections could be due to management protocol, severity of injury or a combination of fractures. Immediate internal fixation of open forearm fractures does not increase infection rates because the major influence on infection is the adequacy of soft-tissue management.

Immediate plating has the advantage of allowing early rehabilitation and thereby maximizing restoration of function. Grace and Eversmann (1980b) found that patients with plated both bone fractures and early active motion regained better forearm movement than those immobilized in a cast after surgery. Most authors consider that the most significant influence on function is the severity of the soft-tissue injury and Grace and Eversmann also noted that open forearm fractures regained significantly less motion than closed injuries. Moed and his colleagues (1986) reported a recovery of >80% of forearm rotation in 43 of the 47 patients who underwent functional assessment and stated that the damage to soft tissues was the most important prognostic indicator. Jones (1991) performed the most rigorous functional testing of all these series measuring wrist and elbow flexion and extension, rotation and grip strength and also noted that restoration of function was most heavily influenced by soft-tissue injury and in particular by nerve injury. One-third of his patients regained <50% of their grip strength, reflecting the severe soft-tissue injuries reported in this series.

At a later stage, refracture of forearm bones after plate removal can occur due to relative bone weakness from stress protection. There is a remarkable variation in the reported incidence of refracture, ranging in adults from 5% (Rosson and Shearer 1991) to 22% (Hidaka and Gustilo 1984). Hidaka and Gustilo recommend delaying plate removal for at least one year, splinting the arm for a few weeks afterwards and protection from strenuous activity for one year. It is suggested by Rosson and Shearer (1991) that only symptomatic plates should be removed in view of the potential complications of removal.

Intramedullary fixation

Theoretically, closed nailing of open long bone fractures is preferable to open internal fixation because less disturbance of any intact periosteum and soft tissues is required. This has proven a successful technique in open long bone fractures of the lower limb (Court-Brown et al 1991, Grosse et al 1993). The specific problem of the forearm related to intramedullary nailing is difficulty in obtaining reduction of the fracture. Developments in intramedullary nailing in the forearm have not kept pace with the lower limb and in particular in the development of interlocking nails. Until recently, intramedullary nails in the forearm required plaster immobilization (Sage 1959,

Caden 1961, Aho et al 1984, Street 1986) postoperatively, thus negating any rehabilitation advantages. Street (1986) reports a union rate of 93% and an infection rate of 1% in a mixed group of patients treated with a square intramedullary nail designed to reduce rotation. Malunion rates were not reported although 31% of the patients lost >25% of the range of forearm rotation.

An interlocking nail for the ulna was first described by Lefèvre et al in 1990 and was subsequently reported by De Pedro et al in 1992. De Pedro and his colleagues' results are rather scanty but they seem to have achieved union with a full range of motion in all 20 patients. This is a technique which requires closer evaluation in both open and closed fractures but potentially may allow these fractures to be treated with intramedullary nailing without cast immobilization.

External fixation

External fixation of both closed and open diaphyseal fractures of the radius and ulna has been advocated by Schuind et al (1991). They reported few general complications in a mixed group of open and closed fractures but a 16.5% malunion rate and a delayed union or non-union rate of 8.5%. All the delayed unions or non-unions had been treated by open reduction. Restoration of the range of forearm rotation was disappointing, with 82% of pronation and 77% of supination regained. There was no deep infection in 25 open fractures.

Smith and Cooney (1990) reported a series of 32 open forearm fractures most of which were Gustilo type III. They recommended external fixation of open forearm fractures as a method of stabilizing the bone and soft tissues until definitive fracture treatment can be performed. The reason for this is a claim that internal fixation of type III open injuries is associated with 'extraordinarily high rates of infection' and 'amputation for overwhelming sepsis is not uncommon'. They do not support the statements with any evidence and they are refuted by other authors' results (Moed et al 1986, Jones 1991). Smith and Cooney did not describe their method of debridement, the adequacy of which is acknowledged as having the major influence on infection rates rather than the method of fixation.

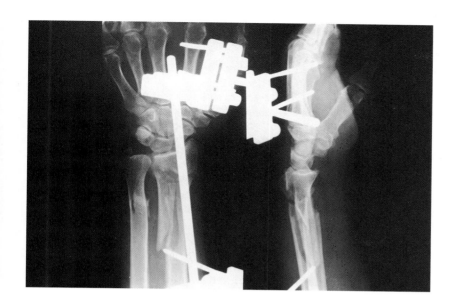

Figure 9.11

An open fracture of the distal radius treated by bridging fixation.

Based on the available evidence, external fixation cannot be recommended in the treatment of open forearm diaphyseal fractures except in situations where internal fixation is not technically possible.

Functional bracing

Non-operative methods are contraindicated for fractures of both forearm bones because of difficulty in obtaining and maintaining reduction. In isolated fractures of the ulna, however, there are some advocates of fracture bracing even in open fractures (Sarmiento et al 1976, Zych et al 1987, Szabo and Skinner 1990) although only fractures with minimal or no displacement were treated. Szabo and Skinner (1990) further recommend that only fractures in the distal two-thirds of the ulna should be managed non-operatively.

In general it is preferable, however, that at the time of wound excision, stabilization of the fracture should be performed in order to allow easy access to the soft tissues and early rehabilitation. The exception to this may be the isolated undisplaced fracture of the ulna with minimal soft-tissue injury.

Fractures of the distal ends of the radius and ulna

As can be seen from the epidemiology of open forearm fractures, open fractures of the distal end of the forearm bones are usually either high-energy articular fractures or low-energy fractures in osteoporotic patients with diaphyseal comminution. In either case, the fracture is unstable and therefore the management of the unstable distal radial fracture will be considered in this chapter.

Unstable extra-articular distal radial fractures

These injuries are usually treated by application of a forearm cast or by external fixation, with occasional use of a small T plate in the extra-articular volar displaced fracture (Keating et al 1994). In open fractures of the distal radius plaster fixation is to be avoided as it does not maintain the radiological position in unstable fractures (McQueen et al 1986, Schmalholz 1989) or allow easy access to the soft-tissue wounds. It may be indicated, however, in the frail elderly patient whose functional demands are low or in the demented patient who is unlikely to tolerate external fixation.

External fixation of the wrist may be used with either bridging fixation, bridging fixation with mobilization of the wrist using a ball joint or peri-articular or metaphyseal fixation.

Bridging the wrist joint is the commonest method. This involves placing two fixator pins in the second metacarpal and two in the proximal radius (Figure 9.11) and depends on traction on the distal fragment through its ligaments or ligamentotaxis to maintain the reduced position.

Bridging external fixation is generally accepted as achieving a good anatomical result with residual dorsal angulation of around 5–8° and radial shortening of a few millimetres (Cooney et al 1979, Kongsholm and Olerud 1989, Howard et al 1989, McQueen et al 1992, Sommerkamp et al 1994, Pritchett 1995, McQueen et al 1996). However, authors who have reported functional results along with radiological results have shown disappointing recovery of hand function in terms of strength, with approximately 60–80% of the normal mass grip strength being regained (Roumen et al 1991, Sanders et al 1991, McQueen et al 1992, 1996, Sommerkamp et al 1994). Overall, the recovery of range of movement is good, with values approaching or exceeding 90% of the range in the opposite unaffected wrist.

Some authors have advocated early mobilization of the wrist using a ball joint within a bridging fixator (Asche 1989). From the evidence available at the present time this does not improve functional results (Sommerkamp et al 1994, McQueen et al 1996).

Complications of bridging fixation are relatively high (Weber and Szabo 1986, Kongsholm and Olerud 1989, Roumen et al 1991, McQueen et al 1992, Sommerkamp et al 1994, McQueen et al 1996), and have been shown to have a direct influence on the functional result (McQueen et al 1992). Another significant negative influence on the functional result is the presence of carpal collapse as defined by Taleisnik and Watson (1984). In a recent series of 120 unstable fractures of the distal radius, carpal collapse was shown to have a significant effect on function (McQueen et al 1996) and it may be that the persistent slight dorsal angulation reported after bridging external fixation allows persistent carpal collapse and explains the

relatively poor restoration of power in the hand. Correction of carpal collapse is dependent on regaining volar tilt, which is very difficult to achieve with bridging external fixation (Bartosh and Saldana 1995).

There are no series of open fractures of the distal radius reported in the literature. Of the 55 patients reported in the epidemiology section in this chapter, treated in the Edinburgh Orthopaedic Trauma Unit, 31 were treated with external fixation. All underwent initial debridement but the antibiotic protocol was inconsistent. Nevertheless, there were no cases of deep infection although six patients (20%) developed pin track infections. The absence of deep infection is likely to be due to the copious blood supply of the metaphyses. The most common complication was malunion, which occurred in a significant number of patients despite bridging external fixation. There was one delayed union in the only type IIIb open injury which had significant bone loss and united after bone grafting.

Other complications of open fractures treated by bridging fixation were related to the fractures rather than the fixation and included carpal tunnel syndrome and one volar compartment syndrome, reflecting the high-energy type of injury common in this series.

Metaphyseal non-bridging external fixation

This is a relatively new technique and can only be used where there is sufficient space in the distal part of the fracture to insert two fixator pins. This usually requires 1 cm of volar cortex and an intact or reconstructed joint surface. Two pins are inserted into the distal fragment under radiographic control using an open technique to avoid tendon injury. The pins are then placed in the radius proximal to the fracture (Figure 9.12).

This technique has yet to be fully evaluated but its advantages are ease of insertion and reliable restoration and maintenance of volar tilt. Free movement of the wrist during the period with the fixator on is possible (Figure 9.13).

Internal fixation

Internal fixation is suitable for both open volar displaced fractures or open fractures with severe articular displacement.

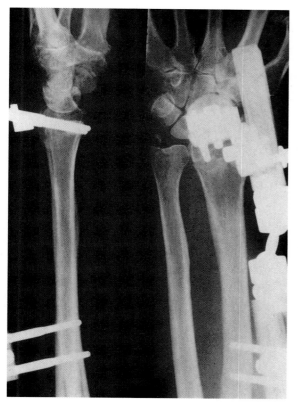

Figure 9.12

Non-bridging external fixation of a distal radial fracture.

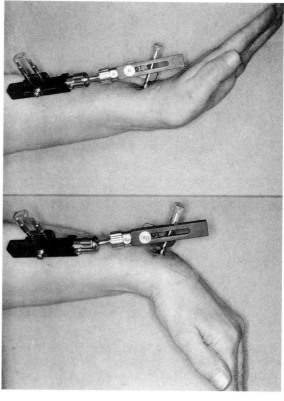

Figure 9.13

The range of movement possible with non-bridging fixation.

In open volar displaced fractures, the distal radius is approached on the volar side taking care not to injure the radial vessel. Pronator quadratus is detached from the radial side of the bone and the fracture exposed. A small AO T plate is suitable for fixation but must be contoured to fit the distal radius, as otherwise a dorsal malunion may result (Keating et al 1994). Functional results with this technique are acceptable although a significant number of cases have persistent weakness (Keating et al 1994).

In open articular fractures of the distal radius, most will be amenable to the treatment methods described above. There will, however, be a small number in whom articular congruity is not restored by these methods and either open or percutaneous reduction of the articular surface should be performed unless the patient is very elderly or the articular surface is so comminuted as to be unreconstructible. In the latter case, it is still important to achieve good extra-articular alignment in order to facilitate possible later wrist fusion.

Where possible, percutaneous techniques should be used. This is facilitated by good visualization of the articular surface, which can be achieved either by tomography or CT scanning (Singer and Pierret 1995) (Figure 9.14). The advent of three-dimensional CT is likely to prove particularly useful in this context.

Overall alignment may first be achieved by bridging external fixation. The joint surface is then assessed by fluoroscopy and if possible percutaneous manipulation of fracture fragments

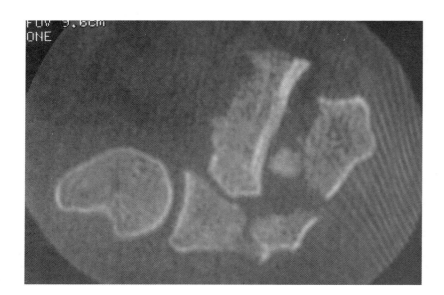

Figure 9.14

CT scan of a severe intra-articular distal radial fracture.

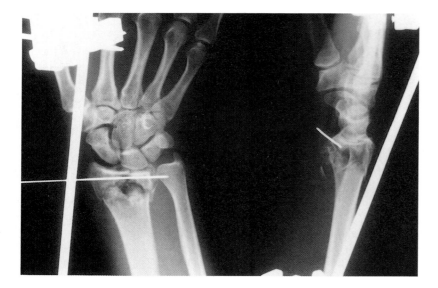

Figure 9.15

Open reduction and K wire fixation of an intra-articular distal radial fracture. Note the bone defect underlying the articular surface.

carried out with a small awl under fluoroscopic control. If this is successful and there is sufficient space in the distal fragment, the external fixator may be converted to a non-bridging fixator, allowing free movement of the joint.

Where percutaneous fixation is not possible, open reduction and fixation of articular fragments is indicated. Pre-operative assessment remains important in order to plan the best approach. Fracture fragments may be held either with K wires or small cannulated screws often in combination with external fixation (Figure 9.15). Bone graft is frequently required to fill underlying metaphyseal defects (Figure 9.16).

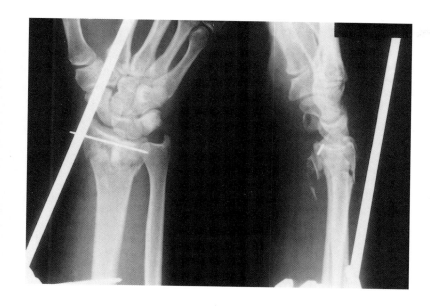

Figure 9.16

The same fracture as in Figure 9.15 with bone graft filling the defect.

The importance of regaining articular congruity in articular fractures of the distal radius is acknowledged (Knirk and Jupiter 1986), particularly to avoid post-traumatic osteoarthritis. Reported results of these techniques are remarkably good (Melone 1986, Fernandez and Geissler 1991, Seitz et al 1991, Jupiter and Lipton 1993), reflecting the skill and experience of the surgeons undertaking the procedures. These can be difficult and demanding fractures to treat and are best dealt with by those with experience of the injury.

References

Aho AJ, Nieminen SJ, Salo U, Luoma R (1984) Antebrachium fractures, *J Trauma* **24**: 604–10.

Anderson LD, Sisk D, Tooms RE, Park WI (1975) Compression plate fixation in acute diaphyseal fractures of the radius and ulna, *J Bone Joint Surg* **57A**: 287–97.

Asche G (1989) The moving fixator in the treatment of wrist fractures. Proceedings of the 13th International Conference on Hoffmann External Fixation, Rochester, p. 143.

Bartosh RA, Saldana MJ (1995) A cadaveric study to determine whether ligamentotaxis restores radiopalmar tilt in intra-articular fractures of the distal radius. In: *Fractures of the Distal Radius*, Saffar P, Cooney WP, eds, pp. 37–40. (Martin Dunitz: London).

Breit R (1983) Post-traumatic radio-ulnar synostosis, *Clin Orthop* **174**: 149–52.

Caden JG (1961) Internal fixation of fractures of the forearm, *J Bone Joint Surg* **43A**: 1115–21.

Calkins MS, Burkhalter W, Reyes F (1987) Traumatic segmental bone defects in the upper extremity. Treatment with exposed grafts of corticocancellous bone, *J Bone Joint Surg* **69A**: 19–27.

Chapman MW, Gordon JE, Zissimos AG (1989) Compression plate fixation of acute fractures of the diaphysis of the radius and ulna, *J Bone Joint Surg* **71A**: 159–69.

Cooney WP, Linscheid RL, Dobyns JH (1979) External pin fixation for unstable Colles' fractures, *J Bone Joint Surg* **61A**: 840–5.

Court-Brown CM, McQueen MM, Quaba AA, Christie J (1991) Reamed intramedullary nailing: its use in type II and III open tibial fractures, *J Bone Joint Surg* **73B**: 959–64.

De Pedro JA, Garcia-Navarrete F, Garcia de Lucas F, Otero R, Oteo A, Stern LL-D (1992) Internal fixation of ulnar fractures by locking nail, *Clin Orthop* **283**: 81–5.

Duncan R, Geissler W, Freeland AE, Savoie FH (1992) Immediate internal fixation of open fractures of the diaphysis of the forearm, *J Orthop Trauma* **6**: 25–31.

Elstrom JA, Pankovich AM, Egwele R (1978) Extra-articular low velocity gunshot fractures of the radius and ulna, *J Bone Joint Surg* **60A**: 335–41.

Fernandez DL, Geissler WB (1991) Treatment of displaced articular fractures of the radius, *J Hand Surg* **16A**: 375–84.

Fyfe IS, Mossad MM, Holdsworth BJ (1985) Methods of fixation of olecranon fractures, *J Bone Joint Surg* **67B**: 367–72.

Gartsman GM, Sculco TP, Otis JC (1981) Operative treatment of olecranon fractures, *J Bone Joint Surg* **63A**: 718–21.

Grace TG, Eversmann WW (1980a) The management of segmental bone loss associated with forearm fractures, *J Bone Joint Surg* **62A**: 1150–5.

Grace TG, Eversmann WW (1980b) Forearm fractures. Treatment by rigid fixation with early motion, *J Bone Joint Surg* **62A**: 433–8.

Grosse A, Christie J, Taglang G, Court-Brown CM, McQueen MM (1993) Open adult femoral shaft fractures treated by early intramedullary nailing, *J Bone Joint Surg* **75B**: 562–5.

Gustilo RB, Anderson JT (1976) Prevention of infection in the treatment of one thousand and twenty-five open fractures of long bones, *J Bone Joint Surg* **58A**: 453–8.

Gustilo RB, Mendoza RM, Williams DN (1984) Problems in the management of type III (severe) open fractures: a new classification of type III open fractures, *J Trauma* **24**: 742–6.

Gustilo RB, Merkow RL, Templeman D (1990) Current Concepts Review. The management of open fractures, *J Bone Joint Surg* **72A**: 299–304.

Hadden WA, Reschauer R, Seggl W (1984) Results of AO plate fixation of forearm shaft fractures in adults, *Injury* **15**: 44–52.

Hicks JH (1961) Fractures of the forearm treated by rigid fixation, *J Bone Joint Surg* **43B**: 680–7.

Hidaka S, Gustilo RB (1984) Refracture of bones of the forearm after plate removal, *J Bone Joint Surg* **66A**: 1241–3.

Holdsworth BJ, Mossad MM (1984) Elbow function following tension band fixation of displaced fractures of the olecranon, *Injury* **16**: 182–7.

Horne JG, Tanzer TL (1981) Olecranon fractures: a review of 100 cases, *J Trauma* **21**: 469–79.

Howard PN, Stewart HD, Hind RE, Burke FD (1989) External fixation or plaster for severely displaced comminuted Colles' fractures? *J Bone Joint Surg* **71B**: 68–73.

Hughston JC (1957) Fracture of the distal radial shaft: Mistakes in management, *J Bone Joint Surg* **39A**: 249–64.

Hume MC, Wiss DA (1992) Olecranon fractures. A clinical and radiographic comparison of tension band wiring and plate fixation, *Clin Orthop* **285**: 229–35.

Jensen CM, Olsen BB (1986) Drawbacks of traction absorbing wiring (TAW) in displaced fractures of the olecranon, *Injury* **17**: 174–5.

Jones JA (1991) Immediate internal fixation of high-energy open forearm fractures, *J Orthop Trauma* **5**: 272–9.

Jupiter JB, Lipton H (1993) The operative treatment of intraarticular fractures of the distal radius, *Clin Orthop* **292**: 48–61.

Keating J, Court-Brown CM, McQueen MM (1994) Internal fixation of volar-displaced distal radial fractures, *J Bone Joint Surg (Br)* **76**(3): 401–5.

Knight RA, Purvis GD (1949) Fractures of both bones of the forearm in adults, *J Bone Joint Surg* **31A**: 755–64.

Knirk JL, Jupiter JB (1986) Intra-articular fractures of the distal end of the radius in young adults, *J Bone Joint Surg* **68A**: 647–59.

Kongsholm J, Olerud C (1989) Plaster cast versus external fixation for unstable intra-articular Colles' fractures, *Clin Orthop* **241**: 57–65.

Langkamer VG, Ackroyd CE (1991) Internal fixation of forearm fractures in the 1980s: lessons to be learnt, *Injury* **22**: 97–102.

Lefèvre C, Nen D Le, Oriot O, Mathevon H, Malingue E, Courtois B (1990) L'enclouage verrouillé de l'ulna, SICOT Meeting Abstracts, Montreal, p. 65.

Macko D, Szabo RM (1985) Complications of tension band wiring of olecranon fractures, *J Bone Joint Surg* **67A**: 1396–401.

McQueen MM, MacLaren A, Chalmers J (1986) The value of remanipulating Colles' fractures, *J Bone Joint Surg* **68B**: 232–3.

McQueen MM, Michie M, Court-Brown CM (1992) Hand and wrist function after external fixation of unstable distal radial fractures, *Clin Orthop* **285**: 200–4.

McQueen MM, Hajducka C, Court-Brown CM (1996) Unstable fractures of the distal radius: a randomised comparison of four treatment methods, *J Bone Joint Surg (Br)* in press.

Melone CP (1986) Open treatment for displaced articular fractures of the distal radius, *Clin Orthop* **202**: 103–11.

Moed BR, Kellam JF, Foster RJ, Tile M, Hansen ST (1986) Immediate internal fixation of open fractures of the diaphysis of the forearm, *J Bone Joint Surg* **68A**: 1008–16.

Moore TM, Klein JP, Patzakis MJ, Harvey JP (1985) Results of compression plating of closed Galeazzi fractures, *J Bone Joint Surg* **67A**: 1015–21.

Pritchett JW (1995) External fixation or closed medullary pinning for unstable Colles fractures? *J Bone Joint Surg* **77B**: 267–9.

Rojczyk M (1984) Results of treatment of open fractures. Aspects of antibiotic therapy. In: Tscherne H, Gotzen L, eds, *Fractures with Soft Tissue Injuries*, pp. 33–8. (Springer Verlag: Berlin).

Rosson JW, Shearer JR (1991) Refracture after the removal of plates from the forearm: an avoidable complication, *J Bone Joint Surg* **73B**: 415–17.

Roumen RMH, Hesp WLEM, Bruggink EDM (1991) Unstable Colles' fractures in elderly patients. A randomised trial of external fixation for redisplacement, *J Bone Joint Surg* **73B**: 307–11.

Sage FP (1959) Medullary fixation of fractures of the forearm, *J Bone Joint Surg* **41A**: 1489–516.

Sanders RA, Keppel FL, Waldrop JI (1991) External fixation of distal radial fractures: results and complications, *J Hand Surg* **16A**: 385–91.

Sarmiento A, Kinman PB, Murphy RB, Phillips JG (1976) Treatment of ulnar fractures by functional bracing, *J Bone Joint Surg* **58A**: 1104–7.

Schmalholz A (1989) Closed rereduction of axial compression in Colles' fracture is hardly possible, *Acta Orthop Scand* **60**: 57–9.

Schuind F, Andrianne Y, Burny F (1991) Treatment of forearm fractures by Hoffmann external fixation, *Clin Orthop* **266**: 197–204.

Seitz WH, Frolmison AI, Leb R, Shapiro JD (1991) Augmented external fixation of unstable distal radius fractures, *J Hand Surg* **16A**: 1010–16.

Singer RM, Pierret G (1995) Evaluation of comminuted intra-articular distal radial fractures with computerised tomography. In: Saffar P, Cooney WP, eds, *Fractures of the Distal Radius*, pp. 143–7. (Martin Dunitz: London).

Slauterbeck JR, Britton C, Moneim MS, Clevenger F (1994) Mangled extremity severity score: an accurate guide to treatment of the severely injured upper extremity, *J Orthop Trauma* **8**: 282–5.

Smith DK, Cooney WP (1990) External fixation of high-energy upper extremity injuries, *J Orthop Trauma* **4**: 7–18.

Sommerkamp TG, Seeman M, Silliman J, Jones A, Patterson S, Walker J, Semmler M, Browne R, Ezaki M (1994) Dynamic external fixation of unstable fractures of the distal part of the radius. A prospective randomized comparison with static external fixation, *J Bone Joint Surg* **76A**: 1149–61.

Street DM (1986) Intramedullary forearm nailing, *Clin Orthop* **212**: 219–30.

Szabo RM, Skinner M (1990) Isolated ulnar shaft fracture, *Acta Orthop Scand* **61**: 350–2.

Taleisnik J, Watson HK (1984) Midcarpal instability caused by malunited fractures of the distal radius, *J Hand Surg* **9A**: 350–7.

Teasdall RR, Savoie FH, Hughes JL (1993) Comminuted fractures of the proximal radius and ulna, *Clin Orthop* **292**: 37–47.

Weber BG, Vasey H (1963) Osteosyntese bei Olecranonfraktur, *Z. Unfallmed Berufski* **2**: 90.

Weber SC, Szabo RM (1986) Severely comminuted distal radius fracture as an unsolved problem. Complications associated with external fixator and pins and plaster techniques, *J Hand Surg* **11A**: 157–65.

Zych GA, Latta LL, Zagorski JB (1987) Treatment of isolated ulnar shaft fractures with prefabricated functional fracture braces, *Clin Orthop* **219**: 194–200.

10
Open fractures of the hand

C.M. Court-Brown and G. Hooper

Open fractures of the hand have received less attention than might be expected given the relative frequency of open phalangeal fractures and the considerable morbidity and expense associated with the treatment and rehabilitation of the patients. There has been a change in the incidence of open fractures of the hand in many parts of the world in recent years due to the decline of heavy industry and the introduction of improved laws regarding industrial safety. Thus, in Edinburgh, mutilating hand injuries involving open carpal fractures and gross soft-tissue damage were not uncommon 10–15 years ago, but the decline of local heavy industry has resulted in an alteration of the incidence of open fractures of the hand with severe fractures being much less common.

Open fractures of the hand can be classified into specific fracture types.

1. Distal phalangeal fracture.
2. Proximal and middle phalangeal fractures.
3. Metacarpal fractures.
4. Soft-tissue injuries with incidental fractures.
5. Carpal fractures.
6. Mutilating hand injuries.

Fractures of the hand are relatively common. About 42% of all upper limb fractures presenting to the Edinburgh Orthopaedic Trauma Unit between 1988 and 1990 involved the hand (see Chapter 3, Table 3.2). As has already been stated, there has been a marked drop in the incidence of severe hand injuries presenting to the unit in the last 10–15 years because of the local decline in heavy industry. This has resulted in a decreased incidence of open fractures of the carpus and mutilating hand injuries. Both metacarpal and phalangeal fractures remain common but although fractures of the phalanges are associated with a relatively high incidence of open wounds, open fractures of the metacarpals are relatively unusual. The only exception to this is seen in the metacarpal heads of the ring and little fingers where impaction fractures secondary to tooth indentation following fist fights or assaults are not uncommon. These are not included in Table 3.2 (Chapter 3) and will be discussed separately in this chapter.

Comparison of the Edinburgh epidemiological data with those of other centres is difficult. The epidemiology of hand injuries is markedly affected by the local social and industrial scene as well as by the numbers and types of hospitals in the areas. In Edinburgh, the proportion of severe crush injuries is low and there are no shotgun wounds included in the data presented in Chapter 3. All the hand injuries in the city present to one unit and therefore the epidemiological data are a reflection of the overall incidence of the different types of hand injuries in the community. In other areas, where hand injuries present to a number of different hospitals, it is possible for the central teaching hospital to be presented with the more difficult injuries while peripheral hospitals receive the less complex problems. Thus the central and peripheral hospitals will deal with different types of hand injuries.

The different spectrum of injuries seen in different areas is reflected in the incidence of open metacarpal fractures. In Edinburgh, this is relatively low but in other centres open metacarpal fractures are more common. In the series of Swanson et al (1991), 34.1% of all open fractures distal to the carpus were metacarpal fractures but a review of all the causes in this series shows a relatively high incidence of gunshot wounds and crush injuries. It is likely that their epidemiological data are more representative of a specialist unit while the Edinburgh data represent that of a more general patient population. Chow et al (1991) analysed 245 open digital fractures with results that are much closer to the Edinburgh experience. In Hong Kong, they had a 6.9% incidence of open metacarpal fractures with open fractures of the proximal and middle phalanges occurring with approximately equal frequency. They found that the commonest finger to sustain an open fracture was the index (30.6%) followed by the middle (23.3%), ring (17.5%), little (17.1%) and thumb (11.4%). They also documented that 51% of open fractures were associated with significant soft-tissue damage with 12.6% of the digits having extensive soft-tissue loss. In the 125 open fractures with significant soft-tissue damage, 20 were associated with flexor tendon damage and 83 with extensor tendon injury.

Barton (1979) analysed 148 phalangeal fractures to assess the outcome of fracture management. He showed that open phalangeal fractures were associated with a poorer prognosis than closed fractures. He also detailed the relative incidence of open fractures in relation to the fracture morphology and location within the phalanx. This is shown in Table 10.1 which indicates that there is an increased incidence of open wounds in association with comminuted fractures. This is not surprising given that fracture comminution is commoner in high-energy injuries. Rotational fractures tended to have a low incidence of soft-tissue injury whereas fractures caused by bending or shearing loads were more often open.

Unlike other open fractures, there is some debate as to who should treat some of the less severe open hand fractures. Obviously there is no debate about the treatment of severe or mutilating hand injuries but there is a school of thought that apparently simple hand fractures can be treated by accident and emergency staff or general practitioners. Davis and Stothard (1990) reviewed the relative success of a British Accident and Emergency Department in treating hand injuries and showed that 27% of finger fractures were treated inappropriately. They also showed that 28% of the patients with open fractures were not prescribed antibiotics and 44% of the intra-articular fractures required secondary operative fixation or later splint adjustment. In particular, the association of nail avulsion and distal phalangeal fractures was frequently missed. There can be no doubt that all open fractures of the hand, and indeed all hand fractures in general, should be referred to a qualified orthopaedic or plastic surgeon who can deal with the condition appropriately. Open hand fractures should be admitted for surgical treatment.

The basic management of open fractures of the hand is the same as that for any other open fracture. There should be a surgical debridement in which all devitalized, dubious or contaminated tissue is removed. Not all fractures will require stabilization but the surgeon should be familiar with the internal and external fracture-fixation techniques that might be required to stabilize an unstable phalangeal fracture. Appropriate antibiotics should be administered and careful consideration given to soft-tissue closure. The vascular supply to the fingers is usually good and infection is uncommon. However, primary closure is practised too often and the basic soft-tissue management advocated in Chapter 5 should be followed.

Post-operatively, the best results are gained by early joint movement. Thus unstable fractures should be fixed so that early motion can be instituted. Non-operative management of open fractures should be reserved for distal phalangeal fractures and those open phalangeal and metacarpal fractures that have a stable configuration.

Open distal phalangeal fractures

There are a number of injuries which affect the fingertips. The commonest problems encountered are those of a closed fracture of the distal

Table 10.1 The incidence of open wounds associated with different fractures of the phalanges and metacarpals (Barton, 1979)

Fracture location	Incidence (%)
Transverse fracture (base of phalanx)	16.1
Transverse fracture (mid-shaft)	29.4
Transverse fracture (neck of phalanx)	33.3
Oblique shaft fracture	37.9
Spiral shaft fracture	9.1
Comminuted fracture (non-articular)	47.6
Comminuted fracture (articular)	55.6

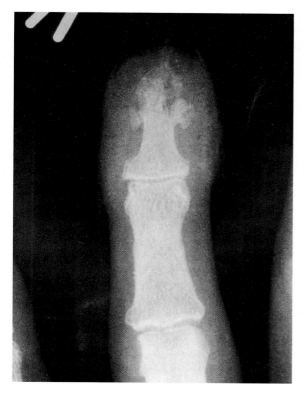

Figure 10.1

An open tuft fracture of the distal phalanx. Damage to the distal phalanx and associated soft tissues is clearly visible.

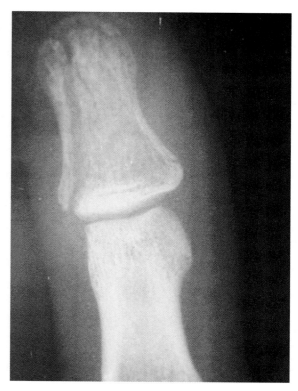

Figure 10.2

A longitudinal fracture of the distal phalanx.

phalanx or open fracture with or without nail-bed involvement. There may also be an amputation of the fingertip, this involving only soft tissue or a combination of soft tissue and bone. Treatment of the latter condition is well described in texts dealing with hand injuries (Foucher 1991, Green 1993) and many different techniques have been described to gain closure of the fingertip defect.

Open fractures of the distal phalanx are relatively common. They commonly involve the thumb or middle finger and are usually divided into tuft or shaft fractures. Tuft fractures (Figure 10.1) are usually secondary to a crushing injury and are frequently associated with an injury to the nail bed. Even in open tuft fractures there may be a subungal haematoma which can be released with a sharp sterile needle or a heated

paper clip. Distal phalangeal fractures rarely require fixation and in open fractures the surgeon should concentrate on treatment of the soft tissues. Frequently no action is required after cleansing and debridement.

If there has been extensive laceration, it is recommended that the fingertips be reconstructed with loosely applied stitches. It should be remembered that there will often be considerable post-operative swelling and the surgeon should not over-tighten the sutures that are used to reconstruct the tip of the finger. Any associated injury of the nail bed should be repaired and the detached nail can be used as a splint.

Fractures of the shaft of the distal phalanx are usually either transverse or longitudinal (Figure 10.2). Undisplaced fractures do not need fixation

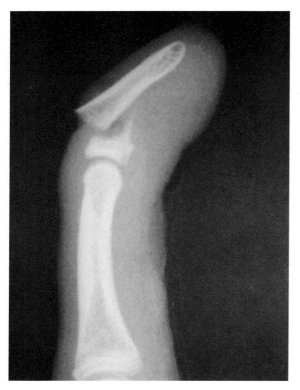

Figure 10.3

An open Salter Harris II fracture of the epiphysis of the distal phalanx. The potential for damage to the nail bed and adjacent soft tissues is obvious.

DaCruz et al (1983) emphasized the relatively poor prognosis for many distal phalangeal fractures. In a series of 110 consecutive patients with non-operatively treated distal phalangeal fractures, they documented a high incidence of fracture non-union, osteolysis, dysaesthesia, abnormal nail growth and loss of dexterity. These problems arise more frequently in fractures of the tuft than fractures of the shaft. They separated the fractures according to location and morphology and presented the results of tuft, shaft, longitudinal and basal fractures. Seventy per cent of the tuft fractures were open compared with 52.9% of the shaft fractures, 45.5% of the longitudinal fractures and 25% of the basal fractures. In general terms the prognosis was worse for the open phalangeal distal fractures than for the closed fractures. At six months a relatively large number of patients with open tuft fractures had symptoms of numbness (50%), hypoaesthesia (26%), cold sensitivity (37%), abnormal sensory distribution (34%), abnormal nail growth (56%), reduced movement (13%) and fracture non-union (29%). The figures for the other distal phalangeal fractures were not dissimilar and point to the need for surgeons to inform the patient of the relatively high morbidity that accompanies these fractures and not to give too benign a prognosis in the short term.

Other phalangeal and metacarpal fractures

After debridement, the surgeon must decide about whether the fractures of the metacarpus or proximal or middle phalanges require stabilization and if so what method is appropriate. The same methods of fixation are available for hand fractures as for any other open fractures, namely plating, external skeletal fixation, intramedullary nailing and various wiring techniques such as the use of Kirschner wires, cerclage wires, interosseus wires or a combination of these techniques. Interfragmentary screw fixation can also be used and there has been a recent interest in the use of the Herbert screw.

Although the state and handling of the soft tissues largely governs the prognosis for all open fractures, this is especially true of phalangeal

after debridement and cleansing but displaced longitudinal fractures may require fixation, this often being performed with a Kirschner wire or bone screw.

Children and adolescents may sustain open Salter type II epiphyseal separations at the base of the terminal phalanx with dislocation of the nail from the proximal nail fold (Figure 10.3). This not uncommon injury is often treated badly. After debridement of the wound the displacement must be reduced carefully and the nail replaced in the fold to maintain reduction. Failure to replace the nail, or even worse, removal of the nail renders the injury unstable and the bone may protrude through the nail bed, resulting in a troublesome infection (Seymour 1966).

that there is a considerable legacy of non-operative management combined with a paucity of good reports detailing the results of this type of treatment. As in other open fractures, open fractures of the hand have not been well classified in the various reports. Many workers have combined stable transverse phalangeal fractures with unstable comminuted fractures when examining the role of different treatment methods.

Surgeons should select the treatment method appropriate for the particular phalangeal or metacarpal fracture based on the fracture morphology and the extent of soft-tissue damage or loss but always keeping in mind that return of maximal hand function is the goal. Although a severely comminuted proximal phalangeal fracture associated with extensor tendon damage may well unite on a splint, the combined effect of malunion, joint stiffness and adhesions between the extensor mechanism and the underlying fracture may render the finger useless. Thus in unstable open fractures it is reasonable to consider operative fixation and to restrict the use of splints or traction to essentially stable fractures without significant soft-tissue damage (Reyes and Latta 1987).

If splintage is selected as a method of management, however, it is important to realize that, as with all non-operative techniques, it is a labour-intensive technique and the surgeon will have to review the patient carefully over the ensuing 2–3 weeks to ensure that there is no fracture malposition. There is a tendency to assume that non-operative management of phalangeal fractures is straightforward but this is not the case. Fitzgerald and Kahn (1984) advocated three weeks' immobilization for comminuted or long oblique fractures and a maximum of four weeks for transverse midshaft or neck fractures. They emphasized that the surgeon should not wait for radiological union before removing the splint and commencing an intensive physiotherapy regime. They documented excellent results but were not specific about the type of fractures that they treated.

Percutaneous pinning

Kirschner wires can be used in a number of ways to stabilize open phalangeal and metacarpal

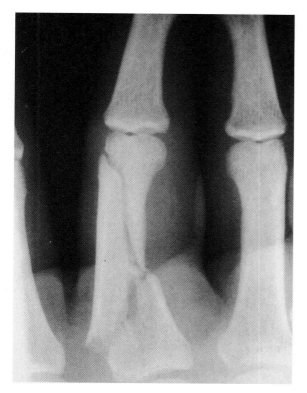

Figure 10.4

A proximal phalangeal fracture showing comminution with a large intermediate fragment. The relative instability of these fractures is demonstrated.

fractures because of the complex nature of the soft tissues and their sophisticated interaction. Barton (1979) has shown that open fractures of the phalanges have a high incidence of comminution (Figure 10.4) and in addition they may well be associated with considerable damage or division of the flexor and/or extensor tendons and neurovascular bundle. Where there is extensive bone comminution associated with tendon transection and neurovascular damage, consideration should be given to primary amputation. However, the majority of phalangeal fractures will not fall into this category and the surgeon will have to choose a method of fracture fixation.

The treatment of open phalangeal fractures mirrors the treatment of other open fractures in

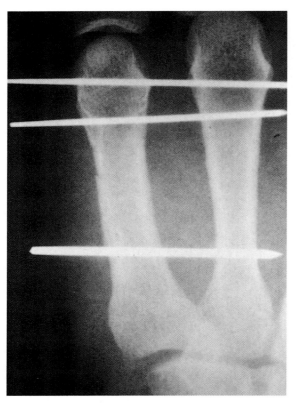

Figure 10.5

Transverse Kirschner wires to immobilize a fracture of the little finger metacarpal.

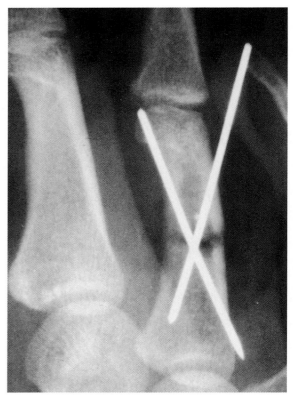

Figure 10.6

Crossed Kirschner wires can be used to immobilize transverse fractures. Care must be taken not to distract the fracture as the wires are passed as the crossed wires prevent subsequent fracture compression.

fractures. In metacarpals they can be passed transversely through the fractured bone to secure the bone to the adjacent intact metacarpals (Figure 10.5). Obviously this technique has no role in the management of open phalangeal fractures but Kirschner wires can be used as intramedullary fixation (see Figure 10.9) or they can be placed across the fracture site. If the latter technique is used it is common to use two crossed Kirschner wires to gain stability (Figure 10.6).

The superficial attractions of the use of the Kirschner wire are obvious. They are cheap and relatively easy to insert. There is little soft-tissue dissection required and they can, in theory, be used by less experienced surgeons. However, the fixation they produce is not rigid and pin loosening often occurs. The lack of rigid fixation means that external splintage may be required. One common problem particularly in the management of closed fractures is distraction of the fracture. This is less common in open fractures where direct compression of the fracture site during wire passage is possible. In addition, great care must be taken in inserting a Kirschner wire as any transcutaneous technique can fix the adjacent soft tissues rendering joint movement impossible.

The relative lack of rigidity of fixation provided by the Kirschner wire coupled with the need for external support suggests that Kirschner wiring of open phalangeal and metacarpal fractures should be restricted to transverse oblique and spiral fractures without associated comminution.

Wiring techniques

Interosseous wiring

Interosseous wiring can be used to stabilize small bone fragments in long-bone fractures (Brunner and Weber 1982). This technique can also be used for hand fractures. Gingrass et al (1980) reported the use of the technique in 51 patients who presented with 72 complex open hand fractures. They advocated the use of 30 gauge wire in comminuted fractures which they passed through drill holes on each side of the fracture. Up to eight wires could be used but on average they found two or three wires sufficient.

In transverse fractures, they recommended the use of 26 gauge wire, the wires being placed through the two cortices on either side of the bone. Where there was doubt about the rigidity of fixation, they added a supplementary Kirschner wire (Figure 10.7), this being particularly useful if there was missing bone. They had no infection in this series but did detail a number of technical problems. Overall, however, the technique was satisfactory but did require considerable attention to detail and for this reason it may not be a suitable technique in inexperienced hands. Other wiring techniques can be employed. Gropper and Bowen (1984) used cerclage wiring to immobilize 21 oblique and spiral fractures. They advocated the use of two to three lengths of 24 gauge stainless-steel wire. They allowed mobilization 10 days after surgery with unlimited use of the hand after six weeks. Seventeen of their patients had no restriction of their range of motion, the remaining four having some loss of finger movement. Although they advocated the technique for oblique spiral or comminuted fractures associated with large fracture fragments, it is probably more useful in spiral and oblique fractures where some soft-tissue stripping has already been caused by the energy associated with the production of the

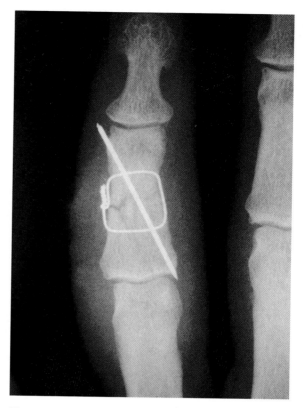

Figure 10.7

A phalangeal fracture immobilized by cerclage wiring with a supplementary Kirschner wire. This is also a useful technique in arthrodesis work.

fracture. The use of cerclage wire without pre-existing soft-tissue stripping may result in the surgeon unnecessarily mobilizing soft tissues from the bone.

Greene et al (1987) reported on the use of tension band wiring techniques in the management of unstable metacarpal and phalangeal fractures. In transverse fractures they supplement cross-Kirschner-wire stabilization with the use of a 26 or 28 gauge figure-of-eight wire loop. Oblique or spiral fractures are treated by placing a transverse Kirschner wire on each side of the fracture, these being joined by a figure-of-eight loop. They listed a number of indications for this technique, one of which was displaced open fractures, and they reported good results in the treatment of a number of patients, stating that non-union, malunion, loss of fixation, infection and tendon rupture had not occurred in over 65 fractures. However, the technique is only applicable in certain cases and is not indicated where there is bone loss or extensive comminution, both of these being commonly seen in open hand fractures.

Interfragmentary screw fixation and plating

Popularization of the use of interfragmentary screws and accompanying plating techniques by the AO group in the 1960s and 1970s quickly extended to an examination of their use in hand fractures (Figure 10.8). The technique certainly had a number of superficial attractions. Rigid internal fixation could be achieved and therefore early mobilization facilitated. Length could be restored or maintained and biomechanical testing (Vanik et al 1984) showed that dorsal plates provided excellent strength with results comparable to those of the best interosseus wire loop techniques and better than those achieved with Kirschner wires. However, there has been disquiet about AO plating of hand fractures, essentially for the same reason as has occurred in other areas of the body. Plating is the most demanding of the standard operative techniques, requiring considerable surgical skill to undertake it properly. Ill-judged soft-tissue dissection is easy and can lead to considerable morbidity. A number of orthopaedic surgeons have examined the usefulness of interfragmentary screws and plates in the management of phalangeal and metacarpal fractures. Ford et al (1987a) examined the use of interfragmentary screws in 38 phalangeal fractures selected because of fracture instability, displacement or rotation. Sixteen fractures were complicated by comminution, skin injury or damage to the extensor mechanism although the open wounds associated with these fractures tended to be fairly minor. They advocate lag screw fixation where there is marked fracture obliquity or a large interarticular fragment. Their results were good but they pointed out that the technique of

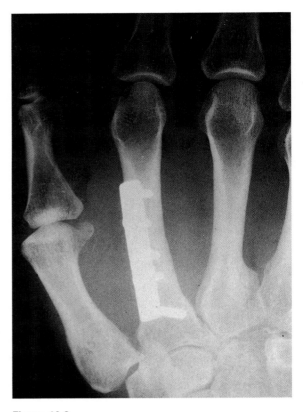

Figure 10.8

A compression plate used to immobilize a metacarpal fracture.

interfragmentary screw fixation in phalangeal fractures is demanding.

The same group, Ford et al (1987b), examined 26 fractured metacarpals treated by internal fixation using AO mini-fragment screws and plates. Nine patients had open fractures. The technique was successful in that the patients regained good function but the authors commented that patients with open fractures showed restricted mobility. Given the relative rarity of open metacarpal fractures, it is likely that the open metacarpal fractures in this series were high-energy injuries; hence the relatively poor results.

Dabezies and Schutte et al (1986) also documented the use of plates and screws in the management of metacarpal and phalangeal fractures. Again fractures were chosen because of instability. They also demonstrated good results but again stressed the need for meticulous operative techniques stating, correctly, that the surgeon could only have one attempt at placing a correct drill hole.

Pun et al (1991) carried out a similar prospective study of the management of 52 unstable fractures of the proximal and middle phalanges of the hand. Unlike the previous authors they did not report good results, stressing the relatively high incidence of implant failure, loss of fracture fixation, non-union and infection. They also compared their series to their earlier similar series of fractures treated with Kirschner wires (Pun et al 1989) and concluded that the results of plating were no better.

Stern et al (1987) have also drawn attention to the complications of using plate fixation in the hand. They documented complications in 67% of their proximal phalangeal platings and 34% of their metacarpal platings. Their overall complication rate was 42%. As with other authors, the complication rates were higher in those fractures in which there was significant soft-tissue damage.

It is interesting to observe that the literature concerned with the plating of phalangeal and metacarpal fractures is following the trend seen with plating of other long bones. There is little doubt that the difference in results between these workers reflects the choice of fractures selected for plating. Most authors have not defined their indications for the use of plating particularly well and have applied the techniques to different fracture types. Plating remains a difficult technique, although with care, good results can be achieved in some fractures. However, when the technique is applied to open fractures associated with comminution or bone loss, the results seem little better than can be achieved with other techniques. In other long bones, the trend has undoubtedly been towards the use of locked intramedullary nailing or external fixation for the management of complex open fractures.

Intramedullary nailing techniques

The usual method for intramedullary fixation of phalangeal or metacarpal fractures has already

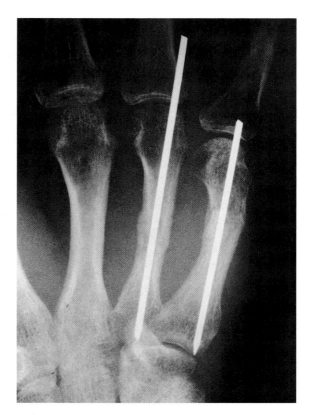

Figure 10.9

Kirschner wires used for intramedullary fixation. The wire in the ring finger is somewhat long.

been mentioned. One or more Kirschner wires can be passed into the phalanx or metacarpal to stabilize the transverse fracture (Figure 10.9). This technique has little application in the fracture configurations commonly associated with open hand injuries and it is probably only of occasional value in the management of open fractures. Other intramedullary techniques have however been described. Grundberg (1981) used an intramedullary rod in 27 fractures of which 23 were open. He estimated the size of the medullary canal with a Steinmann pin and then used a Steinmann pin one size larger to enlarge the medullary canal before passing the rod. A supplementary 30 gauge circumferential wire was used to stabilize the comminuted fragments and rotatary stability was achieved by locking the fracture fragments together as the fracture was impacted. There were no infections but one patient experienced rod migration and one other patient had a non-union which united with exchange nailing and bone grafting. The results were good, but clearly the technique would be difficult if there was extensive comminution.

The size of the hand long bones precludes the use of conventional intramedullary nailing but an experimental intramedullary metacarpal phalangeal nail has been devised (Lewis et al 1987). This is a reamed implant which consists of a fenestrated hollow metal rod which is passed into the bone in its compressed state. Once in the bone, the rod is allowed to expand by removal of a cerclage suture. Thus far there is little documentation on the usefulness of this device but it is likely to be difficult to introduce into all but the most comminuted fractures and probably achieves little hold in the residual intramedullary canals of this type of fracture. This concept of interlocking intramedullary rods or nails is, however, attractive and has proven to be successful in other long bones. Further work needs to be done in this area.

External skeletal fixation

Along with intramedullary interlocking nailing external skeletal fixation can stabilize long-bone fractures without the need for extra soft-tissue stripping (Figure 10.10). It is particularly useful in cases of segmental bone loss and where there is

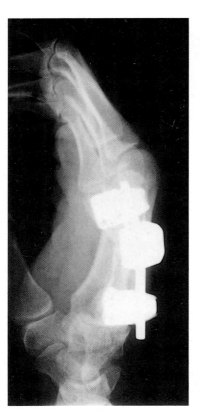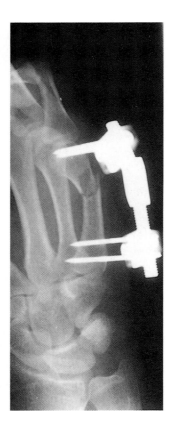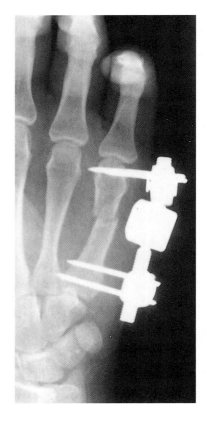

Figure 10.10

The Pennig mini-fixator used to immobilize a little finger metacarpal fracture.

extensive diaphyseal comminution. In addition, it can be used to deal with the problem of infected non-union of phalangeal or metacarpal fractures. Another theoretical advantage of external fixation is that the surrounding soft tissues can be maintained at their correct tension.

As with other types of fixation, the literature dealing with external fixation of the phalangeal and metacarpal fractures consists largely of small retrospective series. Bilos and Eskestrand (1979) used the Anderson frame in the treatment of comminuted gunshot injuries of the proximal phalanx. They used it specifically for the diaphyseal component of these fractures but did not attempt to preserve motion in the joints affected by intra-articular fractures. They documented a 25% diaphyseal non-union rate and suggested that the principal problems were infection, fracture site distraction and scarring of the extensor mechanism.

Parsons et al (1992) undertook a prospective study of 37 unstable or complex metacarpal and phalangeal fractures and stated that there was good or excellent function in 94% of the metacarpal fractures and 85% of the phalangeal fractures by nine weeks. They had no cases of non-union although they stated that delayed union occurred in 8.1%. They had minor problems with pin tract sepsis and malunion.

Shehadi (1991) used a simple frame of Kirschner wires fixed externally with polymethylmethacrylate and reported good results in 30 patients. However, this type of fixation cannot be recommended and it is suggested that if external fixation is used for phalangeal or metacarpal fractures, the basic principles of external fixation described for the tibia and other long bones be applied to the hand bones. Threaded pins should be used and, ideally, there should be two pins above and below the fracture site. Great care should be taken with pin insertion as pin tract sepsis while a nuisance in the tibia may be devastating in the finger as it may further damage the soft tissues. The fixation should be maintained until union or until it is unlikely that there will be significant incidence of malunion. There is no doubt that static external fixation in the tibia is associated with a longer time to union than dynamic external fixation. Currently, however, dynamic external fixation for metacarpal and phalangeal fractures is not possible and therefore as reported by Bilos and Eskestrand (1979) non-union may well be a problem.

As with plating, external fixation of hand fractures is a difficult technique and it is suggested that other techniques may well be easier to use in most hand fractures. However, the obvious role for external fixation in open hand fractures is where there is extensive comminution in the diaphysis or where there is significant diaphyseal bone loss. The use of external fixation under these circumstances will facilitate soft-tissue reconstruction and later bone grafting.

Prognosis of phalangeal and metacarpal fractures

Unfortunately many of the reports detailing the management of open fractures of the hand do not adequately describe the outcome of management. However, McLain et al (1991) studied 146 consecutive cases of open hand fractures in an attempt to identify factors that predicted infection and poor outcome. They had an overall incidence of infection of 11%, finding a positive correlation between the degree of soft-tissue and skeletal injury and the incidence of later infections. They used the Gustilo and Anderson (1976) classification showing that there was a 14% incidence of sepsis in the type III fractures. This rose to 20.5% in grossly contaminated wounds. They found that the functional outcome of the fractures showed a high correlation with the initial fracture type and with the presence of infection. In the 16 patients that they reported to have infected open hand fractures, only three achieved normal function. It is interesting to note that they failed to show any correlation between early debridement and infection rate, the prognosis appearing to relate to the severity of the initial injury rather than to the speed of treatment.

Swanson et al (1991) recorded a relatively high complication rate in the management of 200 open phalangeal and metacarpal fractures. They also noted that the infection rate increased in the presence of wound contamination and they did suggest that a delay of >24 hours was associated with a higher infection rate. They failed to demonstrate any association between immediate wound closure and infection rate and, in fact, recommended primary closure of relatively small wounds. These authors, however, demonstrated a relatively high incidence of malunion, non-union and fixation problems.

Suprock et al (1990) studied 91 patients with open fractures of the fingers with intact digital circulation. Alternate patients were treated with and without antibiotics but all had thorough surgical debridement and wound irrigation. Four patients in each group developed infections and it was concluded that adequate wound treatment was of greater importance than antibiotic treatment in preventing infection in open fractures of the fingers.

The fact that open fractures of the proximal and middle phalanges and the metacarpals are relatively uncommon and often associated with extensive bony and soft-tissue damage suggests that they should be treated by surgeons experienced in their management. We feel that open hand injuries should be transferred quickly to an appropriate hospital where they may receive appropriate care.

Soft-tissue injuries with incidental fractures

Articular impaction fractures

Impaction fractures of the distal articular surface of the metacarpals commonly occur after a blow to the mouth with a clenched fist. They often occur in the metacarpal heads of the ring and little fingers and are associated with damage to the extensor tendons as well as the joint capsule. The impaction fracture is obviously caused by a tooth entering the articular cartilage causing impaction of the cartilage and underlying subchondral bone. Occasionally the fracture will be more severe and Dreyfuss and Singer (1985) documented 26 cases of complete fracture associated with 106 human bites.

The problems associated with human bites have been well described (Mann et al 1977, Dreyfuss and Singer 1985) and consist of infection, articular damage and degenerative arthritis. The primary treatment is that of the soft tissues and the impaction fracture does not need any specific treatment.

Ring avulsion injuries

The other major soft-tissue injury to the finger that may be accompanied by a fracture is the avulsion injury that is commonly caused by catching a ring and thereby avulsing much or all of the soft tissues distal to the ring. In this type of injury, the presence of an open fracture is of secondary importance to the soft-tissue injury but, if present, it suggests that the overall injury has been very severe indeed. Carroll (1974) classified ring avulsion injuries into four classes depending on the extent of the injury.

Class I.   Crushing of the skin with an abrasion or bruise to the finger. Soft-tissue swelling with venous engorgement. Laceration of the skin without neurovascular tenderness impairment. Slight degree of skin avulsion.
Class II. Extensive laceration of the skin. Crushing of skin and soft tissue. Avulsion of skin with damage to one neurovascular bundle. No tendon damage. Bones and joints undamaged.
Class III. Severe crushing of skin, avulsion with laceration, damage to flexor tendons or extensor tendons or both. Damage to both neurovascular bundles.
Class IV. Crushing of skin. Damage to tendons. Loss of neurovascular bundles. Dislocation of joints. Fractures of phalanges.

Class IV injuries may be associated with open fractures of the phalanges and Carroll agrees with other authors that primary amputation is a suitable method for treating ring avulsion injuries of this severity.

Open carpal fractures

Open fractures of the carpus are rare and tend to be associated with major crushing injuries or mutilating injuries to the whole hand. One circumstance in which open fractures of the carpus may well occur is in traumatic axial dislocation of the carpus. This condition was initially described by Oberst (1901) but was well documented by Garcia-Elias et al (1989). These

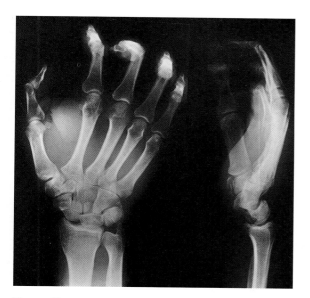

Figure 10.11

A Garcia-Elias IIb carpal dislocation. The lateral view shows the carpal instability and the open fracture of the trapezium.

authors described six common types of axial dislocation of the carpus of which three involved carpal fractures. In the 16 cases described by Garcia-Elias et al 15 had severe associated soft-tissue damage, only one patient presenting with a closed injury. An example of an open carpal fracture is shown in association with a hitherto unpublished case of traumatic axial dislocation of the carpus (Figure 10.11). This illustrates the hand of a 59-year-old man which was caught in a log splitter. He sustained a Garcia-Elias type IIb traumatic axial carpal dislocation and in addition had a fracture of the trapezium. The carpus was reduced, the reduction being held with Kirschner wires. The fracture of the trapezium was not internally fixed. He made an excellent recovery and at final discharge he had returned to full activity, the only problem being a contracture of the first web space.

The treatment of open carpal fractures is the same as for any other open fracture. Usually these uncommon fractures would be internally fixed using either Kirschner wires or a Herbert screw but the choice of fixation will vary with the morphology of the fracture. The carpal tunnel should be formally decompressed.

Mutilating hand injuries

The treatment of mutilating hand injuries will not be discussed in this chapter. These are essentially soft-tissue injuries with incidental fractures. These fractures are treated with the same methods as detailed for metacarpal and phalangeal fractures, the choice depending on the morphology of the fracture and the stage of the soft tissues. In general, the surgeon should choose the simplest method that will stabilize the bones sufficiently to allow soft-tissue reconstruction and early mobilization.

References

Barton NJ (1979) Fractures of the shafts of the phalanges of the hand, *The Hand* **11**: 119–33.

Bilos ZJ, Eskestrand T (1979) External fixator use in comminuted gunshot fractures of the proximal phalanx, *J Hand Surg* **4**: 357–9.

Brunner CF, Weber BG (1982) *Special Techniques in Internal Fixation* (Springer-Verlag: Berlin).

Carroll RE (1974) Ring injuries in the hand, *Clin Orthop* **104**: 175–82.

Chow SP, Pun WM, So YC, Luk KDC, Chiu KY, Ng KM, Ng C, Crosby C (1991) Prospective study of 245 open digital fractures of the hand, *J Hand Surg* **16B**: 137–40.

Dabezies EJ, Schutte JP (1986) Fixation of metacarpal and phalangeal fractures with miniature plates and screws, *J Hand Surg* **11A**: 283–8.

DaCruz DJ, Slade RJ, Malone W (1983) Fractures of the distal phalanges, *J Hand Surg* **13B**: 350–2.

Davis TRC, Stothard J (1990) Why all finger fractures should be referred to a hand surgery service: a prospective study of primary management, *J Hand Surg* **15B**: 299–302.

Dreyfuss UY, Singer M (1985) Human bites of the hand: a study of one hundred and six patients, *J Hand Surg* **10A**: 884–9.

Fitzgerald JAW, Khan MA (1984) The conservative management of fractures of the shafts of the phalanges of the fingers by combined traction-splintage, *J Hand Surg* **9B**: 303–6.

Ford DJ, El-Haddidi S, Lunn PG, Burke FD (1987a) Fractures of the phalanges: results of internal fixation using 1.5 mm and 2 mm AO screws, *J Hand Surg* **12B**: 28–33.

Ford DJ, El-Haddidi S, Lunn PG, Burke FD (1987b) Fractures of the metacarpals: treatment by AO screw and plate fixation, *J Hand Surg* **12B**: 34–7.

Foucher G (ed) (1991) *Fingertip and Nailbed Injuries* (Churchill Livingstone: Edinburgh).

Garcia-Elias M, Dobyns JM, Cooney WP, Linscheid RC (1989) Traumatic axial dislocations of the carpus, *J Hand Surg* **14A**: 446–57.

Gingrass RP, Femring B, Matloub M. (1980) Interosseous wiring of complex hand fractures, *Plast Reconst Surg* **66**: 383–91.

Green DP (ed) (1993) *Operative Hand Surgery* (Churchill Livingstone: New York).

Greene TL, Noellert RC, Belsole RJ (1987) Treatment of unstable metacarpal and phalangeal fractures with tension band wiring techniques, *Clin Orthop* **214**: 78–84.

Gropper PT, Bowen V (1984) Cerclage wiring of metacarpal fractures, *Clin Orthop* **88**: 203–7.

Grundberg AB (1981) Intramedullary fixation for fracture of the hand, *J Hand Surg* **6**: 568–73.

Gustilo RB, Anderson JT (1976) Prevention of infection in treatment of open fractures of long bones: retrospective and prospective analysis, *J Bone Joint Surg (Am)* **58A**: 453–8.

Lewis RC, Nordyke M, Duncan K (1987) Expandable intramedullary device for treatment of fractures in the hand, *Clin Orthop* **214**: 85–92.

McLain RF, Steyer C, Stoddard M (1991) Infection in open fractures of the hand, *J Hand Surg* **16A**: 108–12.

Mann RJ, Hoffeld TA, Baring C (1977) Human bites of the hand: 20 years of experience, *J Hand Surg* **2**: 97–104.

Oberst M (1901) Fracturen und Luxationen der Finger und des Carpus, die Fracturen des Metacarpus und der Vorderarmknochen, *Forstchr Geb Roentg* **5**: 1–21.

Parsons SW, Fitzgerald JAW, Shearer JR (1992) External fixation of unstable metacarpal and phalangeal fractures, *J Hand Surg* **17B**: 151–5.

Pun WK, Chow SP, So YC, Luk KDH, Ip FK, Chan KC, Ngai WM, Crosby C, Ng C (1989) A prospective study on 284 digital fractures of the hand, *J Hand Surg* **14A**: 474–81.

Pun WK, Chow SP, So YC, Luk KDH, Ngai WK, Ip FK, Peng WH, Ng C, Crosby C (1991) Unstable phalangeal fractures: treatment by AO screw and plate fixation, *J Hand Surg* **16A**: 113–17.

Reyes FA, Latta L (1987) Conservative management of difficult phalangeal fractures, *Clin Orthop* **214**: 23–30.

Seymour N (1966) Juxta-epiphyseal fracture of the terminal phalanx of the finger, *J Bone Joint Surg* **48B**: 347–9.

Shehadi S (1991) External fixation of metacarpal and phalangeal fractures, *J Hand Surg* **16A**: 544–50.

Stern PJ, Wieser MJ, Reilly DG (1987) Complications of plate fixation in the hand skeleton, *Clin Orthop* **214**: 59–65.

Suprock MD, Hood JM, Lubahn JD (1990) Role of antibiotics in open fractures of the fingers, *J Hand Surg* **15A**: 761–4.

Swanson TV, Szabo RM, Anderson DD (1991) Open hand fractures: progress and classification, *J Hand Surg* **16A**: 101–7.

Vanik RK, Weber RC, Matloub MS, Sanger JR, Gingrass RP (1984) The comparative strengths of internal fixation techniques, *J Hand Surg* **9a**: 216–21.

11

Open fractures of the foot

M.M. McQueen

Foot injuries are some of the most challenging cases encountered by the orthopaedic traumatologist. Bony reconstruction is difficult because of comminution and the complex nature of foot anatomy. The soft tissues are often the final determinant of outcome and preservation of the specialized tissues on the sole of the foot is crucial. It is mostly upon the foot that a stable normal pain-free gait allowing normal physical, economic and social function depends. Open fractures of the foot can result in significant disability, even leading to amputation, and optimum management is of prime importance.

Epidemiology

In a five-year period from January 1988 to December 1992 65 patients were treated in the Edinburgh Orthopaedic Trauma Unit for open fractures of the foot. Fifty-five (85%) were male and 10 (15%) were female with an average age of 37 years, ranging from 16 to 83 years.

There were 32 open fractures of the toes. During this time, 398 fractures of the toe phalanges were treated, giving an incidence of open fractures of 8%. Thirty-one of these patients were male with an average age of 38 years. Half the fractures occurred as a result of a crushing injury, seven (22%) in a road traffic accident, five (15.5%) due to a laceration often from a rotary mower and four (12.5%) due to falls. Ten of the open toe wounds were Gustilo type I (Gustilo and Anderson 1976) and 18 were Gustilo type II. There were two type IIIa wounds (Gustilo et al 1984), one IIIb and one IIIc injury (Figure 11.1) which resulted in amputation. The rest all healed by secondary closure or granulation except one which required split-skin grafting.

Nine open metatarsal fractures were treated during this period within a total of 982 metatarsal fractures, giving an overall incidence of 0.9% of open metatarsal fractures. The average age of the patients was 33 years and seven of the nine were male. Four of the fractures were caused by crushing injuries, three by road traffic accidents,

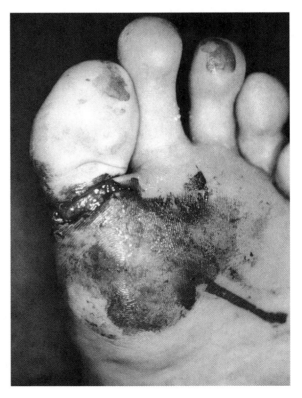

Figure 11.1

A Gustilo type IIIc open fracture of the great toe. The toe was ischaemic and was amputated.

one by an assault and one by a laceration. The majority were Gustilo type II (44%) or III (44%) with only one Gustilo type I injury. Two of the type III open wounds were IIIa and two type IIIb. There were no type IIIc open metatarsal injuries. None required plastic surgery.

Open fractures of the talus are uncommon, with only three being treated during the five-year period. A total of 44 talar fractures were treated during the same period, giving an incidence of 6.8% of open talar fractures. All patients were male with an average age of 33 years. Two fractures were caused by road traffic accidents and one by a crushing injury. There was one Gustilo type II and two type IIIa injuries, one of which required split-skin grafting to achieve soft-tissue cover.

Other authors have reported on the incidence of open talar fractures. In Hawkins' classic paper in 1970, he reported on 57 talar neck fractures, 12 (21%) of which were open. Seventeen of Canale and Kelly's (1978) series of 71 (25%) talar fractures were open. Twenty-one of 85 patients (25%) of Szyszkowitz et al's series (1985) were open, all but two being type II or III soft-tissue injuries. The severity of bone injury was generally matched by the severity of the soft-tissue injury.

Of the 12 open calcaneal fractures, the average age of the patients was 36 years and the majority (67%) were male. Half of the fractures were caused by a fall from a height, four by a road traffic accident, one by a direct blow and one by a crushing injury. There were no Gustilo type I injuries but four type II injuries and eight type III injuries, five being type IIIa and three being type IIIb. Four of the type IIIb injuries required plastic surgery, with three split-skin grafts and one pedicle flap.

The remaining nine tarsal fractures were all severe injuries to more than one of the tarsal bones. Six of the patients were male and three were female, and their average age was 36 years. Five fractures were caused by a road traffic accident, three by a fall from a height and one by a crushing injury. Two were Gustilo type II injuries and the remaining seven were type III injuries, two being IIIa, four IIIb and one IIIc. Plastic surgery was required for four, with two split-skin grafts, one fascio-cutaneous flap and one wound being covered by defatted local skin. The type IIIc injury required amputation.

Overall, open fractures of the foot generally occur in young males due to high-energy injury and result in relatively severe soft-tissue injury but a fairly low requirement for plastic surgery.

Management of the soft tissues

The management of the soft-tissue injury associated with open foot fractures is of prime importance since the integrity of the soft-tissue envelope has a major influence on the outcome of the bone injury and on functional outcome for the patient. In the foot, the heel pad is of particular importance because of its specialized nature and the importance of its sensation.

Open fractures of the foot should be treated in the same manner as open fractures elsewhere in the body. Immediate and aggressive debridement should be carried out, excising all dead and contaminated tissues, including devascularized bone. This may require surgical extension of the open wound to allow adequate exposure. Copious irrigation and antibiotic therapy are important adjuncts to an aggressive debridement (Gustilo et al 1990). The wound should then be left open and a 'second look' procedure performed 24–48 hours later. Further debridement should be carried out as necessary and the wound closed secondarily or covered with split skin or a flap when the excision is deemed complete, preferably within five days.

In open fractures with significant loss of the heel pad several points should be considered. Firstly, normal sensation is important to prevent ulceration, and secondly, damage to the weight-bearing area causes loss of shock-absorbing qualities during walking. Because of this, some authors recommend very careful consideration of below-knee amputation for these very severe injuries (Levin and Nunley 1993). In this respect, the use of the MESS (Mangled Extremity Severity Score) can predict the need for amputation following lower extremity trauma (Johansen et al 1990) although this system was based mainly on severe long bone injury.

Open foot fractures can be complicated by acute compartment syndromes and it is dangerous to assume that the open wound will decompress all the foot compartments, which have been shown to be multiple and complex (Manoli and Weber 1990). Open foot fractures may be particularly at risk because so many are crushing or high-energy injuries. Calcaneal fractures and metatarsal fractures seem to be most at risk (Manoli and Weber 1990, Sherreff 1990). Awareness of the possibility of acute compartment syndrome resulting in prompt decompression will reduce the morbidity of these severe injuries.

Management of the bone injury

Calcaneus

Treatment of fractures of the calcaneus remains a controversial subject, particularly in open fractures, which tend to be severe intra-articular injuries.

The calcaneal fracture not involving the subtalar joint or the undisplaced intra-articular fracture is usually not difficult to treat. There is little dispute that these are well treated by initial elevation followed by non-weight-bearing mobilization for 8–12 weeks (Essex-Lopresti 1951, Giachino and Whithoff 1989). The outcome of these fractures is usually excellent (Essex-Lopresti 1951). The only exception is the displaced 'beak' type of fracture of the tuberosity which should be treated by open reduction and internal fixation.

Displaced intra-articular fractures remain a therapeutic challenge and a source of considerable dispute. Since the majority of open calcaneal fractures fall into this category, it is on these injuries that this chapter will concentrate.

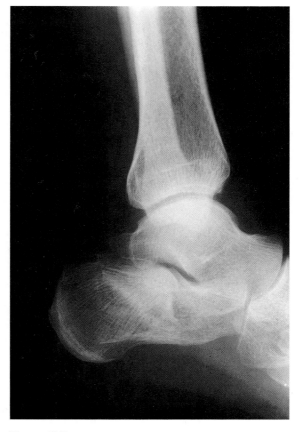

Figure 11.2

A lateral view of a depressed calcaneal fracture showing a decrease in Bohler's angle and an increase in Gissane's angle. This is a joint-depression type of calcaneal fracture.

Assessment

Initial basic assessment of the calcaneal fracture is by plain radiographs with a lateral view of the hind foot, an anteroposterior view of the foot and an axial view of the heel. The lateral view is the most useful, confirming a fracture of the calcaneus and, if present, demonstrating a loss of height of the posterior facet, a decrease in Bohler's angle and an increase in the critical angle of Gissane (Figure 11.2). The lateral view also allows classification into a joint depression or tongue type of fracture (Essex-Lopresti 1951).

The anteroposterior view adds very little whilst the axial view usually demonstrates any loss of height or increase in width. The axial view can allow visualization of the joint surface although it is a difficult view to obtain in the acutely injured foot.

A further useful view to image the subtalar joint is Broden's view (Broden 1949). Koval and Sanders (1993) give a clear description of the method of obtaining Broden's view and recommend this method of imaging when computed tomography (CT) scanning is not available. The advent of CT scanning has revolutionized our understanding and management of calcaneal fractures particularly in the improved visualization

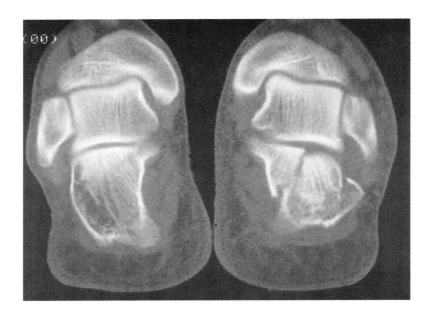

Figure 11.3

A coronal CT scan of a calcaneal fracture.

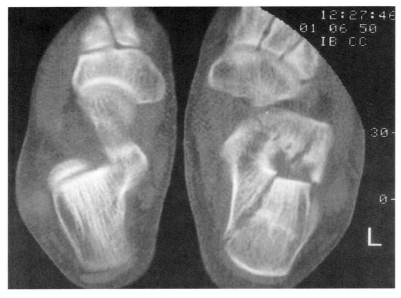

Figure 11.4

A transverse CT scan of a calcaneal fracture.

of the fracture patterns and selection of cases for surgery. Nevertheless, good visualization by plain radiographs is essential in the open fracture since the necessary delay to obtain a CT scan may be contraindicated.

Computed tomography scanning is performed in two planes: coronal (Figure 11.3) and trans-verse (Figure 11.4). The coronal scan gives infor-mation about the state of the posterior facet, the sustentaculum tali, the shape of the heel and the position of the surrounding tendons. The trans-verse scan allows assessment of the calca-neocuboid joint, the sustentaculum tali and the lateral wall.

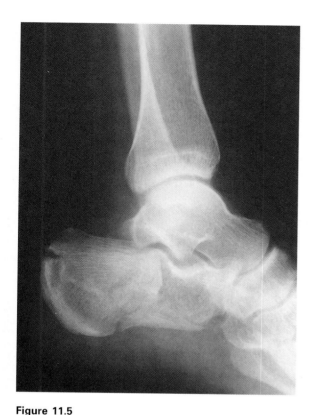

Figure 11.5

A tongue type of calcaneal fracture.

Classification of the calcaneal fracture is now centred on the CT scan, although Essex-Lopresti's classification (1951) is still in widespread clinical use. He described two types of intra-articular fractures of the calcaneus. Both have a primary fracture line which results from the angle of the talus being 'driven like an axe' into the crucial angle. In Essex-Lopresti's tongue type of fracture, the secondary fracture line then runs straight backwards to the posterior border of the tuberosity (Figure 11.5). In his joint-depression type, the secondary fracture line runs vertically across the body (Figure 11.2).

Classification systems based on CT scans concentrate on the amount of damage to the subtalar joint (Crosby and Fitzgibbons 1990, 1993, Sanders et al 1993) to aid in prognosis and

choice of treatment, or on the lateral wall composition and orientations of fragments to aid operative reduction (Eastwood et al 1993).

Closed treatment

Closed treatment varies between acceptance of the initial deformity with or without early mobilization and closed reduction techniques and percutaneous fixation. The former method is at odds with the modern principles of fracture treatment in that these are intra-articular fractures. Pozo and his colleagues (1984) reported on a long-term follow-up of patients with comminuted intra-articular calcaneal fractures treated without reduction and with early active motion and found approximately 25% of patients with significant restrictions in terms of pain and inability to run or walk without restriction on flat ground. All the feet were an abnormal shape. He considered that 20% had poor results. Nade and Monahan (1972) reviewed 101 calcaneal fractures treated by plaster immobilization of which one-third were severe intra-articular fractures. Two-thirds of these injuries had persistent pain and over half had stiffness and weakness; 52% were unable to stand on tiptoe, 67% unable to walk on uneven ground and 36% unable to climb ladders.

Kitaoka et al (1994) studied the gait patterns of 27 patients who had had displaced intra-articular calcaneal fractures treated non-operatively. Seventeen patients had fair or poor results and most patients had gait abnormality showing persistent functional impairment.

Closed reduction techniques rarely obtain accurate reduction of displaced intra-articular calcaneal fractures. Essex-Lopresti (1951) is credited with popularizing the technique of closed reduction with a Gissane spike and a clear description of the technique appears in his article. It is often not appreciated that he recommended open reduction of the subtalar joint in his joint-depression type and indeed states that 'no amount of pulling, pounding, force or manipulation of the os calcis from outside would elevate it into its proper position'. He urges reduction by one of his two techniques in patients under the age of 50 years but concludes that an exact reposition is necessary.

Operative treatment

Many authors consider that displaced intra-articular fractures of the calcaneus can only be
accurately aligned by open reduction (Essex-
Lopresti 1951, Giachino and Whithoff 1989,
Letournel 1993). The lateral approach is used by
many authors (Palmer 1948, Essex-Lopresti 1951,
Eastwood et al 1993, Fernandez and Koella 1993,
Leung et al 1993, Sanders et al 1993, Zwipp et al
1993, Soeur and Remy 1995). The main principles of this approach are dissection down to
bone and elevation of an intact flap to prevent
problems of skin necrosis and mobilization of the
peroneal tendons with an intact sheath to
prevent peroneal tendonitis. The lateral wall is
opened gently with a lever to expose the
depressed talar fragment which is elevated and
held temporarily with Kirschner (K) wires. The
body is then reduced and the fracture held with
lag screws and a plate.

The use of bone graft is controversial, with
some authors feeling bone graft is unnecessary
(Sanders et al 1993, Eastwood et al 1993). In
some cases, a defect is apparent in the calcaneum and provided an accurate reduction is
confirmed may be managed by bone grafting to
increase the stability of fixation.

Although some authors recommend approaching these fractures from the medial side
(McReynolds 1982, Burdeaux 1993), access to the
subtalar displacement is more difficult and the
advent of CT scanning has shown that the main
fragment of the tuberosity is displaced laterally.
Occasionally, a combined approach is required
to achieve reduction (Fernandez and Koella
1993). Although in open fractures the site of the
open wound may influence the choice of
approach it is probably best to use the lateral
approach supplemented occasionally by a
medial approach when required for an accurate
reduction.

The reported outcome of open reduction and
internal fixation is generally favourable (Soeur
and Remy 1975, Leung et al 1993, Sanders et al
1993, Zwipp et al 1993, Fernandez and Koella
1993, Bèzes et al 1993) although most authors
recognize the limitations imposed by the severity
of the original damage to the subtalar joint and
the importance of accurate operative reduction.
These factors led Sanders and his colleagues to
recommend early subtalar arthrodesis for their

type IV injury in which CT scan reveals a high
degree of comminution of the subtalar joint. They
also demonstrate a clear 'learning curve' in this
surgery and recommended two years of experience before the outcome can be predicted. As in
many open fractures, open fractures of the calcaneus are complex injuries which require specialist treatment.

Comparative studies of operative and non-
operative management are rare. Leung and his
colleagues (1993) found significantly better
results in their operated group in terms of pain,
activity, range of movement and return to work
using stable internal fixation and bone grafting:
91% of their operated group were rated as excellent or good compared to 53% of their non-
operated group. Parmar et al (1993) reported on
a prospective randomized study of 56 patients
treated either by surgery or non-operatively.
Surgery was by open reduction and K-wire
fixation of the subtalar joint. No attempt was
made to reduce the tuberosity or to achieve rigid
internal fixation. A plaster cast was used postoperatively. The authors found no significant differences in outcome between the two groups but
their operative protocol would not be recommended by most authorities.

The complications related to surgery are
usually due to wound necrosis, infection or sural
nerve problems and range from 5% to 22%
(Soeur and Remy 1975, Leung et al 1993,
Fernandez and Koella 1993, Sanders et al 1993,
Zwipp et al 1993).

Arthrodesis

Arthrodesis should be considered when CT scan
shows extensive comminution and severe
displacement of the subtalar joint such that it is
not amenable to reduction and fixation (Sanders
et al 1993). If performed early it is essential to
reconstitute the normal shape of the calcaneus
simultaneously. Arthrodesis should be limited to
the subtalar joint unless the scan shows
evidence of significant calcaneocuboid derange-
ment. Substantial numbers of good or excellent
results have been reported for arthrodesis (Zayer
1969, Thompson 1973, Noble and McQuillan
1979) bearing in mind that these are salvage
procedures.

Fractures of the talus

Open fractures of the talus are rare injuries but when they do occur the talar fracture is generally displaced because of the high energy required to produce this injury. Hawkins (1970) classified talar neck fractures into three groups: Group 1 is an undisplaced vertical fracture of the neck of the talus; Group 2 is a displaced fracture with a subluxed or dislocated subtalar joint but a normal ankle joint; Group 3 occurs when the body of the talus is dislocated from both the ankle and subtalar joint (Figure 11.6). Other authors (Szyszkowitz et al 1985), although preserving Hawkins' basic classification, widened it to include peripheral fractures and body fractures. The majority of the open fractures in Szyszkowitz's series were Hawkins Group 3

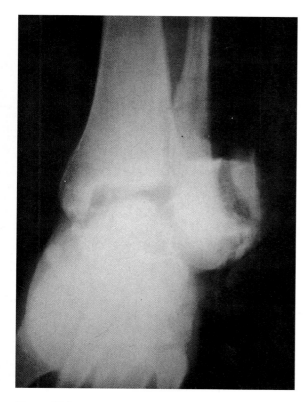

Figure 11.6

A Hawkins Group 3 talar fracture.

fractures and it is therefore on the management and outcome of these severe injuries that this chapter will concentrate.

Management

The anatomy of the talus and its blood supply has a crucial role in the management of talar fractures; 60% of the talar surface is covered by articular cartilage and therefore the majority of fractures are intra-articular. The talus is supplied by three main arteries. The head is supplied by the dorsalis pedis artery and one of its branches, the artery of the tarsal sinus. The body is supplied by the artery of the tarsal canal from which branches course posterolaterally into the body. The body is also supplied by deltoid branches entering medially. A few periosteal branches from the posterior tibial artery enter the posterior tubercle. A displaced fracture will therefore separate the posterior fragment from its blood supply since the posterior periosteal vessels are usually insufficient to supply the whole fragment. This also illustrates the importance of preserving the deltoid ligament and its vessels since they may be the only surviving blood supply to the proximal fragment.

Because of the high incidence of intra-articular fractures and the need to stabilize the fracture to allow the maximum chance for recovery of the bone blood supply it is now acknowledged by most authors that open reduction and internal fixation is the treatment of choice (Penny and Davis 1980, Santavirta et al 1984, Szyszkowitz et al 1985, Comfort et al 1985). Although the approach is influenced by the site of the open wound, in general the anteromedial approach gives the best exposure and allows osteotomy of the medial malleolus if required to increase the exposure. A posterior medial approach parallel to the Achilles tendon may be used if the anterior skin is poor or if entrapment of the tibialis posterior tendon is suspected. Care must be taken to preserve the neurovascular bundle which is often found immediately deep to the skin. After reduction and temporary fixation are confirmed radiologically, definitive fixation with screws may be performed either anterior to posterior or vice versa. Postoperatively, a below-knee cast is applied and weight-bearing is protected either until union occurs or the risk of avascular necrosis diminishes.

Arthrodesis of the ankle can be performed either primarily where the injury to the bone and soft tissues is unreconstructible or secondarily in either the ankle or subtalar joint when disabling posttraumatic arthritis intervenes. Loss of the body of the talus can be treated by tibiotalar arthrodesis (Dennis and Tullos 1980). Despite Gunal et al's (1993) good results, talectomy must be considered a salvage procedure. Amputation is occasionally required for the very severe open fracture of the talus.

Outcome

The prognosis for open talar fractures must be guarded since these are usually high-energy injuries and displaced fractures. Avascular necrosis is the most formidable complication and increases in incidence with increasing fracture severity. Hawkins (1970) considered avascular necrosis to be almost inevitable in Group 3 fractures, with 91% resulting in this complication. Difficulty is encountered in predicting the likelihood of avascular necrosis in the Group 2 fractures, in which Hawkins recorded a 42% incidence. Other authors report varying incidences of avascular necrosis ranging from 17% to 50% in Hawkins Group 2 fractures and from 50% to 100% in Group 3 fractures (Canale and Kelly 1978, Penny and Davis 1980, Grob et al 1985). Open fractures do not appear to have a higher incidence of avascular necrosis than closed fractures (Canale and Kelly 1978). There is some evidence, however, that lower incidences may be expected with open reduction which achieves perfect alignment and rigid fixation (Szyszkowitz et al 1985).

The second disabling complication of open talar fractures is posttraumatic osteoarthritis which can occur in either the ankle or subtalar joint. Malunion, avascular necrosis and high-energy injury all predispose the patient to this complication and fusion of the ankle or subtalar joint is required in 10–45% of patients (Canale and Kelly 1978, Penny and Davis 1980, Santavirta et al 1984, Szyszkowitz et al 1985). It is of utmost importance in these patients to differentiate between ankle and subtalar arthritis as fusing the subtalar joint with a degenerate ankle or vice versa will cause significant progression of degeneration in the unfused joint.

Infection after open fracture of the talus is poorly reported in the available literature. Canale and Kelly (1978) reported five deep infections in 53 Hawkins Group 2 and 3 fractures. Four of these occurred in the total of 17 open fractures in this series. All required fusion. Occasionally, reconstructive procedures after sepsis are unsuccessful and secondary amputation is necessary (Penny and Davis 1980).

Most authors do not discuss union rates of talar fractures. Kenwright and Taylor (1970) reported no non-unions in their severe cases treated by a mixture of closed reduction and open reduction and K-wire fixation. In contrast, Penny and Davis (1980) found non-union to occur in 14% of their Hawkins Group 2 and 17% of their Hawkins Group 3 injuries, again treated by various methods.

Functional outcome is usually assessed on a combination of pain level, gait abnormality and range of movement in the ankle and subtalar joint. It is generally agreed that functional ability at review deteriorates with increasing fracture class, avascular necrosis and inadequacy of reduction (Hawkins 1970, Canale and Kelly 1978, Penny and Davis 1980, Santavirta et al 1984, Szyszkowitz et al 1985, Comfort et al 1985).

Forefoot

Severe open injury of the forefoot is usually caused by machinery of some type, and in particular rotary mowers. The principles of management of open fractures elsewhere in the body should be applied to open fractures of the forefoot with special attention to a thorough and aggressive debridement.

Lawnmower injury is a particularly severe soft-tissue and bone injury to the foot. The majority of the open fractures occur in the metatarsals or toe phalanges and these with the associated severe soft-tissue injury result in a high rate of amputation. Meticulous attention to the soft-tissue injury results in a low infection rate despite a high level of initial contamination of these injuries (Anger et al 1995).

The commonest open injury in the forefoot is to the phalanges of the toes. Internal fixation is

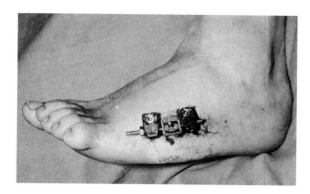

Figure 11.7

External fixation of a fifth metatarsal fracture.

rarely indicated in this situation especially in the lesser toes. Even where articular involvement is evident the small sizes of fragments make internal fixation impossible. Occasionally in fracture of the great toe, the fragments may be large enough to allow internal fixation of articular fragments. Amputation of all or part of a toe may be required when soft-tissue or bony injury is not reconstructible or in Gustilo type IIIc open injuries (Figure 11.1).

Displaced open fractures of the metatarsals are less common than those of the toes but, conversely, are more likely to require fixation. Sherreff (1990) recommends reduction of a metatarsal fracture with >3–4 mm of displacement or >10° of angulation. In open fractures with displacement, fixation should use K wires, screw fixation or external fixation (Figure 11.7) depending on the fracture configuration and soft-tissue injury.

Tarsometatarsal dislocation or fracture dislocation is a severe injury to the forefoot and is commonly open, being reported in seven of 40 cases (18%) of Arntz and his co-authors' series (1988) and six of 66 (9%) of Vuori and Aro's (1993) patients. In the past there was general agreement that reduction of these severe injuries should be anatomical but disagreement on whether reduction should be closed or open (Gissane 1951, Aitken and Poulson 1963, English

1964, Hardcastle et al 1982). Clearly, with open fractures, open reduction should be performed at the time of debridement. Internal fixation is usually achieved with K wires. Arntz et al (1988) believe that K wires caused multiple problems including migration of pins, pin track infections and loss of reduction. They reported excellent maintenance of position using AO screw fixation. Fair or poor results occurred in patients with open injuries or inadequate reduction.

Open fractures of other tarsal bones are rare. The general principles of treatment of fractures should be applied to these injuries, with internal fixation being used for intra-articular fractures (Sangeorzan et al 1989, Sangeorzan and Swiontkowski 1990, Nyska et al 1989). In cases with severe comminution, bone grafting may be required (Sangeorzan and Swiontkowski 1990).

Although the reported results only include a limited number of patients, it appears that functional results are best with the use of open reduction and internal fixation with or without bone grafting rather than closed treatment or primary arthrodesis (Nyska et al 1989, Sangeorzan and Swiontkowski 1990).

References

Aitken AP, Poulson D (1963) Dislocations of the tarsometatarsal joint, *J Bone Joint Surg* **45A**: 246–60.

Anger DM, Ledbetter BR, Stasikelis P, Calhoun JH (1995) Injuries of the foot related to the use of lawnmowers, *J Bone Joint Surg* **77A**: 719–25.

Arntz CT, Veith RG, Hansen ST (1988) Fractures and fracture-dislocations of the tarso-metatarsal joint, *J Bone Joint Surg* **70A**: 173–81.

Bèzes H, Massart P, Delvaux D, Fourquet JP, Tazi F (1993) The operative treatment of intraarticular calcaneal fractures, *Clin Orthop* **290**: 55–9.

Broden B (1949) Roentgen examination in subtalar joint in fractures of the calcaneus, *Acta Radiol* **31**: 85.

Burdeaux B (1993) The medial approach for calcaneal fractures, *Clin Orthop* **290**: 96–107.

Canale ST, Kelly FB (1978) Fractures of the neck of the talus, *J Bone Joint Surg* **60A**: 143–56.

Comfort TH, Behrens F, Garther DW, Denis F, Sigmond M (1985) Long term results of displaced talar neck fractures, *Clin Orthop* **199**: 81–7.

Crosby LA, Fitzgibbons T (1990) Computerised tomography scanning of acute intraarticular fractures of the calcaneus—a new classification system, *J Bone Joint Surg* **72A**: 852–9.

Crosby LA, Fitzgibbons T (1993) Intraarticular calcaneal fractures. Results of closed treatment, *Clin Orthop* **290**: 47–53.

Dennis MO, Tullos HS (1980) Blair tibiotalar arthrodesis for injuries to the talus, *J Bone Joint Surg* **62A**: 103–7.

Eastwood DM, Gregg PJ, Atkins RM (1993) Intra-articular fractures of the calcaneum. Part 1: Pathological anatomy and classification, *J Bone Joint Surg* **75B**: 183–8.

English TA (1964) Dislocations of the metatarsal bone and adjacent toe, *J Bone Joint Surg* **46B**: 700–4.

Essex-Lopresti P (1951) The mechanism, reduction technique and results in fractures of the os calcis, *Br J Surg* **39**: 395–419.

Fernandez DL, Koella C (1993) Combined percutaneous and minimal internal fixation for displaced articular fractures of the calcaneus, *Clin Orthop* **290**: 108–16.

Giachino AA, Whithoff HK (1989) Current concepts review. Intra-articular fractures of the calcaneus, *J Bone Joint Surg* **71A**: 784–7.

Gissane W (1951) A dangerous type of fracture of the foot, *J Bone Joint Surg* **33B**: 535–8.

Grob D, Simpson LA, Weber BG, Bray T (1985) Operative treatment of displaced talus fractures, *Clin Orthop* **199**: 88–96.

Gunal I, Athela S, Arac S, Gursoy Y, Karagoylu H (1993) A new technique of talectomy for severe fracture dislocations of the talus, *J Bone Joint Surg* **75B**: 69–71.

Gustilo RB, Anderson JT (1976) Prevention of infection in the treatment of one thousand and twenty-five fractures of long bones: retrospective and prospective analyses, *J Bone Joint Surg* **58A**: 453–8.

Gustilo RB, Mendoz RM, Williams DN (1984) Problems in the management of type III (severe) open fractures: a new classification of type III open fractures, *J Trauma* **24**: 742–6.

Gustilo RB, Merkow RL, Templeman D (1990) Current concepts review. The management of open fractures, *J Bone Joint Surg* **72A**: 299–304.

Hardcastle PH, Reschauer R, Kutcsher-Lissberg E, Schoffman W (1982) Injuries to the tarsometatarsal joint. Incidence, classification and treatment, *J Bone Joint Surg* **64B**: 349–56.

Hawkins LG (1970) Fractures of the neck of the talus, *J Bone Joint Surg* **52A**: 901–1002.

Johansen K, Daines M, Howley T, Helfet D, Hansen ST (1990) Objective criteria accurately predict amputation following lower extremity trauma, *J Trauma* **30**: 568–73.

Kenwright J, Taylor RG (1970) Major injuries of the talus, *J Bone Joint Surg* **52B**: 36–48.

Kitakoa H, Schaap EJ, Cuao EJ, An K (1994) Displaced intraarticular fractures of the calcaneus treated nonoperatively, *J Bone Joint Surg* **76A**: 1531–40.

Koval KJ, Sanders R (1993) The radiologic evaluation of calcaneal fractures, *Clin Orthop* **290**: 41–6.

Letournel E (1993) Open treatment of acute calcaneal fractures, *Clin Orthop* **290**: 60–7.

Leung KS, Yuen KM, Chan WS (1993) Operative treatment of displaced intraarticular fractures of the calcaneum, *J Bone Joint Surg* **75B**: 196–201.

Levin LS, Nunley JA (1993) The management of soft tissue problems associated with calcaneal fractures, *Clin Orthop* **290**: 151–6.

Manoli A, Weber TG (1990) Fasciotomy of the foot: an anatomical study with special reference to release of the calcaneal compartment, *Foot Ankle* **10**: 267–75.

McReynolds IS (1982) The case for operative treatment of fractures of the os calcis. In: Leach RE, Hoaglund FT, Riseborough EJ, eds, *Controversies in Orthopaedic Surgery*, pp. 232–54 (Philadelphia: WB Saunders).

Nade S, Monahan PRW (1972) Fractures of the calcaneum: a study of the long-term prognosis, *Injury* **4**: 200–7.

Noble J, McQuillan WM (1979) Early posterior subtalar fusion in the treatment of fractures of the os calcis, *J Bone Joint Surg* **61B**: 90–3.

Nyska N, Margulies JY, Barbarawi M, Muschler W, Dekel S, Segal D (1989) Fractures of the body of the tarsal navicular bone: case reports and literature review, *J Trauma* **29**: 1448–51.

Palmer L (1948) The mechanism and treatment of fractures of the calcaneus, *J Bone Joint Surg* **30A**: 2–8.

Parmar HV, Triffitt PD, Gregg PJ (1993) Intraarticular fractures of the calcaneum treated operatively or conservatively. A prospective study, *J Bone Joint Surg* **75B**: 932–7.

Penny JN, Davis LA (1980) Fractures and fracture-dislocations of the neck of the talus, *J Trauma* **20**: 1029–37.

Pozo JL, Kirwan EOG, Jackson AM (1984) The long-term results of conservative management of severely displaced fractures of the calcaneus, *J Bone Joint Surg* **66B**: 386–90.

Sanders R, Fortin P, DiPasquale T, Walling A (1993) Operative treatment in 120 displaced intraarticular calcaneal fractures, *Clin Orthop* **290**: 87–95.

Sangeorzan BJ, Swiontkowski MF (1990) Displaced fractures of the cuboid, *J Bone Joint Surg* **72B**: 376–8.

Sangeorzan BJ, Benirschke SK, Mosca V, Mayo KA, Hansen ST (1989) Displaced intra-articular fractures of the tarsal navicular, *J Bone Joint Surg* **71A**: 1504–10.

Santavirta S, Seitsalo S, Kiviluoto O, Myllynen P (1984) Fractures of the talus, *J Trauma* **24**: 986–9.

Sherreff MJ (1990) Fractures of the forefoot, *Instr Course Lect* **39**: 133–40.

Soeur R, Remy R (1975) Fractures of the calcaneus with displacement of the thalamic portion, *J Bone Joint Surg* **57B**: 413–21.

Szyszkowitz R, Reschauer R, Seggl W (1985) Eighty-five talus fractures treated by ORIF with five to eight years of follow-up study of 69 patients, *Clin Orthop* **199**: 97–107.

Thompson KR (1973) Treatment of comminuted fractures of the calcaneus by triple arthrodesis, *Orthop Clin N Am* **4**: 189–91.

Vuori J-P, Aro HT (1993) Lisfranc joint injuries: trauma mechanisms and associated injuries, *J Trauma* **35**: 40–5.

Zayer M (1969) Fractures of the calcaneus, *Acta Orthop Scand* **40**: 530–42.

Zwipp H, Tscherne H, Thermann H, Weber T (1993) Osteosynthesis of displaced intraarticular fractures of the calcaneus, *Clin Orthop* **290**: 76–86.

12
Open fractures of the pelvis

J.N. Powell

This chapter may be paraphrased to read 'the lethal pelvic fracture'. In patients with this particular injury, a mortality rate of near 50% has been reported and is significantly higher than the mortality rate (10–15%) for closed pelvic fractures (Perry 1980, Tile 1984).

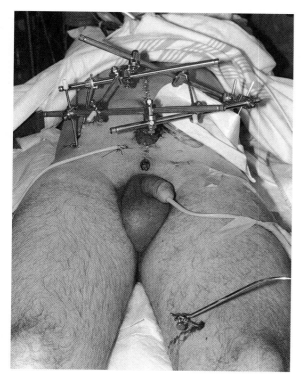

Figure 12.1

This patient was transferred to our trauma unit one week following an open pelvic fracture. He had a rectal laceration and underwent a diverting colostomy. As well, he had a urethral injury which had been treated by a suprapubic tube, a Foley catheter from below and insertion of a suction drain. The fixator pins were loose.

Two recent reports from major trauma centres, Sacramento (Hanson et al 1991) and Toronto (Jones et al 1990) have reported mortality rates which demonstrate that the open pelvic fracture remains a lethal injury, with a 25–30% mortality rate in these series.

By definition, an open pelvic fracture is a fracture which communicates with the rectum, vagina, or through a break in the skin. Contamination of the fracture site, by an infected urinary tract or by gastrointestinal tract contents, is common. The soft-tissue injury is often accompanied by a significant disruption of the pelvic ring. Raffa and Christensen (1976), as noted below, suggested that this injury is often the first stage in a traumatic hemipelvectomy. The mechanism of the injury is either hyperabduction of the lower extremity of the affected hemipelvis ('wishbone') or vertical shear. The pelvic floor is disrupted. As a consequence, this leads to a loss of tamponade and greater difficulty in controlling haemorrhage.

The high-energy nature of these injuries is reflected in the high injury severity score which averaged 29 in the combined series, including the University of Toronto (Jones et al 1990). The management of patients with recognized open pelvic injuries, therefore, requires attention to the basics of resuscitation as a first step and then specific measures to be outlined below.

Clinical picture

Any patient with a laceration in the region of the perineum (Figures 12.1 and 12.2) or gluteal area, associated with the clinical signs and symptoms of a pelvic fracture, should be considered to have an open pelvic fracture, until proven otherwise. Anterior lacerations over the iliac crest are generally obvious.

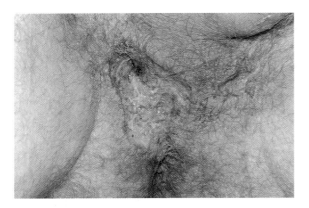

Figure 12.2

This perineal wound communicated with the retropubic space.

Delayed diagnosis may occur in the 'hidden' open injury, with laceration of either the vagina or rectum. Spicules of bone may perforate either the vaginal or the rectal mucosa. Haemorrhage from the introitus and blood on the examining finger following a vaginal examination or rectal examination, in the presence of a pelvic fracture, mandate further examination. A speculum examination is mandatory with vaginal bleeding and a proctoscopic/sigmoidoscopic examination is mandatory to investigate the cause of the rectal bleeding.

As in all patients with pelvic fractures, the posterior soft tissues must be examined carefully, looking out for both evidence of a shear injury to the soft tissues and evidence of a laceration.

Management

General management, resuscitation and haemorrhage control

Immediate resuscitation measures must be initiated. We follow the general principles of resuscitation, as outlined in ATLS protocols (1989). After an airway has been secured, and the patient's ventilatory status is determined to be satisfactory, attention is paid to haemodynamic parameters.

Two large-bore intravenous catheters are established and if the patient is hypotensive, red cell transfusion initiated immediately. Uncross-matched O Rh-positive blood is initiated in cases of life-threatening haemorrhage, when time does not permit a full cross-match. O Rh-negative blood will be used in female children and female adults of child-bearing age. A Foley catheter is inserted early in the resuscitative phase of the patient's care, after the integrity of the genito-urinary tract has been established by clinical and, if necessary, radiological criteria. Important in the radiological investigation of these patients is a urethrogram in all male patients. A cystogram should be performed in all patients with a high-energy pelvic injury, to confirm that the bladder has not ruptured. Contraindications to Foley-catheter placement on a clinical basis include a high-riding prostate, a scrotal haematoma and blood at the tip of the urethral meatus of the penis.

The principles of haemorrhage control are:

1. Packing of open pelvic wounds, using pressure dressings.
2. Reduction of a displaced hemipelvis, if vertically displaced, by the application of traction to the limb through a tibial traction pin.
3. By further measures, to reduce the volume of the pelvis, including rotational reduction with stabilization using an external fixator.

A high percentage of patients with major pelvic fractures have major intra-abdominal injuries, mostly splenic tears and liver lacerations. This potential for injury must be sorted out early by peritoneal lavage, computed tomography scan, or more recently, by the use of abdominal ultrasound. Clearly, if an intra-abdominal injury of significance is identified, laparotomy will be necessary.

The decision regarding the priority of laparotomy versus reduction and external fixation must be individualized. Consultation between the orthopaedic service and general surgical service is necessary. Angiographic embolization is generally considered only after the stabilization and a laparotomy (where necessary) have been performed. In exceptional circumstances, open packing of the pelvis in an attempt to provide a greater tamponade has been effective.

Richardson et al (1982) have reported on two patients who underwent hemipelvectomies, in desperate circumstances, to control haemorrhage. Both of these patients survived.

Antitetanus prophylaxis and broad-spectrum antibiotics are recommended. Particularly, if bowel contamination has occurred, a triple antibiotic regime for a minimum of 48 hours is appropriate.

Control of sepsis

The principles of open fracture management as stated for elsewhere in the body (see Chapter 5), need to be applied in the pelvis as well. The wound requires careful cleansing, followed by a meticulous debridement, instituted once the patient is haemodynamically stable. All wounds are packed open to prevent the development of gas gangrene.

The presence of a rectal laceration is an absolute indication for an immediate diverting colostomy. When perineal wounds occur, each must be judged by location for the potential to contaminate the fracture and the retroperitoneal haematoma. Generally, in any situation where a perineal wound has occurred, it is appropriate for a colostomy to be performed and consultation with the general surgical service should be obtained. Most centres now accept that a distal loop washout is appropriate.

Urethral injuries are generally managed conservatively either by primary re-alignment or a suprapubic tube. The treatment of intraperitoneal bladder injuries is generally operative by direct repair, whereas extraperitoneal ruptures are often managed by urethral catheter drainage alone. Where possible, the use of suprapubic tubes is to be discouraged if surgery is going to be necessary through an anterior approach to either the pelvic ring or the acetabulum. The urological service at Sunnybrook Health Science Centre (Toronto) has been successfully able to repair extraperitoneal ruptures and drain the bladder by urethral catheterization when a formal plating of the pubic symphysis has been done.

Fracture management

The location of the soft-tissue injury and the degree of contamination will be a factor in the decision-making regarding pelvic fracture stabilization. In general, if the wound is an anterior wound along the crest of the iliac wing, then internal fixation can be considered, using lag screw and plating techniques. Pubic symphyseal disruptions can be managed by primary plating, often done at the time of a laparotomy. Controversy exists as to whether this should be done in the presence of a bladder rupture and when a rectal laceration has occurred. Primary plating is being used more frequently now.

In injuries with a perineal or buttock wound, further dissection for lag screw and plating techniques is not generally recommended. In these situations, the provisional stabilization is generally achieved by application of an external fixator and where the fracture is potentially vertically unstable, by the use of a skeletal traction pin. On occasion, this becomes the definitive method of treatment.

Internal fixation of open pelvic fractures can be recommended early in the course of treatment in two situations. The first is when a soft-tissue injury is such that the dissection has already been done. An example would be the application of lag screws across a disrupted sacro-iliac joint in the presence of a buttock wound where a traumatic dissection has already taken place.

Secondly, in pelvic ring injuries, with either a sacro-iliac dislocation or a sacral fracture, the use of a percutaneous lag screw can be recommended. This represents one and probably the best indication for percutaneous fixation of the pelvic ring (Figures 12.3–12.6).

Biomechanically, iliosacral lag screw fixation has been shown to be one of the strongest methods of fixation of the posterior pelvic ring (Hearn et al 1992, Kraemer et al 1994). The benefits of early stable internal fixation include patient comfort, facilitation of nursing care, and maintenance of the reduction of the pelvic-ring disruption with elimination of traction. Two screws can be solidly placed into the ala of the sacrum, or preferably the body of S1 (Kraemer et al 1994) depending on the actual posterior injury.

These screws should only be used by trained pelvic surgeons in trauma centres as they are very technically demanding and potentially dangerous.

Stabilization of the anterior pelvic injury either internally or with an external fixation should be

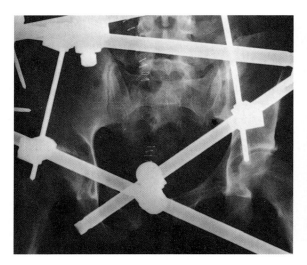

Figure 12.3

These are the radiographs of the patient in Figures 12.1 and 12.2. This is the anteroposterior radiograph showing the vertical displacement of the left hemipelvis through the left sacro-iliac joint (see arrow). Also evident is the diastasis at the pubic symphysis.

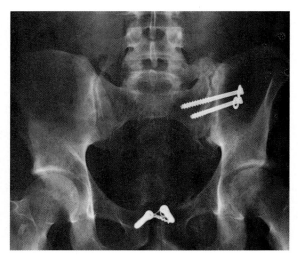

Figure 12.5

Percutaneous stabilization was chosen for a number of reasons. The colostomy was near the usual incision site for an anterior approach to the sacro-iliac joint. The fixator pins were loose and contaminated. This is the anteroposterior radiograph showing percutaneously placed iliosacral lag screws placed into the ala of the sacrum, after the pelvic ring had been stabilized anteriorly.

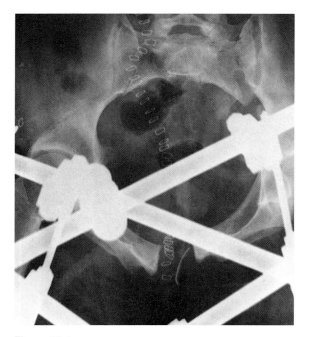

Figure 12.4

This is the inlet view showing the posterior displacement of the hemipelvis.

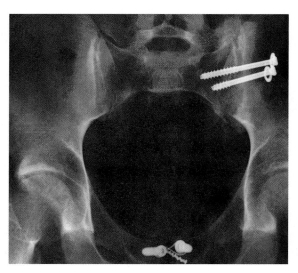

Figure 12.6

This is the inlet view showing the reduction and stabilization achieved. Note fusion of the sacro-iliac joint.

used even if posterior ring fixation has been accomplished. This will improve the overall stability of the pelvic ring.

Aftercare for these injuries will obviously vary, dependent upon the specific soft-tissue injury complex. In general, patients will require repeat examination of the wound in the operating room at 48 hours post-injury. If an infection ensues, aggressive wound care will be necessary at 24–48 hour intervals. This may necessitate many trips to the operating room, but in the early care of the patient, these wounds cannot be managed in any other fashion. The open wounds are generally managed by allowing them to granulate if there is any evidence of sepsis. If no evidence of sepsis ensues, then these wounds can be closed at 5–7 days. On closing the wounds, attempts must be made to eliminate dead space and the use of suction drains is recommended.

Outcome

Raffa and Christensen (1976) described 26 patients with open pelvic fractures. Of the 16 patients with injury caused by blunt, high-energy trauma, eight died, giving a mortality of 50%. In seven cases, the death was directly related to sepsis, and in the other, to massive haemorrhage. The high-energy nature of this injury is reflected by the presence of genito-urinary injuries in 12 of 16 and gastrointestinal lesions in seven of 16 patients.

In the series of Raffa and Christensen, 13 of 16 soft-tissue injuries were either perineal or gluteal, two were into the rectum and one into the vagina. Aside from sepsis, massive haemorrhage, often uncontrollable, was common with nine of 16 patients requiring more than 20 units of blood. The authors related the high mortality from sepsis to either a delayed colostomy or no colostomy at all. In the 14 patients who had immediate faecal diversion, only one death occurred, whereas in those who had no diversion or in whom it was delayed, seven of 12 patients died.

Perry (1980) reported on 31 patients with open pelvic fractures. The mortality for the patients with open pelvic fractures was 42%, compared to 10.3% for the remaining 707 patients with closed pelvic fractures. The major causes of death from open pelvic fractures were again noted to be haemorrhage and sepsis.

Hanson and co-authors (1991) reported the experience in Sacramento from 1984 to 1988. Their series reported on 43 patients retrospectively. They noted 3.1 additional injuries per patient, with only two isolated open pelvic injuries. The average injury severity score for those who died was 40.

An attempt to classify the fractures using mechanistic classification proved difficult, with 13 of 43 patients having fracture patterns which did not fit into the classification. The patients were generally treated by the principles outlined above. Two patients required hip disarticulation, two required a hemipelvectomy and one required a gracilis flap for coverage.

The two important factors in mortality were age and the mechanism of injury. The most significant factor was the age of the patient: those over 40 years of age had a 78% mortality as compared with 18% of those who were under 40. The mortality rate for the overall series was 30%. They found no significant correlation between fracture pattern and the wound type or location.

A combined report, including patients treated in three trauma centres, including Sunnybrook Health Science Centre in Toronto (Jones et al 1990), reported on 39 patients with open pelvic fractures. The average injury severity score was 29.

Treatment was generally by the established ATLS protocols, with irrigation and debridement of wounds and identification and treatment of associated injuries. Diverting colostomies were performed in each of nine patients with rectal lacerations. However, only five patients in this series underwent diverting colostomy within 48 hours. One of the five in whom diverting colostomy was performed in the initial 48 hours died, while three of the four who underwent a delayed colostomy died of sepsis. A total of 10 patients had an open reduction and internal fixation. The anterior stabilization was performed acutely in four patients. The six posterior stabilizations were performed on a delayed basis. One of the patients in the posterior fixation group became infected.

Ten of 39 (25%) of the patients in this series died. All of the patients who died sustained unstable Tile type B or C pelvic fractures. All the patients who died from sepsis had an associated rectal tear. In this series, instability of the pelvic fracture showed a statistically significant association with mortality.

Conclusion

The open pelvic fracture remains an injury with an associated 30% mortality. It is critical to search diligently in all patients with a pelvic ring disruption for any of the signs of an open injury, including obvious lacerations as well as signs on a careful examination of the vagina and rectum.

The principles of management include the general principles of management of haemorrhage. It is important in patients with pelvic fractures to reduce any displacement and stabilize the pelvis. Early use of a traction pin and a simple external fixator are important in haemorrhage control. Packing of open pelvic wounds can be life-saving.

The wound must be cared for by a meticulous debridement and irrigation with large amounts of saline. A colostomy is mandatory when a rectal tear occurs and for all perineal wounds. The use of a suprapubic tube should be avoided where possible.

We favour stabilization of the pelvic ring to facilitate management of these patients and generally recommend external fixation anteriorly. In trauma centres, use of percutaneous iliosacral fixation is indicated.

References

Advanced Trauma Life Support Instructor Manual (1989) (American College of Surgeons: Chicago).

Hanson P, Milne J, Chapman M (1991) Open fractures of the pelvis, *J Bone Joint Surg (Br)* **73**: 325–9.

Hearn TC, Tile M, DiAngelo D, Schopfer A, Vrahas M, Powell JN, Willett K (1992) Mechanics of the pelvic ring in relation to ligamentous loading and the stability of internal fixation. Presentation at the Combined Orthopaedic Societies of the English-Speaking World, June 9 1992, Toronto, Ontario.

Jones A, Kellam JF, Powell JN, Dust W, McCormack R (1990) Open pelvic fracture. Presentation at the American Academy of Orthopaedic Surgeons, February 13 1990, New Orleans, Louisiana.

Kraemer W, Hearn TC, Tile M, Powell JN (1994) The effects of thread length and location on extraction strength of iliosacral lag screws, *Injury* **25**: 1: 5–9.

Perry JF (1980) Pelvic open fractures, *Clin Orthop* **151**: 41–5.

Richardson JD, Harty J, Amin M (1982) Open pelvic fractures, *J Trauma* **22**: 533–8.

Raffa J, Christensen NM (1976) Compound fractures of the pelvis, *Am J Surg* **132**: 282–6.

Tile M (1984) *Fractures of the Pelvis and Acetabulum* (Williams and Wilkins: Baltimore).

13

The relationship between plastic surgery and orthopaedic trauma surgery

C.M. Court-Brown and A.A. Quaba

Given the obvious relationship between plastic surgery and orthopaedic traumatology it is somewhat surprising that we know little about the requirement for plastic surgery in the management of open fractures. Just as orthopaedic traumatologists have been mainly interested in the differences between implants that are commonly used to fix fractures, so plastic surgeons have concentrated mostly on the mechanics of flap cover and both sets of surgeons have neglected to investigate just how important each is to the other's clinical practice. There is perhaps some excuse for the apparent lack of communication between plastic surgeons and orthopaedic traumatologists in many parts of Great Britain and other countries. For historical reasons, many orthopaedic trauma units do not have plastic surgery units in the same hospital. In a recent report, the British Orthopaedic Association (1992) estimated that only 26% of orthopaedic trauma units have ready access to plastic surgery and the situation concerned both the British Orthopaedic Association and the British Association of Plastic Surgeons enough to stimulate the production of a booklet entitled *The Early Management of Severe Tibial Fractures: The Need for Combined Plastic and Orthopaedic Management*. This booklet, published in 1993, emphasized the need for close communication between the specialities, but was unable to reproduce epidemiological information regarding the interrelationship between the two specialities as little information existed at the time of its production.

In an effort to address the problem of the lack of epidemiological data, the 1000 cases detailed in Chapter 3 have been further analysed to examine the requirement for plastic surgery and the type of plastic surgical procedure used to close the soft tissues. It must be emphasized that we are not seeking to dictate how plastic surgeons should close a particular defect but instead are trying to estimate what proportion of patients require plastic surgery in their management and also to help to establish what proportion of plastic surgery time might be utilized in the management of orthopaedic trauma cases. We further accept that the Edinburgh Orthopaedic Trauma Unit makes considerable use of distally based fasciocutaneous flaps in cases where free flaps provide a viable alternative and might well be used in other centres. Thus, the proportion of local flaps to free flaps detailed in this chapter may be somewhat different from that encountered in other units. We do not believe that this is a problem and suggest that surgeons look beyond the particular flaps detailed in this chapter and concentrate more on the requirement for plastic surgery than the relative proportions of split-skin grafts, local fasciocutaneous flaps, local muscle flaps and free flaps.

Analysis of the 1000 cases detailed in Chapter 3 shows that 754 fractures did not require any plastic surgery in their management. However, it should be noted that a number of these fractures had very major soft-tissue defects or had occurred in patients who were seriously injured and the reason that plastic surgery was not undertaken was that a primary amputation was performed or the patient died within 48 hours of admission. However, in the vast majority of the

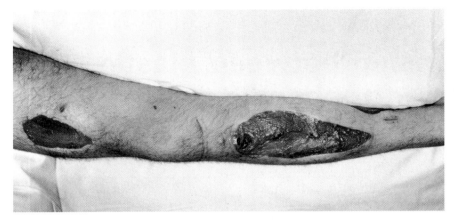

Figure 13.1

Split-skin grafting is used in two principal ways for the management of soft-tissue defects associated with trauma. The type IIIb open femoral fracture has been treated with the application of a skin graft. This patient also has an ipsilateral type IIIb open tibial fracture with considerable bone loss and this has been treated with a latissimus dorsi free flap with an overlying split-skin graft.

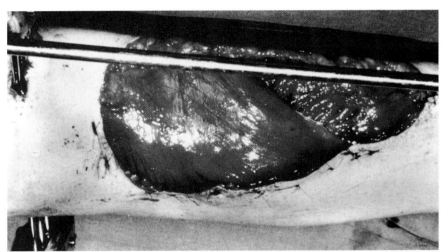

Figure 13.2

Gastrocnemius muscle flap used to cover a type IIIa open tibial fracture situated at the junction of the proximal and middle thirds of the diaphysis.

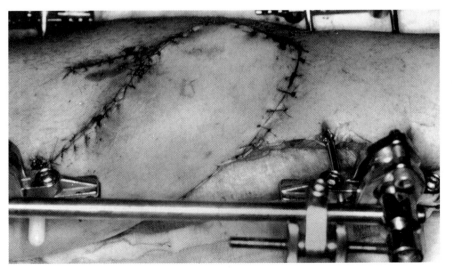

Figure 13.3

A proximally based fasciocutaneus flap used to cover a type IIIb fracture of the tibial diaphysis.

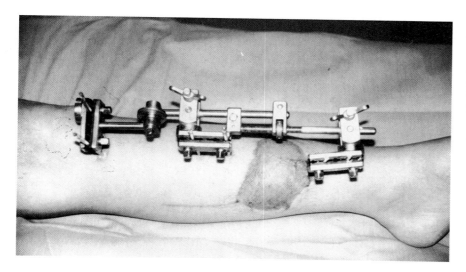

Figure 13.4

Free rectus abdominis flap used to cover a type IIIb fracture of the tibial diaphysis. Figure 13.1 illustrates the use of a free latissimus dorsi flap.

754 cases, it was considered that plastic surgery was not required in the management of the fracture. A further 141 open fractures required split-skin grafting (Figure 13.1), 13 required local muscle flaps (Figure 13.2), 77 required other local flaps, these mostly being proximally and distally based fasciocutaneous flaps (Figure 13.3), and the remaining 15 open fractures had distant flaps (Figure 13.4). The average age of the whole group was 42.5 years and there was no difference in the average ages of the sub-group that required no plastic surgery (42.2 years), the split-skin sub-group (40.6 years) and the local muscle flap group (41.9 years). The other local flap sub-group was somewhat older at 48.6 years and the distant flap sub-group somewhat younger at 36.2 years. This latter figure probably reflects the relatively young age of the group of patients who have severe Gustilo type IIIb open fractures of their long bones.

Further analysis of the other local flap sub-group showed that 70 of the 77 patients had proximally or distally based fasciocutaneous flaps. The remaining seven local flaps comprised two metacarpal artery flaps, two forearm flaps, one fascial flap, one island sural flap and a pedicle foot flap. The 11 muscle flaps were mainly gastrocnemius flaps (nine) although there was one trapezius flap and one soleus flap. The 15 distant flaps were made up of six latissimus dorsi free flaps, five rectus abdominis free flaps, two radial forearm flaps and two groin flaps.

The age distribution of these five different patient sub-groups is shown in Figure 13.5. It can be seen that the distant flap sub-group has a marked peak between 20 and 29 years with the

Table 13.1 The requirement for plastic surgery in different open fractures. Finger fractures are not included as, despite their relative frequency, few open finger fractures need plastic surgery

Location	n	Incidence (%)	Plastic surgery (%)
Ankle	40	4.0	55.0
Tibial diaphysis	244	24.4	54.9
Tibial plafond	11	1.1	54.5
Carpus	15	1.5	46.6
Tarsus	30	3.0	40.0
Tibial plateau	10	1.0	30.0
Distal femur	10	1.0	30.0
Femoral diaphysis	62	6.2	29.0
Forearm diaphyses	41	4.1	19.5
Patella	27	2.7	18.5
Metacarpus	16	1.6	12.5
Distal radius/ulna	78	7.8	10.3
Proximal forearm	16	1.6	6.2
Humeral diaphysis	18	1.8	5.5
Hand phalanges	297	29.7	2.6
Foot phalanges	42	4.2	2.4
Distal humerus	17	1.7	0
Metatarsus	11	1.1	0
Proximal femur	1	0.1	100
Clavicle	2	0.2	50
Proximal humerus	5	0.5	20
Pelvis	6	0.6	0
Scapula	1	0.1	0

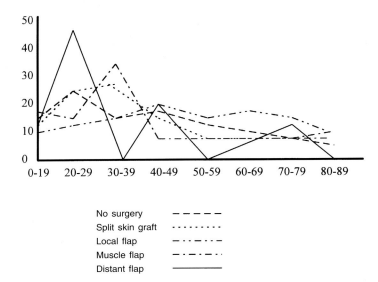

Figure 13.5

The age distribution of the different types of plastic surgery procedures. It is obvious that most of the free flaps were done in younger patients. There is a tendency in all types of plastic surgery procedures for a reduction in the requirement for plastic surgery in later years.

muscle flap peak being a decade later. The other sub-groups of patients, those requiring no plastic surgery as well as those needing split-skin grafts and local flaps, do not show a marked peak in the early decades but unquestionably there is a slight drop in incidence as the patients get older.

Table 3.1 (see page 23) shows the prevalence of open fractures in the population. A listing of the open fractures based on the requirement for plastic surgery shows a somewhat different pattern (Table 13.1) with some of the less common open fractures having a relatively high requirement for plastic surgery. The most interesting aspect of Table 13.1 is the need for plastic surgery in fractures of the tibial diaphysis, tibial plafond and ankle. Each of these areas has a similar requirement for plastic surgery and there is no doubt that serious injuries to the leg and hindfoot present the greatest combined challenge to the orthopaedic traumatologist and plastic surgeon.

It is also interesting that fractures of the femoral diaphysis, distal femur and tibial plateau also have a similar incidence. However, not only is the incidence less than that of the leg and hindfoot but the requirement for flap cover is also less. Common open fractures such as those of the distal radius and the hand phalanges have a relatively low requirement for plastic surgery. In the case of the distal radius few fractures are severe, most being caused by low energy injuries in the elderly. One might argue that more flap procedures could be performed in open hand fractures but most of the patients sustaining these injuries in this series were manual workers and fingertip injuries were usually treated by terminalization to facilitate a rapid return to work, an essential requirement in most countries.

The humerus is obviously well protected from the requirement for plastic surgery. Open proximal humeral fractures are extremely rare, but even the commoner diaphyseal and distal humeral fractures require little plastic surgery and if it is required split-skin grafting is usually satisfactory. The last group of open fractures in Table 13.1, those of the proximal femur, clavicle, proximal humerus, pelvis and scapula, will not be considered further. The low numbers of these fractures and the high energy nature of the trauma required to produce them makes the figures for incidence of plastic surgery meaningless.

Specific fractures

Ankle fractures

The greatest requirement for plastic surgery was seen in open fractures of the ankle, tibial plafond and tibial diaphysis. In all of these fractures there is obviously a tendency towards increased plastic surgery in the more severe fractures. Thus in the five Gustilo type I open ankle fractures, no plastic surgery procedures were used. In the 18 open type II ankle fractures, however, eight (44.4%) of the fractures required plastic surgery with six defects being closed by split-skin grafting and two by fasciocutaneous flaps. Twelve (80%) of the Gustilo IIIa open ankle fractures needed plastic surgery with nine having split-skin grafting and three having fasciocutaneous flaps. Both of the type IIIb open fractures needed flap cover, one with a fasciocutaneous flap and the other with a latissimus dorsi free flap.

Tibial diaphyseal fractures

Of the 244 open tibial diaphyseal fractures, 134 required plastic surgery techniques to facilitate soft-tissue closure. As mentioned earlier, a number of patients had primary amputations and several patients died, usually of severe neurological damage in the 48 hours after admission. Thus the figure of 54.5% requirement for plastic surgery might be considered an underestimate in some other centres in the world, but we believe that the figure gives a reasonable estimate of the average requirement for plastic surgery in the management of tibial diaphyseal fractures.

Fifty-five of the patients required split-skin grafting to close their wounds. A further 58 required local flaps with 56 of these being proximally or distally based fasciocutaneous flaps. In addition, there was one fascial flap and one pedicle foot flap was performed in a type IIIb fracture treated by amputation. There were ten muscle flaps used of which nine were gastrocnemius flaps, one being a soleus flap. The remaining 11 fractures were treated with distant flaps. All were free flaps with five latissimus dorsi, five rectus abdominis and one radial forearm flap being used. There were nine type

Table 13.2 The requirement for plastic surgery procedures in open fractures of the tibia.

Parameter	I	II	IIIa	IIIb
Number	59	53	55	68
No plastic surgery	86.4%	56.6%	32.7%	5.9%
Split-skin graft	10.2%	22.6%	36.3%	23.5%
Local flap	3.4%	17.0%	27.3%	45.6%
Local muscle flap	0	1.9%	3.6%	10.3%
Distant flap	0	1.9%	0	14.7%

IIIc fractures in the study. One received a fasciocutaneous flap and one had a temporary split-skin graft applied, but all of these patients were treated by amputation either primarily or as a secondary procedure. We believe that with increasing awareness of the role of amputation in the management of type IIIc tibial diaphyseal fractures the need for plastic surgery in these difficult problems will diminish.

The requirement for plastic surgery in the remaining 235 open tibial fractures is shown in Table 13.2. It is self-evident that the need for plastic surgery increases with increasing severity of fracture as assessed by the Gustilo classification. Only 13.6% of type I open tibial diaphyseal fractures required plastic surgery techniques to close the soft tissues, whereas only 5.9% of the Gustilo type IIIb fractures did not. Of the four patients who make up this figure, one had a primary amputation and a second died soon after surgery. Thus, in effect, only two Gustilo type IIIb fractures did not have plastic surgery.

Split-skin grafting is used increasingly up to fractures of grade IIIa in severity. It is clearly less useful in IIIb fractures where the highest incidence of local and distant flaps were seen. It is likely that other centres might use more free flaps, but we have found the combination of distally based fasciocutaneous flaps and locked reamed intramedullary nails to be particularly useful in the management of tibial diaphyseal fractures (Keating et al 1994).

Tibial plafond

The only other fracture where more than 50% of the patients required plastic surgery was the tibial plafond or pilon fracture. Open pilon fractures are much less common than open ankle and tibial diaphyseal fractures, but their location ensures a high incidence of Gustilo type III fractures with significant soft-tissue defects. In this series, both the type I open fractures were treated without plastic surgery and the Gustilo type II fracture had a split-skin graft. Three of the type IIIa open fractures did not require plastic surgery. All these three fractures occurred in older patients where low-velocity injuries often result in a skin laceration of >5 cm without significant underlying soft-tissue damage. The remaining two Gustilo type IIIa fractures had fasciocutaneous flaps as did all three of the type IIIb fractures.

Carpal fractures

As with open tibial plafond fractures the incidence of open carpal fractures is low. However, the need for plastic surgery is relatively high, suggesting a high percentage of type III open fractures. Analysis of the data confirms that this is the case with only two type I fractures and one type II fracture being found in the study period. None of these fractures required plastic surgery. Of the ten type IIIa fractures, five did not require plastic surgery and three only needed a split-skin graft. One fracture had a local flap, the remaining one being treated by a distant groin flap. Both of the type IIIb fractures required plastic surgery, one being treated by a radial forearm flap and the other with a split-skin graft.

Tarsal fractures

The vulnerability of the leg and foot to severe open fractures is highlighted by the relatively high requirement for plastic surgery in the management of open tarsal fractures. Of the 30 tarsal fractures, nine were Gustilo type II in severity and none required plastic surgery. Four of the eleven type IIIa tarsal fractures also had no plastic surgery, with six of the remaining seven fractures being treated with a split-skin graft. One fasciocutaneous flap was used. Three

of the seven type IIIb fractures did not have plastic surgery with three more having a split-skin graft and one a fasciocutaneous flap. One of the three type IIIc fractures had a temporary skin graft, but all of the type IIIc fractures were eventually treated by amputation. The distribution of plastic surgery procedures between the three types of fractures involving the tarsus, and those of the calcaneus, talus and the other tarsal bones is very similar. The striking difference between the open tarsal fractures and those of the tibia, pilon and ankle is that despite the relatively high incidence of plastic surgical procedures that are required to treat open tarsal fractures, few flaps are required. Only two (6.6%) of the open tarsal fractures required flap cover whereas nine (30.8%) of the combined open tibial diaphysis, tibial plafond and ankle group required flap cover.

Tibial plateau fractures

As with the tibial plafond fractures, the prevalence of open tibial plateau fractures is relatively low, but the requirement for plastic surgery is such that 30% of the open fractures required plastic surgery to gain soft-tissue closure. None of the three Gustilo type I or four Gustilo type II fractures required plastic surgery, but all of the type III fractures did. There were two type IIIa fractures, both of which required a gastrocnemius muscle flap, and one type IIIb fracture where a local island sural artery flap was used to close the soft tissues.

Distal femur

The adjacent fracture to the tibial plateau, that of the distal femur, had the same incidence of plastic surgery but the techniques required to close the soft tissues were simpler. Only three of the ten fractures required plastic surgery, all being successfully closed with split-skin grafting. Only two of the six type IIIb fractures required split-skin grafting. No flaps were required. The remaining two required split-skin grafts. There was one further split-skin graft performed in a type I open distal femoral fracture.

Femoral diaphyseal fractures

A similar pattern of plastic surgery requirement is seen in femoral diaphyseal fractures. These are relatively common injuries; it was illustrated in Chapter 3 that 12.1% of all femoral diaphyseal fractures are open. In addition, the incidence of type III fractures is also high with 63.9% of the open femoral fractures being type III in severity. However, despite this no flaps were required and only 18 (29.5%) of 62 open femoral fractures needed split-skin grafting. The remainder did not need plastic surgery at all. A breakdown of the plastic surgery required according to the different Gustilo fractures types shows that 16.6% of type I, 42.8% of type II, 66.6% of type IIIa and 45% of type IIIb fractures had split-skin grafting. All of the seven type IIIc femoral fractures were amputated. In this series, all of the IIIc femoral diaphyseal fractures occurred in road traffic accidents and in all cases the thigh musculature was extensively crushed, precluding limb reconstruction.

Forearm diaphyseal fractures

The forearm diaphysis shows a similar spectrum of plastic surgery requirement to the femoral diaphysis, although in the forearm three flaps were used, one in a type II open ulna fracture and two in IIIb fractures of both the radius and ulna. However, of the 20 type I open fractures, only one (5%) required a split-skin graft. Seven of the nine type II fractures had no plastic surgery, with one split-skin graft and one fasciocutaneous flap being performed. Three of the four type IIIa fractures had split-skin grafts performed, the fourth not requiring plastic surgery. Two of the seven type IIIb fractures had distant flaps, with one radial forearm and one groin flap being used. The remaining IIIb fractures had split-skin grafts. The one type IIIc fracture patient who was treated had an amputation. There was no significant difference in the plastic surgery requirement for single or both bone fractures of the forearm.

Patella fractures

It is interesting to observe that the spectrum of plastic surgery requirement for patella fractures was similar to that of the distal femur and proximal tibia. Of the 27 patella fractures that were treated in the group only five required split-skin grafting, with no flaps being used at all. One of the five type I patella fractures required a split-skin graft. In addition, one of 13 type II and three of eight type IIIa fractures also required split-skin grafting.

Metacarpal fractures

Of the 16 metacarpal fractures treated in this series, only two required split-skin grafting. The remaining 14 fractures needed no plastic surgery at all.

Distal radial and ulnar fractures

Table 3.1 (see page 25) indicates that open fractures of the distal radius and ulna are not uncommon. However, the requirement for plastic surgery in these injuries is low. Most open fractures of the distal forearm occur in simple falls in elderly patients. Thus of the 51 type I fractures that were encountered, only three required split-skin grafting. There were 20 type II fractures and only one of these required a split-skin graft. The seven type III fractures tended to occur in younger patients, but even then only four of the seven patients required split-skin grafts. No flaps were performed for this particular open fracture.

Proximal forearm fractures

As with other fractures in the upper limbs, the requirement for plastic surgery procedures in proximal forearm fractures is low. There were 16 proximal forearm fractures in this series, of which 15 involved the olecranon. Only one split-skin graft was performed in a type II fracture. None of the other fractures required plastic surgery.

Humeral diaphysis

As with fractures of the proximal forearm the requirement for plastic surgery of humeral diaphyseal fractures is very low. There were 18 fractures in this series and only one patient who had a type IIIb open humeral diaphyseal fracture required split-skin grafting. No other plastic surgery was required.

Hand phalanges

Open fractures of the hand phalanges are the most common open fractures that orthopaedic traumatologists will be called upon to treat (see Chapter 3). Despite this, the requirement for plastic surgery is fairly low. Five of the fractures had split-skin grafting, with three further fractures being closed by local flaps. Two of these involved dorsal metacarpal artery flaps and the third made use of a cross-finger flap.

It could be argued that more flaps should have been employed in the management of these fractures but, as previously stated, many of the patients who had open fractures of their hand phalanges were manual workers and it was felt important that they should be returned to work quickly. Obviously other units with a different patient population may consider making more use of plastic surgery in the treatment of open hand phalangeal fractures.

Foot phalanges

Foot phalanges are also spared from the necessity of plastic surgery. There were 12 type I fractures in this series, none of which required plastic surgery. Of the 22 type II fractures treated, only one required a split-skin graft and none of the eight type III fractures required plastic surgery.

A review of the data presented here suggests that there is an important relationship between plastic surgery and orthopaedic traumatology. Many of the operations required to close soft-tissue defects relate to severe fractures of the long bones, and take a considerable amount of time, particularly if free-flap techniques are employed. As success in the management of these fractures is gained by early soft-tissue closure, it is clear that the requirement to perform a considerable number of plastic surgery operations may have a considerable impact on the workload of plastic surgeons. The data also suggest that it is important for plastic surgery units to employ a surgeon or surgeons with a particular interest in post-traumatic flap cover.

The data presented here cover a period of six years and three months, but the practice of clinical orthopaedic traumatology is dynamic and there is little doubt that the requirement for plastic surgery closure of soft-tissue defects in Edinburgh has increased over the period analysed in this study. However, we believe that our information provides a good database on which both orthopaedic traumatologists and plastic surgeons may assess their requirement for plastic surgery in the management of open fractures.

References

British Orthopaedic Association (1992) *The Management of Skeletal Trauma in the United Kingdom* (BOA: London).

British Orthopaedic Association, British Association of Plastic Surgeons (1993) *The Early Management of Severe Tibial Fractures: The Need for Combined Plastic and Orthopaedic Management* (BOA: London).

Keating JF, Court-Brown CM, Quaba AA (1994) *Open Tibial Fractures* (American Academy of Orthopaedic Surgeons: New Orleans).

14
Anatomy of the skin and soft tissues

G.C. Cormack

Definitions vary, but for the purposes of this chapter we will regard the integument as composed of skin, subcutaneous fat and deep fascia. The structure and physiology of these tissues are well covered in standard texts, but information about the vascular anatomy is generally harder to find. This chapter will concentrate on the blood supply of these structures particularly as it relates to the effects of trauma and the application of reconstructive techniques.

The skin

The skin is supplied from two vascular plexi, the dermis from a subdermal plexus which in turn feeds the subpapillary plexus lying beneath the epidermis. Veins have a similar arrangement except that they have an additional plexus in the dermis. Our concern in the context of trauma is not so much with these plexi as with how blood gets to them and how these feeding vessels may be compromised.

The subcutaneous tissues

Subcutaneous tissues consist of the fatty layer or panniculus adiposus containing vestiges of the panniculus carnosus. This adipose tissue has its own vascular system and in this respect is different from the perivascular fat grouped around vessels which do not relate specifically to the fat cells but to their associated tissue or organ (e.g. mesenteric fat). The adipose tissue is made up of delicate lobules separated by fibrous septa which are histologically connected both with the dermis and the deep fascia and which contain cutaneous nerves and vessels. Each lobule consists of hundreds, even thousands, of fat cells, and is vascularized through a single pedicle entering the centre of the lobule and is drained to a vein on the periphery. The capillaries are therefore located within each lobule, rather than in the connective-tissue septa around them. It is the surrounding septa which confer on these very delicate structures a surprising mechanical resistance, and it is this system of supporting tissue that is in proportion to the expected mechanical stresses, the heel pad area being the most extremely developed example of this.

The blood vessels which feed the subdermal network arise in the tissues beneath the deep fascia and ascend through the subcutaneous fat in either a vertical or a horizontal–linear fashion (Figure 14.1). In areas with thin layers of subcutaneous fat, the lobules are vascularized largely by descending branches from the wide-meshed subdermal plexus, while in thicker fat layers the deeper lobules are supplied by branches coming directly from the ascending arteries. In these areas of thick fat, the subcutaneous adipose tissue receives blood from two directions, the superficial layer from above and the deep layer from below, with a connective-tissue septum frequently lying between the two and containing a further vessel plexus at this level (Pearl and Johnson 1983). The existence of two such relatively autonomous layers is relevant to the raising of adipofascial flaps in which the deeper layer of fat is moved with the deep fascia, while the skin and superficial fat nourished through the subdermal plexus remains at the donor site.

The ascending branches from the deeper structures may have either a largely vertical course through the subcutis to the skin, in which case the area of skin supplied is small, or alternatively they may run more obliquely, first on the superficial surface of the deep fascia and then through

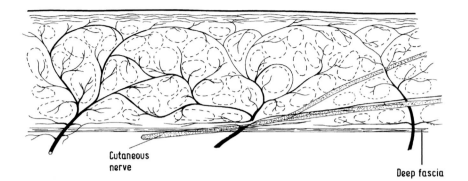

Figure 14.1

Schematic diagram to show the vascular plexi and their supply from ascending vessels. Also demonstrated are the plexi on the deep fascia.

the subcutaneous tissues, giving off branches to the subdermal plexus as they go and supplying a longer strip of skin. The predominating direction of these vessels may be termed their 'axiality' and on the limbs this is generally found to be directed longitudinally. A clue to understanding why this is so is provided by the fact that

arterial branches often accompany cutaneous nerves. Frequently these vessels are reinforced at intervals along the nerve by branches of other ascending vessels, thereby forming what might be termed a 'relay' artery alongside a nerve. These vessels are not 100% constant but Figures 14.2 and 14.3 show good examples from the

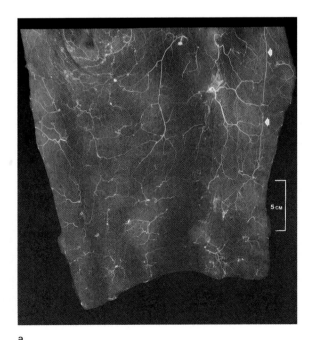

a

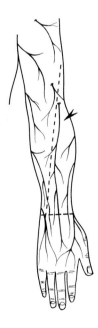

b

Figure 14.2

(a) Radiograph of part of injected forearm skin preparation showing relay artery along the posterior cutaneous nerve of the forearm. (b) Site of radiograph, showing cutaneous nerves.

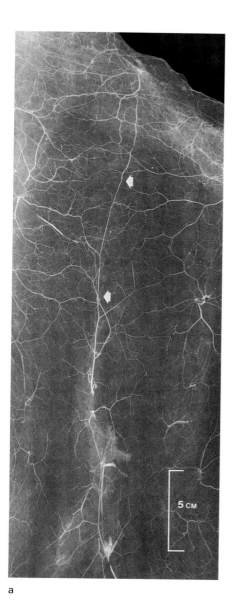

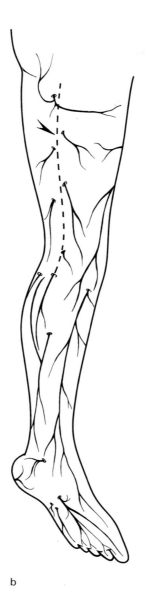

Figure 14.3

(a) Radiograph of the injected posterior thigh skin preparation showing the relay artery along the posterior cutaneous nerve of the thigh. (b) Site of radiograph, showing cutaneous nerves. The subfascial part of the posterior cutaneous nerve of the thigh is shown by an interrupted line.

a

b

forearm and thigh. Similarly, on the lower leg, vessels accompany the superficial peroneal, the medial sural and the peroneal communicating cutaneous nerves. It is these vessels that to some extent account for the predominating longitudinal axiality of the vessels of the fascial and subcutaneous vascular plexi.

The deep fascia

The deep fascia is of two distinctly different types. On the trunk it consists of a well-developed epimyseal surface covering on the muscles. This is elastic in the sense that it is capable of permitting expansion of the abdominal viscera and increase in the diameter of the chest and is therefore very different from the deep fascia on the limbs which is altogether a more rigid structure. The deep fascia on the limbs is continuous with the intercompartmental fascial septa. It not only encloses the muscle groups but also acts in places as a point of origin for muscle fibres (e.g. over tibialis anterior) and near the joints it forms part of the retinacular system restraining the tendons and preventing bowstringing. It is not surprising that the vascularization of the so-called 'deep fascia' is therefore different on the trunk compared with the limbs. On the trunk, the vascularization is tied into the anatomy of the underlying flat muscles and there are no specific fascial plexi with the exception of the area over the scapula. On the limbs the deep fascia is vascularized from vessels passing up along the fascial septa between muscles. These vessels contribute to the formation of two vascular plexi. One is on the undersurface of the fascia and the other on the superficial surface. The deep plexus is made up of tiny branches of the ascending vessels before they perforate the fascia. The superficial plexus is more extensive and made of larger vessels, again originating from the ascending perforators but only after they have pierced the fascia. These two layers are effectively separate except for the ascending ('perforating') vessels themselves and some tiny capillaries which connect them through the fascia (Lang 1962).

The actual structure of the deep fascia on the limbs is also of interest. The fascia is made up of inextensible collagen fibres and has already been described as relatively rigid yet at the same time we are able to observe that, for example, on plantar flexion of the foot there is an increase in girth of the proximal calf as the muscles contract and move proximally. How are these apparent contradictions to be reconciled? The explanation is that in the lower leg, the structure of the deep fascia is an anisotropic lattice web, made up of two lamellae of deep fascia running at an angle to each other (Figure 14.4). The lamellae arise from the medial tibial plateau and from the area over the head of the fibula. Fibres fan out posteriorly over the two heads of gastrocnemius and extend across the midline to pass round the sides of the lower leg and gain insertion into the anterior subcutaneous surface of the tibia. On the lateral side, the more anterior

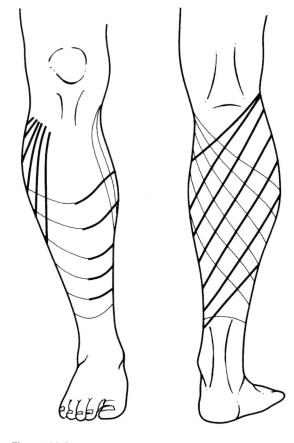

Figure 14.4

Arrangement of the deep fascia on the lower leg (see text for explanation).

fibres pass over the peroneal compartment while the posterior fibres pass over gastrocnemius, generally deep to those from the medial tibial plateau. On the medial side, the fan of fibres crosses the calf and then the peroneal compartment, where some of the fibres pass into the anterior and posterior peroneal septa, and the fibres then cross over the anterior compartment and insert into the tibia. Over the calf muscles a web of rhomboids results which is able to accommodate an increase in bulk in the proximal calf at the same time as a reduction in girth of the distal part. However, horizontal fibres over the anterior tibial compartment limit expansion and render this compartment particularly prone to compression syndromes. In the forearm, a similar lack of extensibility over the forearm flexor compartment may contribute to the generation of compartmental ischaemia and Volkman's contracture; hence the need for anterior fasciotomy in severe forearm and wrist injuries. On the lower leg, the attachment of the deep fascia directly to bone and the blending of fibres of the deep fascia with fibres in the intercompartmental septa creates a deeply tethered structure. Shearing forces applied to the integument therefore tend to separate the much less firmly attached subcutaneous fat from the deep fascia. Characteristically, this is the plane of the 'degloving injury' in which the ascending vessels to skin, be they fasciocutaneous or musculocutaneous perforators, are disrupted. The subcutaneous plexus is deprived of its arterial input and further compromised by underlying haematoma with the result that skin necroses over most, if not all, of the degloved area.

Blood supply to the skin, subcutis and deep fascia

The vessels which pass through the deep fascia to reach the subcutaneous and subdermal plexi have been described as 'ascending vessels'. Other terms which may be used when referring to these vessels up to the point at which they pierce the deep fascia are 'conductors' and 'perforators'. The sources of origin of these vessels now need to be identified and their anatomy described (Table 14.1). At the outset, it must be stated that there is some controversy over how these vessels should be designated and this is a matter that can occupy many hours of fascinating but fruitless discussion. It seems to the author that a simple tripartite division of the vessels supplying the integument on the basis of their anatomy is a very adequate solution. The three types of vessel are as follows:

1. Direct cutaneous arteries. These emerge from deeper vessels and run in a horizontal–linear fashion for some distance in the subcutis. Many of these emerge in the axillae and groins, for example superficial inferior epigastric artery, superficial and deep external pudendal arteries, superficial circumflex iliac artery and superficial thoracic artery, but also at other sites such as on the anterior chest where the cutaneous branches of the internal thoracic artery emerge through the anterior ends of the intercostal spaces and run laterally over the chest in the subcutis.
2. Musculocutaneous perforators. These emerge from the surfaces of muscles to supply the integument.
3. Fasciocutaneous perforators. These pass along an intermuscular or intercompartmental fascial septum to reach the deep fascia.

Latterly a new term, 'septomuscular', has been coined (Schusterman et al 1992) to describe a

Table 14.1 Some terms used to describe the ascending vessels to the integument

Plexus	Fed by arteries described as	Anatomically subdivided as
Subpapillary plexus Subdermal plexus Subcutaneous plexus Superficial fascial plexus Deep fascial plexus	ascending vessels or conductor arteries or perforators	direct cutaneous arteries musculocutaneous perforators fasciocutaneous perforators

Table 14.2 Tripartite classification of the blood supply to skin

Period of discovery	Anatomical system	Category of flap
1940–1970	Direct cutaneous vessels	Axial pattern cutaneous flaps
1970–1980	Musculocutaneous perforators	Musculocutaneous flaps
1980–1990	Fasciocutaneous perforators	Fasciocutaneous flaps

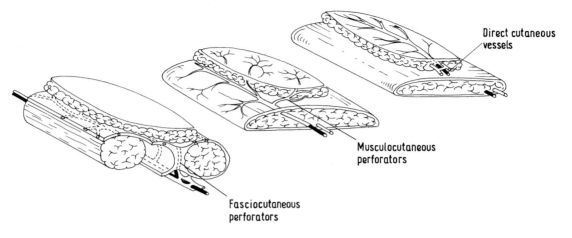

Direct cutaneous vessels

Musculocutaneous perforators

Fasciocutaneous perforators

Figure 14.5

General scheme of direct cutaneous arteries, musculocutaneous vessels and fasciocutaneous vessels.

vessel which emerges along a septum but may be closely adherent to and even pass through the edge of a muscle which is attaching to that septum. This has some validity and is a relevant concept for those already well versed in the details of cutaneous vascular anatomy but for a newcomer to the field it probably is only a distraction.

The general scheme of direct cutaneous vessels, musculocutaneous vessels and fasciocutaneous vessels is shown in Figure 14.5. In historical terms, this tripartite classification also has validity since the clinical development of the concept of flaps can be identified as very roughly having three phases which coincide with the elucidation of these three systems of supply (Table 14.2).

Furthermore, when it comes to describing flaps, the same terms as were used to describe vessels can—with little modification—be used to describe flaps (Table 14.2), thereby not only imparting information about the mode of vascularization, but also giving an indication of the likely tissue constituents of the flap (although this is not invariably so; see below). A note of explanation is perhaps required on the use of the term 'musculocutaneous' since other words that appear in the literature to describe the same entity are myodermal and myocutaneous. Myodermal is derived from the Greek, and musculocutaneous from the Latin; the purist will resist the mixing of Latin and Greek in 'myocutaneous' but this does appear to be the favoured form in the American literature.

Concept of territories

Irrespective of how it gets there, each vessel ascending through the subcutis feeds into the subdermal plexus over a certain area whose boundaries are not absolutely fixed. This has led to the concept of each vessel having a 'territory' or to be more accurate, each vessel may have up to three different territories depending on the circumstances under which the territory is assessed. These have been termed the 'anatomical', 'dynamic' and 'potential territories' (Cormack and Lamberty 1986a,b) (Figure 14.6):

1. The anatomical territory of a vessel is defined by its structure and is delineated by the physical limits to which that vessel branches out before anastomosing with branches of vessels from adjoining territories.
2. The dynamic territory of a vessel is that which is indicated by injection studies of that vessel in intact cadavers. In this situation, the intravascular pressure in adjoining territories is zero and a medium injected into one

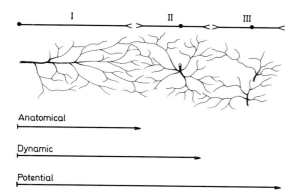

Figure 14.6

The concept of territories (see text for explanation).

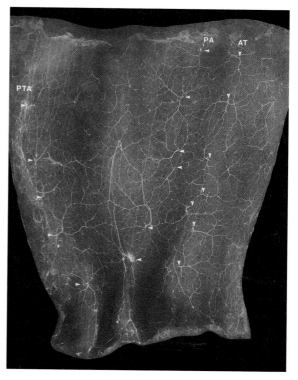

Figure 14.7

Radiograph of injected lower leg skin and deep fascia showing fasciocutaneous perforators. AT = from anterior tibial artery; PA = from peroneal artery along posterior peroneal septum; PTA = along medial side of leg from posterior tibial artery.

ascending vessel will pass, via anastomoses at the periphery of the anatomical territory, through into surrounding territories. Here the medium will pursue the path of least resistance which generally means back into major vessels by retrograde flow down other ascending vessels.

3. The potential territory can only be defined by clinical flap elevation. Here the ascending vessels of adjacent territories are divided and ligated and the blood flows through the anastomotic connections across more than one territory. How many territories the blood will flow through depends on a variety of factors which vary from site to site and patient to patient. These territories are only defined by clinical experience.

Anatomy applied to reconstruction

Design of axial cutaneous flaps

The problem with these flaps is that they are all individual in their anatomy and therefore it is hard to define general principles. The questions that must be answered in planning an axial pattern flap are:

- Where is the vessel?
- What is its territory?
- What is the venous drainage of the area?

The course of the vessel concerned can usually be identified with a Doppler ultrasound probe with an 8.5-MHz transducer but judging the extent of the territory that can be raised is a matter of experience. These flaps are largely confined to the head and trunk, in which regions venous drainage is towards the neck, axillae and groins. Since several of the direct cutaneous arteries emerge from the groins or axillae, this makes for a fortunate arrangement in which the draining veins run countercurrent to the arteries, but in areas where the subcutaneous network drains away from the base of the flap, for example in the deltopectoral flap, the venae comitantes of the artery form the only route for venous drainage.

Table 14.3   Septa containing fasciocutaneous perforators

Region	Vessel of origin	Location of septum
Shoulder girdle	Circumflex scapular A	Teres major/teres minor*
Arm	Middle collateral A—interosseous recurrent A	Triceps, lateral head/brachialis/brachioradialis†
	Radial collateral A—radial recurrent A	Brachioradialis/brachialis*
	Superior ulnar collateral A—posterior ulnar recurrent A	Coracobrachialis/triceps, medial head†
Forearm	Radial A	Brachioradialis/flexor carpi radialis*
	Ulnar A	Flexor carpi ulnaris/flexor digitorum superficialis*
	Posterior interosseous A	Extensor carpi ulnaris/extensor digitorum communis*
	Anterior interosseous A	Abductor pollicis longus/extensor pollicis brevis/extensor pollicis longus*
Hand	Dorsal metacarpal A	Between extensor tendons
Thigh	Superficial femoral A	Around sartorius
	Saphenous A	Around sartorius
	Descending branch of lateral circumflex femoral artery	Vastus lateralis/rectus femoris*
	'Adductor' artery	Around gracilis
	Inferior gluteal A	Biceps femoris/semitendinosus*
	Profunda femoris, lateral branches	Vastus lateralis/biceps femoris†
	Profunda femoris, posterior branches	Biceps femoris/semitendinosus/semimembranosus*
	Popliteal A	Vastus lateralis/biceps femoris†/semitendinosus*
Leg	Anterior tibial A	Extensor digitorum longus/peroneus longus and brevis†
		Tibialis anterior/extensor hallucis longus*
	Posterior tibial A	Flexor digitorum longus/soleus*
	Peroneal A	Peroneus longus/soleus†
Foot	Medial plantar A	Around abductor hallucis brevis
	Lateral plantar A	Around abductor digiti minimi
	Dorsalis pedis A	Extensor hallucis longus/extensor digitorum over 1st intermetatarsal space*

*Ordinary intermuscular fascial septum.
†Intercompartmental fascial septum.

Design of fasciocutaneous flaps

These vessels reach the integument by passing along intermuscular and intercompartmental fascial septa where these exist which is generally between long narrow muscles on the limbs (see Table 14.3 and Figure 14.7). Over the scapula there is also a fasciocutaneous supply, which is not so odd if one considers that these vessels reach the surface by passing between teres major and teres minor, which are developmentally limb musculature which approximately conforms to long and narrow proportions. Fasciocutaneous perforators at all these sites form a vascular network whose axiality is predominantly longitudinal as illustrated in Figure 14.8.

Planning a fasciocutaneous flap requires a consideration of the following:

- Where are the fasciocutaneous perforators located?
- Is there a fascial plexus?
- What is the axiality of the vascular plexus?

In designing fasciocutaneous flaps, the vascular anatomy of the perforators can be exploited in basically three different ways. These different

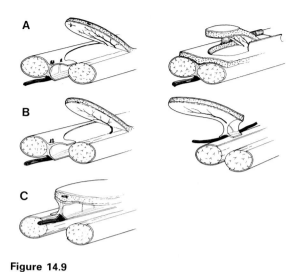

Figure 14.9

Fasciocutaneous flaps of types A, B and C (see text for explanation).

Type A flap. This is dependent for its blood supply on the branches of several fasciocutaneous perforators in its base. This type of flap is always used as a local pedicled flap.

Type B flap. This is supplied by a single perforator and it may be a pedicled, islanded or free flap.

Type C flap. This is removed in continuity with a segment of a compartmental artery and is supplied by several perforators from that artery.

Design of adipofascial flaps

The vascular basis of these flaps, which are intended for local pedicled use, is similar to that of the fasciocutaneous flap types A and B. Thin skin flaps are dissected off the subcutaneous tissue which is then raised with the deep fascia to constitute the flap. The skin flaps are replaced to cover the donor-site defect and survive on their subdermal plexus while the adipofascial flap takes the major share of the vessels of the integument. The flap then requires to be split-skin grafted. Even the principal proponents of these flaps admit that healing time is often prolonged, necessitating

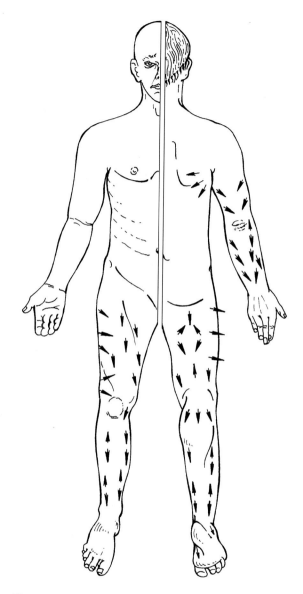

Figure 14.8

Approximate axiality of branches of fasciocutaneous perforators.

types of flap have been classified as types A, B and C (Cormack and Lamberty 1984) and are illustrated in Figure 14.9.

2–6 weeks of immobilization with elevation of the limb (Gumener et al 1991).

The muscles

Vascular anatomy of muscles

The two aspects of muscle anatomy which are of interest in the context of trauma and reconstruction are the vascular supply to the muscle and the supply (if any) from the muscle to the overlying skin.

As long ago as 1919, Campbell and Pennefather considered various examples of infarction of muscles following injury to their blood supply and classified muscles from the point of view of their vascular supply. Blomfield (1945) developed these ideas further with particular regard to the muscles of the lower limb and delineated five types of intramuscular pattern. Blomfield further suggested that the '. . . relative vulnerability of muscles to necrosis and clostridial infection' was related to several vascular factors in addition to the intramuscular pattern of its vessels, viz. the site of entry and source of the main nutrient arteries, the number of arteries derived from independent sources, the efficiency of the intramuscular anastomoses and the relationship between the size of the main nutrient vessel(s) and the size of its anastomotic connections.

Almost precisely the same considerations are relevant to the raising of musculocutaneous flaps and many of them are incorporated in the classification devised by Mathes and Nahai (1981). This simplified the concepts of the earlier workers and is concerned primarily with the *number* of vascular pedicles entering the muscle and their relative *dominance* within the muscle as assessed from the internal angiographic patterns demonstrated in cadaver material. The definitions of the types I to V are contained in Table 14.4 together with examples of typical muscles from each group.

The vascular connections between muscles and overlying skin can be best described by the generalization that broad flat muscles give off perforators to the skin whereas long narrow ones rarely do. As always, there are exceptions and rectus abdominis, which could by its shape fall into either category, is quite definitely a muscle which has perforators to skin.

The perforators which emerge from the surface of a muscle are accompanied by venae comitantes. Another feature is that they may exhibit some axiality in that many musculocutaneous perforators run in a particular direction and give off smaller branches in a manner analogous to direct cutaneous arteries but on a smaller scale. Other musculocutaneous perforators diverge into two, three or more main

Table 14.4   Vascular anatomy of muscles classified into five types according to the scheme of Mathes and Nahai

Type I	*One vascular pedicle*	
	Anconeus	Tensor fasciae latae
	Gastrocnemius*	Vastus intermedius
Type II	*One dominant vascular pedicle usually entering close to the origin or insertion of the muscle with additional smaller vascular pedicles entering the muscle belly*	
	Biceps femoris	Semitendinosus
	Gracilis	Soleus
	Peroneus longus and brevis	Trapezius
	Rectus femoris	Vastus lateralis
Type III	*Two vascular pedicles, each arising from a separate regional artery*	
	Gluteus maximus	Rectus abdominis
	Serratus anterior	Semimembranosus
Type IV	*Multiple pedicles of a similar size*	
	Flexor digitorum longus	Extensor digitorum longus
	Flexor hallucis longus	Extensor hallucis longus
	Tibialis anterior	Sartorius
Type V	*One dominant vascular pedicle and several smaller secondary segmental vascular pedicles*	
	Pectoralis major	Latissimus dorsi

*Each head is regarded as a separate muscle in this context.

branches which each supply their own small irregular territory. The knowledge that musculocutaneous perforators at some sites conform to an axial pattern may influence the design of certain flaps.

Anatomy applied to reconstructive surgery: Design of musculocutaneous flaps

Although many a successful flap has probably been raised simply by following a cookbook-style set of directions, there is no doubt that a true appreciation of the underlying anatomy gives confidence, allows intra-operative modifications when confronted with abnormal anatomy, enables one to create modifications of existing flaps and permits the search for improved designs of flap. A thorough appreciation of this anatomy requires a knowledge of many factors as shown in Table 14.5 but to have this sort of understanding of each muscle is overly ambitious for most people.

For a pedicled muscle flap, the most important points are the *number of vascular pedicles* entering the muscle and their *dominance within the muscle*. The *sources of the pedicles* and their *locations* in relation to the origin and insertion of the muscles then become important because these features determine the centre of the arc of rotation of any pedicled muscle or musculocutaneous flap. Knowledge of the pattern of perforators emerging from the surface of the muscle and their axiality, if any, will allow planning of any skin island that may be required on the muscle. These are the basics and were largely established during the decade 1970–1980.

During the 1980s, knowledge concerning the blood supply of musculocutaneous units progressed to a level where a greater understanding of the intramuscular arrangement of the vessels enabled several modifications of basic musculocutaneous flaps. These resulted from the fact that the segmental morphology which exists in several muscles, and which is reflected by a consistent branching of the neurovascular structures, enables each segment to be surgically separated from other segments by dissections along anatomical planes. There are several possible applications of this but in

Table 14.5 Musculocutaneous flap planning

Aspect	Important points to consider
Vascular pedicles	Source
	Position
	Size
	Constancy
Intramuscular anatomy of vessels	Relative dominance of pedicles
	Branching pattern and constancy
	Size and number of anastomoses
Anatomy of the perforators	Number
	Axiality
	Individual territory size
	Anastomoses with other vessels

the context of lower-limb trauma, the most important advantage is that knowledge of the intramuscular anatomy in some instances allows one to take only as much of the muscle as is required for the reconstruction whilst at the same time permitting preservation of function. This is in marked contrast to what usually happened in the early days of musculocutaneous flap application when the whole muscle would be raised irrespective of how much was actually required. For example, in the case of latissimus dorsi it allows only part of the muscle to be harvested as a free flap on the thoracodorsal pedicle while the remainder of the muscle remains on the chest wall in a functional state because it is supplied by intercostal perforators, is connected to the tendon of insertion and has an intact nerve supply.

Even when the vascular anatomy is not segmental, the intravascular arrangement may be exploited in the creation of small local muscle flaps. For example, in the early period of muscle flap development tibialis anterior, a type IV muscle with no dominant pedicle and no significant connections with the overlying skin, was thought rather poor material for a local muscle flap. However, the muscle has an interesting structure with a central tendon and an encircling vascular network. This was subsequently exploited in the design of broadly based muscle flaps raised from the medial surface of the muscle and left attached on an anterior pedicle of muscle carrying vascular input. This muscle flap is useful for covering small defects over the anterior aspect of the tibia (Møller-Larsen and Petersen 1984).

Soft-tissue connections with bone

Bone has long been regarded as being supplied by two systems of blood vessels; indeed the presence of a circulus vasculosus articuli around the epiphyseal plate was described by William Hunter in 1743. These two systems are:

1. Nutrient vessels entering nutrient foramina which are located in the midshaft and metaphyseal regions of developing long bones, and—in immature bones prior to closure of the growth plate—in a ring around the epiphysis. In the limbs, these vessels are branches of the principal compartmental arteries.
2. A network of much smaller arteries lying on the periosteum in regions of heavy fascial attachment, these being largely the sites of origin or insertion of muscle fibres, or attachment of intermuscular fascial septa.

Classically, the flow of blood through the cortex connecting these two systems was thought to be centripetal but more recent evidence suggests a centrifugal pattern of flow. In areas of loose soft-tissue attachment to the periosteum, the flow is probably centrifugal through the full thickness of the cortex whereas at sites where the attachment is strong, probably the outer third of the cortex is supplied from the periosteal vessels (Rhinelander 1974). This is represented diagrammatically in Figure 14.10. Since the flow is centrifugal, the majority of the foramina penetrating the surface of the bone are occupied by thin-walled veins rather than arteries. At certain points on bones, such as near the ends of long bones, the proportion of foramina occupied by arteries will be higher, and it is these metaphyseal and epiphyseal arteries that are able to maintain perfusion of the medullary cavity when the contribution from the diaphyseal nutrient artery has been obliterated either naturally or surgically.

In the skeletally immature, the blood supply of the bone is more complex because of the presence of the epiphyseal plate. Cross-anastomosis between the epiphyseal and metaphyseal circulations is the exception rather than the rule. Such transphyseal vessels may be found in the large epiphyses (Crock 1967), near their periphery, and become less frequent as the secondary ossification centre enlarges. Perichondrial

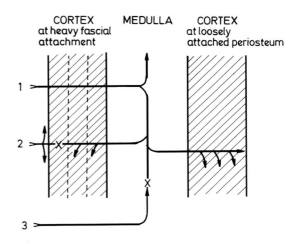

Figure 14.10

Blood flow through cortical bone (after Rhinelander 1974). 1 = nutrient artery of diaphysis; 2 = periosteal vessels; 3 = metaphyseal perforators; X = sites of anastomoses.

vessels supply the epiphysis and by their connections with the periosteal vessels are a further possible communication between the epiphyseal and metaphyseal circulations.

In a manner analogous to that in which the skin may be regarded as being supplied by three different systems, so the periosteal plexus of arteries appears to be fed by three routes. These may be designated as direct periosteal, musculoperiosteal and fascioperiosteal (Figure 14.11). Direct periosteal vessels arise from nutrient arteries entering foramina and come directly from segmental (trunk) or compartmental (limb) arteries without passing through muscles first; musculoperiosteal vessels arise from arteries within muscles; fascioperiosteal arteries pass along intermuscular fascial septa generally from the same vessels as supply fasciocutaneous perforators to overlying skin.

Anatomy applied to reconstructive surgery

Vascularized bone transfer

The improved understanding of the blood supply to bone has allowed reconstructive techniques to

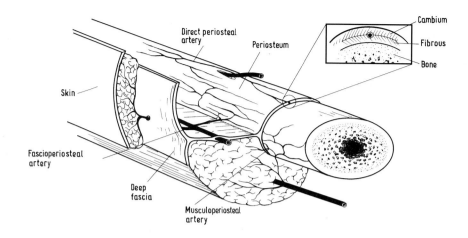

Figure 14.11

Blood supply to periosteum. Insert shows the different layers of the periosteum.

be developed which have moved on a long way from the traditional idea that vascularized bone grafts have to be attached to portions of muscle. The majority of microvascular bone grafts still rely on musculoperiosteal vessels or on nutrient arteries but fascioperiosteal bone transfer is increasingly used and the use of pieces of periosteum as loco-regional pedicled transfers is another development.

Musculoperiosteal vessels are small and lack robustness and their connections with the vessels of the muscle may be further narrowed by tension on the muscle. Indeed, many such grafts probably derive as much benefit from lying within their bed of vascularized muscle as they do through putative connections between the vascular systems of the muscle and the periosteum. By contrast, the fascioperiosteal vessels fed by arteries travelling along relatively inextensible intercompartmental fascial septa may provide a more robust means of carrying a segment of that bone. The combination of a skin flap with a segment of bone supplied by fascioperiosteal perforators from the same compartmental artery (Figure 14.12) provides an elegant anatomical example of how knowledge of these two systems of vessels can be used in the design of a clinically successful composite osteofasciocutaneous flap, for example on the lateral side of the upper arm based on the middle collateral artery.

Vascularized periosteal transfer

The osteogenic potential of periosteum has been recognized since Ollier in 1867 concluded that transplanted periosteum and bone could, under certain circumstances, become osteogenic. This classical study was later re-evaluated and developed by Scandinavian surgeons (Skoog 1965, Ritsilä et al 1972). Successful free-vascularized periosteal transfer has been demonstrated clinically and experimentally although contradictory views exist concerning osteogenic capability with warnings that, without stress, bone formation is unreliable. Local pedicled transfer has also been demonstrated anatomically by Crock in the lower limb and applied clinically to a tibial fracture (Crock and Morrison 1992). Crock has shown that a periosteal flap may be raised on the lateral surface of the middle third of the tibial shaft where the periosteum receives a blood supply from several branches of the anterior tibial artery. A 'flap' of periosteum attached to the anterior tibial vascular bundle may be transferred either distally to the foot (retrograde flow in vessels) or proximally to the knee (orthograde flow).

Conclusion

A simplified view of the vascular anatomy of the soft tissues has been presented and related to

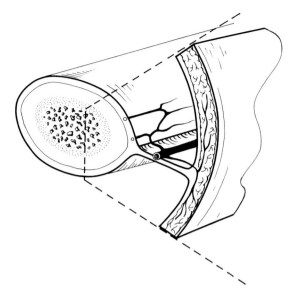

Figure 14.12

One of several methods whereby skin and bone may be carried on a common blood supply. Examples of this type of osteofasciocutaneous transfer would be (i) lateral supracondylar ridge of humerus and lateral arm skin carried on the middle (posterior) collateral artery and (ii) lateral radius and volar forearm skin carried on the radial artery.

the effects of trauma. A classification of flaps based on this anatomical approach has been described. However, there are limitations in this approach, mainly because plastic surgery is complex and getting ever more so, with the aim being not simply to fill a hole but to achieve an elegant reconstruction. The optimal reconstruction has complete reliability based on perfect and consistent blood supply, a perfect match to the requirements of the donor site in terms of volume, colour, shear resistance etc., and an invisible donor site. Clearly, all these criteria are never met and therefore some means of ranking all these parameters must be made, if only in one's own mind, so as to allow a composite and compromise decision to be made. Furthermore, ranking of parameters cannot be absolute; for example, when bone is included in a composite iliac crest free flap, this bony aspect of the musculocutaneous flap is equal in importance to

the nature of its blood supply. Similarly, flaps with a functioning re-innervated muscle transfer are more than just simple musculocutaneous flaps. Finally, for some flaps, geometry can be as important as the vascular supply. The final choice of flap requires a multifactorial decision with only one aspect being the vascular anatomy; however, unless the surgeon gets the blood supply right, there is little point in worrying about the others.

References

Blomfield LB (1945) Intramuscular vascular patterns in man, *Proc R Soc Med* **38**: 617–18.

Campbell J, Pennefather CM (1919) An investigation into the blood supply of muscles, with special reference to war surgery, *Lancet* **i**: 294–6.

Cormack GC, Lamberty BGH (1984) A classification of fasciocutaneous flaps according to their patterns of vascularisation, *Br J Plast Surg* **37**: 80–7.

Cormack GC, Lamberty BGH (1986a) *The Arterial Anatomy of Skin Flaps* (Churchill Livingstone: Edinburgh).

Cormack GC, Lamberty BGH (1986b) Cadaver studies of correlation between vessel size and anatomical territory of cutaneous supply, *Br J Plast Surg* **39**: 300–6.

Crock HV (1967) *The Blood Supply of the Lower Limb Bones in Man* (Churchill Livingstone: Edinburgh).

Crock JG, Morrison WA (1992) Case report: A vascularized periosteal flap: an anatomical study, *Br J Plast Surg* **45**: 474–8.

Gumener R, Zbrodowski A, Montandon D (1991) The reversed fasciosubcutaneous flap in the leg, *Plast Reconstr Surg* **88**: 1034–41.

Lang J (1962) Über die Textur und die Vascularisation der Fascien, *Acta Anat* **48**: 61–94.

Mathes SJ, Nahai F (1981) Classification of the vascular anatomy of muscles: experimental and clinical correlation, *Plast Reconstr Surg* **67**: 177–87.

Møller-Larsen, F, Petersen NC (1984) Longitudinal split anterior tibial muscle flap with preserved function, *Plast Reconstr Surg* **74**: 398–401.

Ollier L (1867) *Traité Expérimental et Clinique de la Régénération des Os et la Production Artificielle du Tissu Osseux*. Part I, p. 79; Part II, p. 461 (Masson: Paris).

Pearl RM, Johnson D (1983) The vascular supply to the skin: an anatomical and physiological reappraisal. Part 1, *Ann Plast Surg* **11**: 99–105.

Rhinelander FW (1974) Tibial blood supply in relation to fracture healing, *Clin Orthop* **105:** 34–81.

Ritsilä V, Alhopuro S, Rintala A (1972) Bone formation with free periosteum, *Scand J Plast Reconstr Surg* **6**: 57–60.

Schusterman MA, Reece GP, Miller MJ, Harris S (1992) The osteocutaneous free fibula flap: is the skin paddle reliable? *Plast Reconstr Surg* **90**: 787–93.

Skoog T (1965) The use of periosteal flaps in the repair of the primary palate, *Cleft Palate J* **2**: 332.

15
Planning of soft-tissue surgery

A.A. Quaba

There are many similarities between the planning of soft-tissue surgery for trauma patients and for those patients who have elective soft-tissue problems. Obviously the plastic surgeon may be faced with similar soft-tissue defects in both types of patients and it must be remembered that he or she only has four basic techniques available for the management of both types of problem, namely direct skin closure, split-skin grafting, local flap cover or distant flap cover, no matter what type of problem is being dealt with. However, there are certain differences inherent in the management of the post-trauma patient and it may be that the number and severity of other injuries in multiply injured patients preclude the plastic surgeon from performing the ideal technique for soft-tissue closure in a particular case. It is therefore important that those surgeons who manage post-traumatic soft-tissue defects be experienced in all types of plastic surgery.

Multiply injured patients account for about 5% of admissions in the average Orthopaedic Trauma Unit. However, for obvious reasons there is a disproportionately large number of open fractures associated with multiply injured patients and therefore in the trauma situation plastic surgeons will be asked to review soft-tissue defects in a disproportionately higher number of multiply injured patients. When planning soft-tissue surgery it is important that they are aware of the nature and extent of all of the patient's injuries and how these injuries are going to affect both the medical and surgical management of the patient. Obviously the presence of other injuries will affect the timing and type of soft-tissue reconstruction procedures that might be performed.

In addition, it is important that the plastic surgeon be aware of the overall state of the patient. Advancing age is not a contraindication to complex reconstructions but advancing age is often accompanied by increased medical pathology and the surgeon should be aware of the presence of a co-existing diseases such as diabetes, peripheral vascular disease and autoimmune diseases which may well affect the vascular supply of the limbs. The plastic surgeon should also be aware of the extent of any injuries that may be present in potential donor sites and in consultation with the orthopaedic surgeon he or she should select a donor site which causes minimum post-treatment morbidity. Thus, while the surgeon might elect to use a latissimus dorsi free flap in an isolated open distal tibial fracture, a rectus abdominis free flap might be more appropriate if the patient has injuries that will necessitate the use of crutches post-operatively. It cannot be overemphasized that both the orthopaedic surgeon and plastic surgeon should cooperate from the time of initial patient assessment so that correct decisions about the planning of soft-tissue cover can be made at a very early stage. The plastic surgeon should be aware of what treatment method the orthopaedic surgeon proposes to use. Good advice can be given to the orthopaedic surgeon on the planning of skin incisions based on the requirement for later flap cover. This is particularly useful if plating is to be used as the method of bone stabilization. If external fixation is chosen by the orthopaedic surgeon advice on the placement of fixator pins in relation to perforating septocutaneous vessels may well be helpful. Attention to detail at this stage may well make soft-tissue cover easier at a later stage.

Just as the orthopaedic surgeon only has a limited number of basic operative techniques available, so the plastic surgeon only has four types of surgery available for soft-tissue cover. As noted, these are direct skin closure, split-skin grafting, local flap cover and distant flap cover. These are often portrayed as a reconstructive

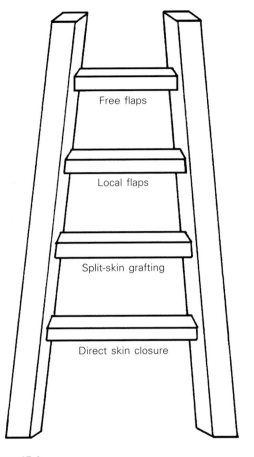

Figure 15.1

The reconstructive ladder. This is a useful diagrammatic representation of the different types of soft-tissue closure available to the plastic surgeon.

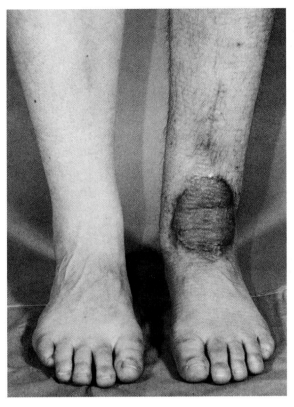

Figure 15.2

The use of a rectus abdominis free flap in the management of a Gustilo type IIIb open distal tibial fracture in a 22-year-old female.

ladder (Figure 15.1). This is a helpful way of considering soft-tissue cover in that the surgeon is moving from the lower rung of direct skin closure serially up the ladder towards more difficult and demanding techniques. Unfortunately, the use of the ladder analogy also suggests that the surgeon should perhaps travel through the simpler techniques before attempting the more difficult techniques and this is not the case. However, the use of the ladder analogy does help the surgeon to plan management and an example of its usefulness is given in Figure 15.2.

Here the end result of the management of a Gustilo IIIb tibial pilon fracture is illustrated. This occurred in a 22-year-old female who was involved in a road traffic accident. It is quite clear that the size of the initial post-operative defect combined with any post-operative swelling that occurred would preclude direct closure. If the surgeon then moves onto the second rung of the ladder and considers skin grafting he or she should then consider the base of the wound on which the skin graft is to be placed. This particular patient was treated by bone plates and there was also exposed tendon in the base of the wound. Clearly, split-skin grafting would be an inappropriate choice for wound closure.

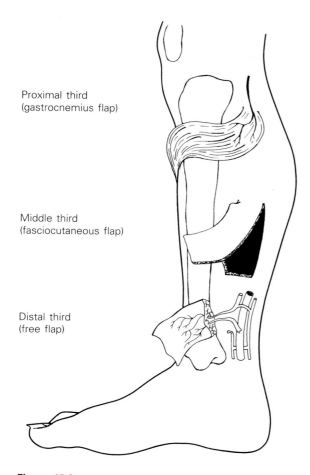

Proximal third
(gastrocnemius flap)

Middle third
(fasciocutaneous flap)

Distal third
(free flap)

Figure 15.3

Topographic division of the tibia into thirds. The use of different flaps to cover soft-tissue defects in the proximal, middle and distal thirds is illustrated.

The third rung of the ladder is local flap cover. A local flap from the calf could be transposed and would adequately cover the defect. This would be acceptable treatment in many patients and Chapter 13 illustrates that it is often used. However, in patients sensitive about the long-term cosmetic aspects of their skin graft, a local flap is unacceptable because of the conspicuous donor site scar. Therefore, the surgeon moves to the top rung of the ladder and uses a latissimus dorsi or a rectus abdominis free flap. In this case Figure 15.2 shows an acceptable result from the use of a rectus abdominis flap.

Chapter 13 illustrates that the open tibial fracture is the most common open fracture which the plastic surgeon will be called on to deal with. A useful aid in planning soft-tissue reconstruction after open tibial fractures is to divide the lower leg into thirds. Options for reconstruction of each third can be considered separately. This is illustrated in Figure 15.3. The upper third of the leg is relatively easily covered by a gastrocnemius flap whereas a fasciocutaneous flap is normally employed for the middle third. Although fasciocutaneous flaps can also be employed for the distal third many surgeons elect to use a free flap for the lower third of the tibia especially if the defect is large.

Although the reconstructive ladder and the topographic division of the tibia into thirds are useful guides in selecting a method for soft-tissue reconstruction, the surgeon's interpretation should not be rigid and as has already been suggested the final management decision will be based on many factors including the physical state and potential requirements of the patient. Planning should begin with an initial combined orthopaedic and plastic surgery evaluation of the injury in the emergency theatre. It is suggested that both surgeons consider the following points of particular relevance to soft-tissue reconstruction.

Important aspects of soft-tissue reconstruction

Skin degloving

Degloving of the skin is not uncommon in elderly patients. Its presence alters the potential for local flap cover and while degloving may not necessarily result in skin devascularization, its extent and location may certainly suggest to the plastic surgeon that a combination of a free flap and split-skin grafting is more appropriate than local flap cover. Degloving is examined in detail in Chapter 18.

Vascular pedicles

The state of the vascular pedicles of potential muscle flaps should always be considered.

Orthopaedic surgeons can be somewhat cavalier in their approach to intact blood vessels in the proximity of the fracture site but they must remember that ill-advised coagulation or ligation of intact vessels may remove the possibility of transferring a particular flap. It is therefore vital that the orthopaedic surgeon understands the local vascular anatomy and consults with the plastic surgeon if there is any dubiety about the requirement for particular blood vessels. In particular, the integrity and location of septocutaneous perforators adjacent to the site of injury should be determined. These are usually well protected within the tough fascial septae and can be the main vascular pedicles for islanded fasciocutaneous flaps. The major neurovascular structures may also be explored and their suitability to receive possible free-tissue transfers assessed.

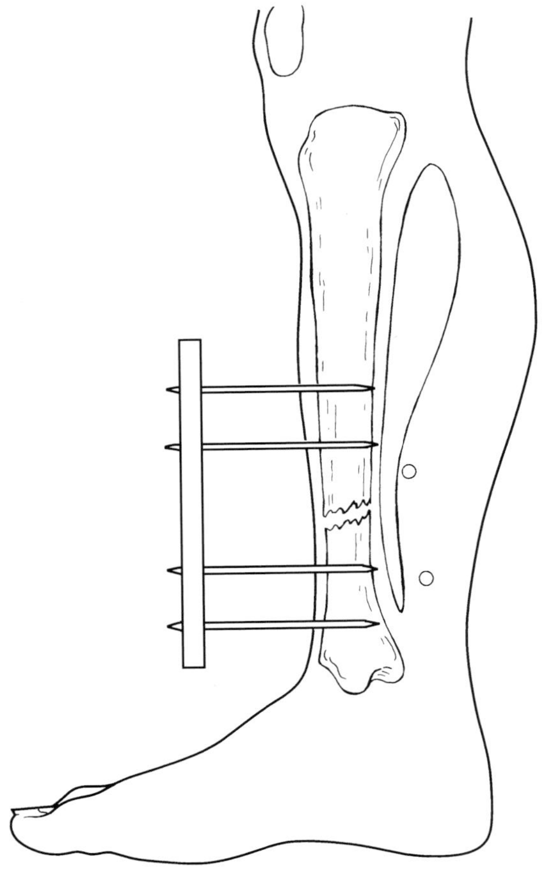

Siting

Fasciotomy incisions

Compartment syndromes and fasciotomies are discussed extensively in Chapter 20. Although the orthopaedic surgeon may understandably wish to decompress a compartment syndrome as an emergency, it is important to consider the local vascular anatomy and to remember that the skin incision on the medial side should be so placed that it avoids the distal septocutaneous perforators which are usually situated 6 cm and 12 cm above the medial malleolus. These perforators may well act as the vascular pedicle for a fasciocutaneous flap at a later stage. The relationship between the fasciotomy wound and the distal two septocutaneous perforators is illustrated in Figure 15.4.

External fixation devices

Chapter 7 has illustrated the use of external fixation devices in the management of open tibial fractures. The data presented in Chapter 7 illustrate that multiplanar external fixators are not associated with improved results compared with unilateral devices and therefore unilateral external fixators are recommended. If such a device is to be used for the tibia, it is suggested

Figure 15.4

The relationship of a medial fasciotomy wound to the 6 cm and 12 cm septocutaneous perforators. It is important that the fasciotomy incision does not damage these perforators. A diagrammatic external fixator is illustrated and it is obvious how easily the fixator pins can damage the septocutaneous perforators if inappropriately placed.

that it be placed on the anteromedial border not just because there is no muscle transfixion if this location is used but because if the external fixator is placed in any other location it can interfere with the design and transfer of local and distant flaps and the pins can also damage the septocutaneous perforators (Figure 15.4). It is very important that the orthopaedic surgeon be aware of the location of the septocutaneous perforators and avoid damage to these vessels when inserting external fixator pins.

Timing

Primary surgical closure of the wound associated with an open fracture should not be carried out as there is a significant risk of infection. Primary flap closure of a wound is theoretically safer as skin tension can be avoided but as suggested in Chapter 5 it is wise to re-examine the wound 36-48 hours after the initial debridement to ensure that the original operation has been adequate. The continuing argument has therefore concerned the optimal timing at which soft-tissue cover should be performed. In recent years there has been a tendency for surgeons to recommend earlier cover.

In a prospective review of open tibial fractures, Byrd et al (1985) advocated radical bone and soft-tissue debridement with flap coverage in the first 5–6 days after injury. If fractures are not covered in this time, the wound enters a subacute, colonized infected phase that extends from approximately one to six weeks after injury. Following that, a chronic phase begins, characterized by granulation of the wound, adherent soft tissue and localized areas of infection. Godina (1986) favoured soft-tissue cover within the first 72 hours of injury and reported a flap failure rate of 0.75% in 134 patients. Higher failure rates were reported in patients who underwent flap cover between 72 hours and three months of the injury (see Chapter 16). Other surgeons such as Yaremchuk (1986) advocated serial debridement procedures to allow all tissues to declare their viability. He subsequently provided microvascular free-flap cover at a later date. Apart from the arguments relating to flap survival and the incidence of infection, early cover shortens hospital stay and decreases the discomfort associated with dressing changes. Many surgeons have now accepted that a good compromise is to undertake soft-tissue cover at the time of the relook procedure, this usually being 36–48 hours after the initial debridement. However, the decision as to when the wound should be covered should be taken jointly by the attending orthopaedic surgeon and

plastic surgeon and should be dictated by the state of the soft tissues at successive relook procedures.

Methods of wound closure and repair

Direct closure

The elective surgical incision

Direct closure is most easily and successfully achieved with fresh tidy wounds of which the most common is a deliberate surgical incision through skin that is free of infection, contusion or degloving. Healing of such a wound should be the rule rather than the exception. However, surgeons are constantly 'testing' the limits of repair with more extensive procedures as well as with incisions into contaminated, ischaemic or infected tissue. In addition, orthopaedic surgeons are tending to use more internal fixation techniques for the management of open fractures. It is, therefore, not surprising that directly closed surgical wounds occasionally break down. Breakdown of an elective surgical incision can be due to factors such as poor surgical technique, rough tissue handling, deep-seated infection, patient malnutrition or disease, or failure to assess the adequacy of the local circulation prior to surgery. It is not unusual for a limb which has sufficient vascularity to survive under normal circumstances to be unable to sustain a surgical incision. This particularly occurs in atherosclerotic patients or after radiotherapy. The failure of healing in such wounds is more likely to happen when surgical technique is rough, leading to 'energy crisis' with the body defences expended in coping with surgical debris rather than focused on the healing process.

Untidy, traumatic and contaminated wounds—the case for delayed primary repair

Wounds that are lacerated or contused or contain foreign material can be rendered fit for surgical closure. This may be achieved by thorough exploration, removal of foreign bodies, excision of all tissue of dubious viability, copious irrigation and the use of appropriate systemic antibiotics. However, it is an established fact that in the presence of contamination and necrotic tissue the wound's innate ability to resist infection can be hampered by suturing. Therefore, if the adequacy of the surgical toilet of a wound is in question as it is in all wounds associated with open fractures, it should be left completely open for a few days. After this time its suitability for closure can usually be decided with confidence. Direct closure or plastic repair can be used as easily and successfully as immediately after the injury.

Skin grafts

A skin graft is transplanted by completely detaching a portion of skin from a donor site and transferring it to a raw bed where it must acquire a new blood supply within 2–3 days to ensure viability. A skin graft consisting of epidermis and part of the dermis is termed a partial or split-thickness skin graft. When the entire thickness is included, then it is a full-thickness or Wolfe graft. It is termed a 'skin autograft' if it is transferred from a donor to a recipient site within the same individual and an 'allograft' ('homograft') if it is transferred between genetically different individuals of the same species.

Selection of skin graft

The choice between split-thickness and full-thickness skin grafts depends on an understanding of the biology of grafts.

1. Split-thickness skin grafts require less ideal conditions for survival and can tolerate less vascularity than full-thickness grafts.
2. The donor site for split-skin grafts can heal spontaneously by epithelialization. If necessary, more split-skin grafts can be harvested from the same site. This is an important consideration in patients with extensive skin loss.
3. Limitations and disadvantages of split-skin grafting include contraction, lack of growth in children, abnormal pigmentation and occasional lack of durability. This is to be

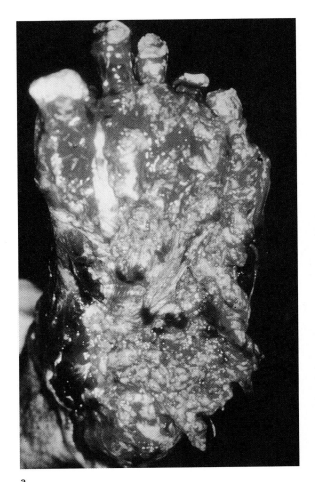

a

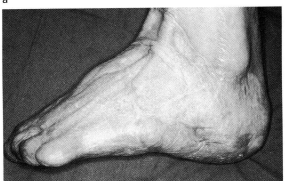

b

Figure 15.5

(a) A severely degloved foot. This was successfully treated by the application of a full-thickness graft taken from the degloved skin. (b) The late result.

contrasted with the fact that full-thickness grafts resist contraction, grow in children and have a texture and pigment appearance more similar to that of normal skin.

Wounds of questionable circulation or large size should thus always be covered with split-skin grafts. Full-thickness grafts need excellent wound vascularity for survival and are therefore used on fresh, non-contaminated wounds of a small size. Usually these are facial or palmar skin defects created by excision of skin lesions or release or scars and contractures. In the trauma situation, full-thickness skin grafts harvested from degloved tissue can be used to cover the anterior aspect of the leg and the sole of the foot. An example of full-thickness skin grafting of the foot is shown in Figure 15.5. Here the degloved skin was defatted and the full-thickness graft used to resurface the foot. After four years' follow-up, the skin remains stable and the foot functional. However, this is not always the case and a further example is shown in Chapter 18 where amputation was eventually required.

Selection of split-skin graft donor sites should consider scar visibility as well as colour match. Where possible, split-thickness skin grafts should be taken from hidden areas such as the inner thigh or lateral buttock. These grafts tend to have a brown-yellowish hue and ideally should not be used on the face, where the scalp or supraclavicular areas are preferred donor sites. The upper inner arm rather than the more accessible forearm is recommended as a split-skin graft donor site for dorsal hand reconstruction.

Full-thickness grafts of the face are often taken from the post-auricular area, the upper eyelid in elderly patients or the supraclavicular region. Large areas of full-thickness skin can be obtained from the groin for palmar hand cover. When this donor site is used in children, extra care must be taken to place the donor site laterally to avoid pubic hair growing in an unwanted visible location. Most full-thickness donor sites are closed directly.

Split-skin grafts

Harvesting split-skin grafts

Cutting split-skin grafts is very painful. If a general anaesthetic is used, the anaesthetist

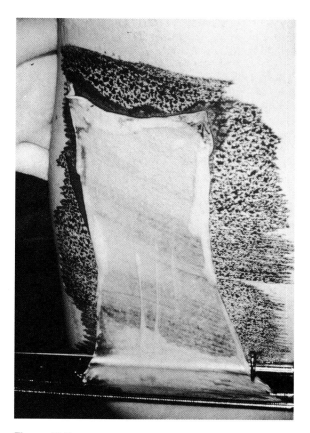

Figure 15.6

A split-thickness skin graft of appropriate thickness. The punctate dermal bleeding is obvious. If too thick a graft is taken, there is less bleeding.

should be alerted before cutting is commenced as a lightly anaesthetized patient may move. Regional block (for example, the lateral cutaneous nerve of the thigh), local infiltration or anaesthetic cream applied for not less than 60 minutes can be used. Most split-skin grafts are cut with a free-hand knife, this commonly being the Watson modification of the Humbie knife. A roller is attached to the knife and the distance between the roller and the blade can be varied by means of a calibration device to permit the cutting of skin grafts of various thickness. Calibration may vary from one knife to another and therefore it is essential that the surgeon visually checks the distance between the roller and the blade keeping in mind that when a medium-thickness split-skin graft is required the slit should be just enough to admit a number 10 surgical blade, a readily available thickness gauge. Graft thickness can also be judged by the type of bleeding observed at the graft donor site (Figure 15.6). Skin grafts leave multiple small bleeding points, whereas deeper cutting leaves fewer bleeding points. Exposure of fat means that a full-thickness graft has inadvertently been taken. Skin varies in thickness depending on the region, age and sex of the patient. A given thickness of split-skin graft harvesting may represent only a small proportion of the total skin thickness on the back of an adult male, whereas on the thigh of an elderly emaciated female it could mean almost the entire thickness of the skin. This fact should be remembered whenever skin grafts are cut.

Split-skin grafts should be used as sheets wherever possible and ideally one sheet should cover the whole defect. Grafts can be meshed by placing them on a disposable plastic sheet that can be advanced through a special graft mesher. Meshed grafts are particularly useful in situations where there is a limitation of the number of donor sites. This may occur in massive degloving injuries or burns. They also allow free drainage in wounds which are expected to ooze and they are very useful when covering an irregular surface.

Preparation of split-skin graft beds

Adequate preparation of the recipient bed onto which a split-skin graft is to be placed is essential. Haemostasis is essential for graft survival. Haematoma acts as a barrier between the graft and its bed, preventing vascularization. Minor oozing usually stops following the application of a split-skin graft and a few strategically placed perforations in a sheet of split-skin graft can be helpful. However, if profuse bleeding persists despite adequate pressure and the judicious use of a bipolar coagulator, then the wound should be dressed with wet saline soaks and skin grafting deferred for 48 hours.

The vascularity of the recipient bed is also important. Tissues with a limited blood supply such as bare bone, cartilage or tendon do not accept grafts. If such a bed is to be covered, it is strongly recommended that a flap be used. The use of split-skin graft on bare cortical bone is one of the commonest causes of post-traumatic osteomyelitis. The vascularity of radiation beds and that of ulcers due to vasculitis associated with autoimmune diseases can be very deceptive. In the former condition, flaps should be used and aggressive medical management for the latter condition should be considered.

Where there is granulation tissue in the recipient bed, this must be free of pus and should have a healthy pink-to-beefy red appearance. Epithelial migration at the edges of the granulating surface may be a sign that the wound is ready for grafting. All granulating tissues contain bacteria, but not all are infected. However, the isolation of β-haemolytic *Streptococcus* group A is a contraindication for skin grafting. Failure also follows the application of skin grafts to beds with heavy growths of other pathogenic bacteria. Unhealthy granulating wounds can be quickly and safely prepared by shaving them with a Watson skin-grafting knife and cutting them back to a healthy base. Shaving also results in a reduction of bacterial load.

Split-skin graft application

Close immobile contact is essential for graft survival. When split-skin graft is applied to a healthy bed, it adheres very quickly due to the conversion of wound fibrinogen into fibrin by tissue factors. Stitching may not be necessary when the whole defect is covered by a single sheet of graft with overlap of the edges. The use of metal clips is a quick method of fixation when extensive grafting is undertaken. Dissolvable sutures may also be used.

Grafts may be left exposed or dressed. In the closed method Vaseline gauze and fluffed gauze are applied followed by circumferential compression with crêpe bandages in the extremities and tie over dressings in awkward places such as the axilla. The delayed exposure technique may be used in cooperative patients as limited movement may be allowed. Complete failure of grafting despite an adequate recipient bed and close immobile contact should suggest a possibility that the graft has been placed upside-down. Mobilization of patients with leg grafts is usually permitted after 7–10 days. Earlier mobilization may be associated with blistering or haematoma formation under the graft and may result in failure.

Donor site care and causes of delayed healing

After a split-skin graft is cut, damp pads are applied to control oozing. The site is then covered with a fine mesh Vaseline gauze or Kaltostat which may be soaked in 0.5% marcaine with adrenaline. Generous amounts of fluffed gauze or Gamgee are secured on top of this by crêpe bandages. Patients must be warned that split-skin graft cutting, particularly of thick grafts, may leave scars that are permanently visible. The more superficial the graft, the faster the donor site will heal. A median-thickness split-skin graft donor site takes 10–12 days to epithelialize. It is essential to remember that the new epithelium on a split-skin graft donor site is not durably attached to the underlying dermis in the early stages and removal of the dressings can easily tear the fragile epithelium.

Changes in skin grafts following a successful 'take'

There are a number of changes which occur in skin grafts following a successful take on a recipient bed. These include graft contraction. Here the covered wound bed contracts and the graft follows. Contraction is less when the wound is relatively immobile such as on the shin or skull periosteum. Contraction can be reduced by using full-thickness grafts or including a thick dermal component in a split-skin graft. It can also be reduced by applying a split-skin graft to a fresh, rather than an actively granulating, wound with a high population of myofibroblasts. In addition, contraction is less if the graft site is splinted for 4–6 months. However, in the trauma situation this may well interfere with joint function.

Split-skin grafts often develop significantly dark pigmentation especially in dark-skinned patients. Exposure to sunshine during the first six months post-operatively should be avoided. In addition, both donor and graft sites may scale and remain itchy and dry for many months because the lubricating sebaceous glands have been temporarily devitalized. Lubrication with a bland aqueous or E45 cream should be recommended for six months after the operation.

In contrast to full-thickness grafts which grow successfully in children, the growth of split-skin grafts may be limited and therefore revisions and releases may be necessary. Protective sensation is recovered as early as 1–2 months after 'take' but grafts placed on muscles and periosteum do not acquire satisfactory sensation.

Flaps

A flap, in contradistinction to a split-skin graft, contains a pedicle attachment to the body receiving its sustenance via a network of blood vessels. Because of its independent blood supply, a flap can be used to reconstruct skin and soft-tissue defects irrespective of the vascularity of their beds. Because of this, it is the most common method of closing the soft-tissue defects associated with severe open fractures of the lower leg, ankle or hindfoot.

For half a century flaps were raised without any precise knowledge of the vessels on which they were based. Their design was restricted by a set of rigid length to width ratios calculated for different regions of the body. During the past two decades, there has been an intensive reappraisal of the vascular anatomy of the integument following publication of previously described maps of vascular territories and additional knowledge gained from injection studies in cadavers, some of which is detailed in Chapter 14. This knowledge has stimulated a dramatic increase in the number and types of flaps available to the reconstructive surgeon and has caused a revolution in the use of flaps which has resulted in a jargon which is particularly confusing to non-plastic surgeons. The following *aide-mémoire* provides a simplified approach to this problem.

The five C's of a flap

A flap may be described by five C's. This is illustrated in Figure 15.7. The five C's detail the flap's anatomical Component, Circulatory pattern,

Component

Circulatory Pattern

Configuration

Contiguity

Conditioning

Figure 15.7

The five C's of a skin flap.

Configuration, Contiguity to the defect and whether it has been Conditioned prior to elevation to tolerate ischaemia or perform a particular task.

Component

Although most defects can be reconstructed using a simple skin flap, the choice has now been broadened to include fasciocutaneous, muscle, myocutaneous and composite flaps (Figure 15.8). This enables the surgeon to reconstruct more complex skin and soft-tissue defects in one stage with minimal donor site morbidity. The use of muscle flaps represents a major breakthrough in reconstructive surgery. A muscle may be detached at one end away from the vascular hilum and transposed to cover, for example, an exposed joint or fracture site. The muscle itself is then covered with a partial-thickness skin graft

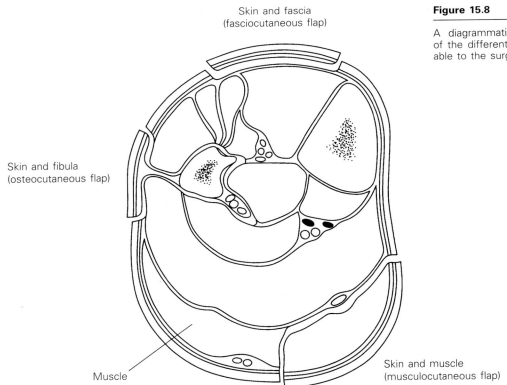

Skin and fascia
(fasciocutaneous flap)

Skin and fibula
(osteocutaneous flap)

Muscle

Skin and muscle
(musculocutaneous flap)

Figure 15.8

A diagrammatic representation of the different flap types available to the surgeon.

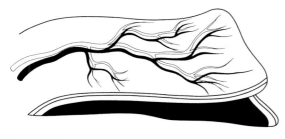

Figure 15.9

An axial pattern flap.

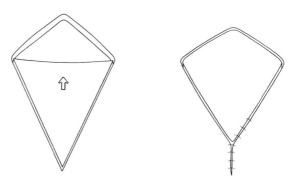

Figure 15.11

A basic V–Y advancement flap.

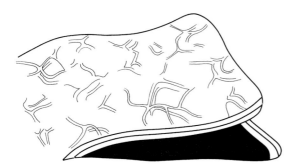

Figure 15.10

A random pattern flap.

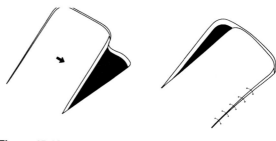

Figure 15.12

A basic transposition flap.

achieving satisfactory cosmesis with minimal donor site morbidity. It is worth remembering that muscle flap viability may be compromised in the severely traumatized limb either by direct damage to the muscle belly or through disruption of the proximal vascular pedicle.

The principle of the muscle flap has been extended by including the overlying skin. Myocutaneous flaps are reliable but leave a conspicuous donor site deficit unless this can be directly closed as with the latissimus dorsi and tensor fascia lata free flaps. The viability of lower limb skin transfer can be enhanced considerably by including the deep fascia in the transfer, this being called a 'fasciocutaneous flap'.

Circulation

An understanding of the cutaneous vascular patterns is essential in the planning of the skin flap. The skin receives its blood supply from the subdermal plexus which in turn is perfused from a number of sources including direct cutaneous as well as perforator vessels from the underlying muscles. A flap is said to have an axial pattern (Figure 15.9) when there is an anatomically recognizable set of vessels which provide input and outflow. This system courses parallel to the skin providing numerous side branches. The high vascular reserve of such a flap makes it safer, more robust and capable of coping with adverse circumstances. A flap which receives its blood supply through the cutaneous subdermal plexus and has no focal point where arterial input and venous outflow are recognizably concentrated is called a random pattern flap (Figure 15.10). The perfusion pressure at the distal end of such a flap is critical and the flap is subject to limitations in its dimensions.

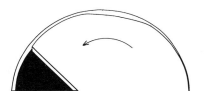

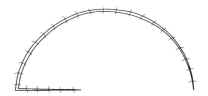

Figure 15.13

A basic rotation flap.

Configuration

The shape of a flap dictates its movement. For example, a V–Y flap can be advanced into a defect by moving it directly forward without any lateral movement (Figure 15.11). A transposition flap is rectangular and is adjacent to, and extends beyond, the defect to ensure movement without tension (Figure 15.12). The donor site is usually closed by a skin graft. This is the standard design of a proximally based fasciocutaneous lower-leg flap. A rotation flap is semicircular and rotates about a pivot point (Figure 15.13). To ensure primary closure of a donor site, the flap should be quite large with a circumference of about six times the width of the defect. Correct design of these flaps is crucial to avoid tension. They should always be planned with a margin of reserve as skimping may create difficulties. An axial patterned flap can be completely islanded by skeletonizing its vascular pedicle and therefore offering a wider arc of movement and better inset. An island flap can be transferred by microsurgical means to a distant site.

Contiguity

Flaps can be divided into local or distant flaps on the basis of the proximity of donor and recipient sites. Local skin flaps composed of tissues lying adjacent to the defect usually match the skin at the recipient site in terms of colour, texture, thickness and hair type. Flaps transferred from a distance can be divided into direct, tube or free. A *direct flap*, such as a cross leg flap, allows approximation of the donor and recipient sites. If the two sites cannot be approximated the alternative is either *tube flap migration* or a *microvascular free flap*. Recent advances in microvascular surgery have enabled the transfer of *free axial patterned skin* and muscle flaps from a distant site in one operation and this has largely superseded other methods of distant flap transfer. Successful free-flap transfer offers the ultimate challenge and requires flawless decision making to ensure a high success rate.

Conditioning

The ischaemic insult suffered by the flap because of elevation can cause considerable metabolic problems. Despite the increased sophistication of flap design a significant number of skin flaps show signs of ischaemia. With random pattern flaps the small safety margin can be increased by 'conditioning the flap' to tolerate the ischaemic insult of elevation by using the delay principle. This is achieved by surgically outlining the flap a week prior to its actual transfer. In theory flap robustness can also be increased by pharmacological manipulation of the cutaneous circulation.

Indications for flap repair

As with other types of surgery, indications for a particular technique in traumatic plastic surgery are frequently relative. However, there are a number of situations where flaps should be used in preference to other methods of soft-tissue closure.

1. Flaps are indicated for the repair of defects associated with poor vascular beds such as wounds overlying the tibia, exposed fractures in other locations, exposed metal plates, bare bone and tendons, bone defects and open joints.
2. They should be used if delayed bone or soft-tissue reconstruction is proposed. This is particularly important if bone grafting or tendon transfer will be required at a later date as these procedures cannot be carried out under split-skin grafts.

3. They provide padding over bony prominences such as the shin or plantar surface of the heel.
4. Flap transfer allows for complex reconstructions such as the use of a neurovascular island flap to restore sensation and the use of composite osteomyocutaneous flaps to facilitate closure of a large bone defect.

Flap selection

The choice of a particular flap will depend on a number of parameters including:

1. Robustness and reserve of safety.
2. Ease of surgical dissection.
3. Cosmetic and functional donor site morbidity.
4. Logistics.

These concepts will be discussed further in Chapters 16 and 17, but if the example of an open fracture of a tibia is used (Figure 15.2), a fasciocutaneous flap is easy to execute and has a good vascular reserve but leaves a very conspicuous donor site deficit. A rectus abdominis free flap is technically more demanding but the flap may be contoured to give an excellent cosmetic result with minimal scarring in the donor site area.

Flap necrosis and prevention

Partial or complete loss of a flap is not uncommon. Poor flap choice and design is probably the most common cause of flap necrosis. Underestimating the size of the defect results in an inadequate flap with unacceptable tension on inset. The elevation of previously irradiated or degloved skin could decompensate a precarious local circulation. Other causes of flap loss include intra-operative technical errors, especially where flaps require complex anatomical dissections, and post-operative external compression by dressings, kinking of the flap pedicle, haematomata and vessel thrombosis.

References

Byrd HS, Spicer TE, Cierny G (1985) Management of open tibial fractures, *Plast Reconstr Surg* **76**: 719–28.

Godina M (1986) Early microsurgical reconstruction of complex trauma of the extremities, *Plast Reconstr Surg* **78**: 285–92.

Yaremchuk MJ (1986) Acute management of severe soft tissue damage accompanying open fractures of the lower extremity, *Clin Plast Surg* **13**: 621–32.

16
Local flaps

A.A. Quaba

It was a common experience of the early pioneers of plastic surgery that flaps that survived well elsewhere on the body commonly failed when applied to soft-tissue defects on the leg, particularly when the skin defects were associated with difficult problems such as open fractures or chronic osteomyelitis. For several decades, the traditional advice was to avoid the use of local flaps below the knee unless the defects were small and the surgeon prepared to use special techniques such as delay incisions (Bowen and Meares 1974). When treating any sizeable defect below the knee, the reconstructive surgeon had to rely on cross-leg flaps and flaps transferred from a distance using the tube pedicle technique. In experienced hands, it was possible to get good results (Morris and Buchan 1978) but the disadvantages, particularly in the trauma situation, can be easily appreciated. In an excellent review article, Dawson (1972) analysed the complications encountered in 99 cross-leg flap procedures. He documented local flap necrosis in 40% and infection in 28% of the flaps.

Ger (1970, 1971) introduced and popularized the use of split-skin grafted transposed muscle flaps for reconstruction of the lower extremities. By the early 1980s, a large variety of these muscle flaps were in use not only in the lower extremities but for reconstructions all over the body (Nahai and Mathes 1982). Unfortunately, the area least well served by these muscle flaps is the lower third of the leg. In this area many muscles become tendinous and the muscle bulk available for transposition is small.

The fasciocutaneous flap was reported by Ponten (1981) who suggested that long narrow flaps could be raised safely from the knee down to the foot as long as the deep fascia was included. Ponten's flaps were not based on specific perforators and therefore could not be islanded. Following extensive use, it was soon realized that this flap was unsuitable for the management of difficult soft-tissue defects in the lower third of the leg. Chatre and Quaba (1987) reviewed the results of 100 Ponten fasciocutaneous flaps used between 1981 and 1986 for the management of soft-tissue defects in the leg. Sixteen per cent of the flaps were used for proximal third defects, 52% for middle third defects and the remaining 32% for distal third defects. It was found that the overall flap necrosis rate was 8% but the necrosis rate of flaps raised to cover defects in the lower third of the leg was 25%. This is clearly unacceptable and demonstrates the fact that the Ponten flap is inappropriate in this location.

The paucity of muscles available for transfer in the lower third of the leg coupled with the unreliability of local proximally based fasciocutaneous flaps meant that free flaps came to dominate the scene in reconstructions of the lower third of the leg, ankle and hindfoot. In the 1980s, free-flap transfers became more reliable for a number of reasons. Surgeons discovered the usefulness of easily dissected flaps with large and predictable pedicles such as the latissimus dorsi and rectus abdominis flaps. These flaps were much easier to use than the groin flaps popularized in the 1970s. In addition, advances in microsurgical techniques allowed surgeons to perform microsurgical repairs outside the zone of injury with its associated intimal damage, and the use of clinically proven end-to-side anastomoses coupled with improved pharmacological management reduced the incidence of vessel spasm and flap necrosis. Surgeons also discovered the importance of performing early free-flap cover before the wounds became heavily colonized or infected.

Despite the obviously excellent results reported by Godina (1986), Yaremchuk et al (1987) and others who showed that free-tissue transfer for complex lower extremity trauma could be carried out successfully, it is accepted that consistently good results depend on dedicated highly skilled teams, special instrumentation, open unscheduled theatre time and a steady flow of cases. It is therefore not surprising that the search for easier and safer lower third flaps continues.

Ponten's description of fasciocutaneous flaps stimulated great interest in the cutaneous circulation of the lower extremities (Chapter 14) and in alternatives to the rigid traditional flap design. Of particular significance were the description of the septocutaneous vessels (Carriquiry et al 1985) and the extension of the concept of the distally based flap (Song et al 1982) to the leg. Two types of distally based fasciocutaneous flaps were described and used. The first type was a distally based fasciocutaneous flap comparable to the radial forearm flap described by Song et al (1982). This relies on a major artery for its blood supply and the effect is to reverse the direction of blood flow in the flap (Figure 16.1). Obviously the sacrifice of one of the major arteries of a limb is associated with a number of disadvantages and the use of this type of flap was soon curtailed. The second type of distally based fasciocutaneous flap is based on a single distal perforator of the tibial or peroneal vessels and therefore the vascular axis remains intact and the normal direction of blood flow is maintained (Figure 16.1). These flaps can be rotated up to 180° with the perforator as the axis of rotation (Amarante et al 1986, Masquelet et al 1988). This flap has now become a viable alternative to microvascular reconstruction in the lower third of the leg, ankle and hindfoot.

Local flaps have a number of obvious advantages over free flaps. They can be performed expeditiously and this is of particular advantage in the management of soft-tissue defects in the multiply injured, elderly and patients with bilateral open leg or hindfoot fractures. In addition, there is no need for special instrumentation and no requirement for transfer of the patient to a specialist centre. This point is of particular importance in countries such as the United Kingdom where the majority of plastic surgery units are located distant to the principal trauma centres. In addition local flap surgery limits the scars and morbidity to one extremity.

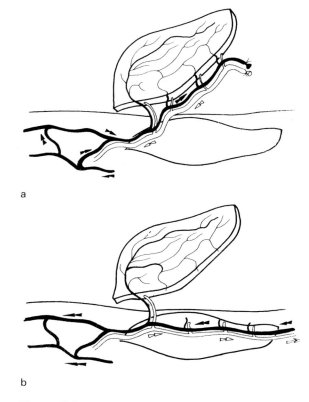

a

b

Figure 16.1

Distally based flaps. (a) The radial artery forearm flap type. The whole vascular axis is incorporated within the flap, the proximal ends of the artery and its accompanying veins being ligated. There is reversed flow within the vessels. This type of distally based flap sacrifices a major artery and its use is limited. (b) The more common type of distally based flap. Here the direction of blood flow is normal and the flap receives its blood supply through a perforator or a direct cutaneous branch which enters the flap at its distal end. Modified from Quaba and Davison (1990).

There are, however, a number of criticisms which can be levelled at the use of local flaps for the management of major soft-tissue defects in association with open fractures. The principal criticism is that the flap is raised within the zone of injury and therefore the vascular pedicle on which the flap is based could already have been damaged, risking flap failure. However, better knowledge of the vascular basis of local flaps and adequate assessment of degloving minimizes this risk. In addition local skin flaps may well interrupt superficial veins and cutaneous veins, leading to oedema and neuromata.

Free flaps can be tailored to suit massive or irregular skin defects but the design of a local flap tends to be limited by the local anatomy, availability of skin and wound orientation. In addition there is a significant deficit related to the donor site which is difficult to camouflage. With distant flaps the donor site can be hidden much more easily.

In Edinburgh the first choice of flap for reconstructing any extremity defect irrespective of its size and site is a local flap when this option is available. However, free flaps are used for massive defects, particularly those associated with degloving injuries, composite reconstructions of bone and soft tissue and also when the donor site scarring of a local flap would be unacceptable. A review of the plastic surgery management of 1000 consecutive open fractures (see Chapter 13) shows that, of the 246 patients who required plastic surgery, only 15 had to have a free flap carried out. In 77 patients, a local flap was used, this usually being either a muscle flap or a fasciocutaneous flap. The two most commonly used local flaps in Edinburgh, namely the distally based fasciocutaneous flap and the gastrocnemius flaps, will be discussed in detail. It is accepted that other surgeons will of course make use of other local flaps but these two flaps will serve to cover most soft-tissue defects in the leg, ankle and hindfoot.

Gastrocnemius muscle flaps

The gastrocnemius flap has been well described by McGraw et al (1977), Dibbell and Edstrom (1980) and Arnold and Mixter (1982). It is one of the easiest and safest flaps to raise and it is certainly the commonest flap used for covering soft-tissue defects around the knee and upper tibia. The functional deficit following its use is probably acceptable provided only one of its two heads is used in the presence of an intact soleus muscle. The gastrocnemius is usually used as a muscle flap and is subsequently covered by split-skin graft. Cosmetically this is a much more elegant reconstruction than the alternative myocutaneous version. The only advantage of

including the overlying skin is extension of the flap reach but the donor site defect is very considerable and there is a risk of loss of the distal cutaneous part of the flap.

The muscle receives most of its blood supply at the level of the knee and has no significant segmental vascular input. The medial and lateral muscle bellies receive independent supplies which enable them to be raised separately. The pedicles are well protected and unlikely to be damaged unless the injury is very considerable such as a serious fracture dislocation of the knee. However, the muscle bellies can be damaged through direct injury.

The medial boundary of the medial head of the gastrocnemius muscle is the medial border of the tibia. The medial gastrocnemius flap can therefore be raised as far medially as the medial border of the tibia and as far laterally as the midline posteriorly. The lateral flap is narrower and shorter than the medial since the lateral belly of the muscle is smaller. Its lateral boundary is the fibula and medially it again extends to the midline posteriorly. The decision as to whether to use a medial or lateral flap depends on the size and position of the defect. In general, the medial flap is more mobile and long enough to close defects even on the lateral side of the knee and is therefore preferable. Mobilization of the lateral head can be difficult due to restriction by the lateral popliteal nerve where it passes over the pedicle.

The flap should be raised under tourniquet. The easiest and most direct approach to dissection is through a midline posterior incision with the patient in the prone position. The incision may extend from the popliteal skin crease to the junction of the middle and lower thirds of the leg. Alternatively the flap may be raised while the patient is in the supine position through an appropriate extension of the existing post-excision or post-traumatic wound (Figure 16.2a). The hip should be externally rotated to facilitate dissection. The free anterior border of the flap is identified and the muscle belly separated from the soleus by sweeping a finger up and down this relatively avascular plane. The next important step is to separate the posterior border of the flap which is fused to the adjacent muscle belly. The sural nerve and accompanying artery lie roughly where the two muscle bellies need to be separated. The nerve should be freed and

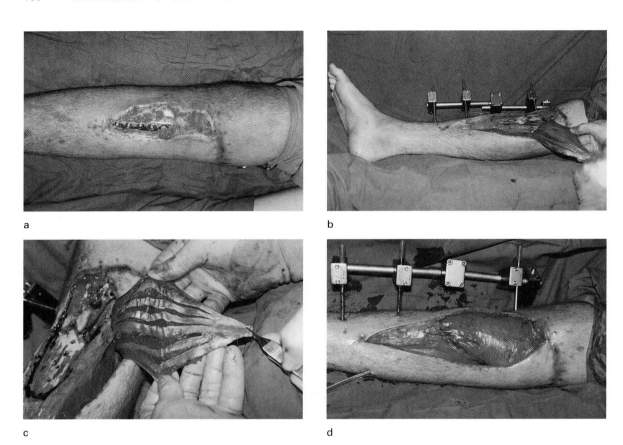

a

b

c

d

Figure 16.2

(a) The use of the medial head of the gastrocnemius flap to cover a soft-tissue defect of the proximal third of the tibia. In this patient a plate has been used to treat an open fracture of the proximal third of the tibia. (b) The initial dissection of the medial head of the gastrocnemius has been undertaken through a posterior approach, the patient having been placed in the conventional supine position on the operating table. The medial gastrocnemius has been passed through a subcutaneous tunnel to allow access to the soft-tissue defect. The fracture was stabilized with a unilateral external fixator. (c) The gastrocnemius muscle is prepared to fit the defect. This is done by scoring the fascia to allow for greater width of the muscle. (d) The defect has been covered by the medial head of the gastrocnemius muscle which has been sutured to the surrounding skin. Split-skin grafting was used to cover the flap.

pushed to one side and separation is achieved by sharp dissection starting from between the two heads of the muscle and working downwards using bipolar coagulation to seal potential bleeding points as required. The distal aponeurotic part of the muscle is separated from the Achilles tendon, freeing the lower part of the flap. Gentle finger dissection is continued superiorly to mobilize the pedicle. Occasionally, the neurovascular leash is identified to enable the femoral bony attachment of the muscle to be divided if more length of either the medial or the lateral head of the muscle is required. Some surgeons also divide the nerve to avoid undesirable muscle contraction during and after healing. The flap may be transposed directly to cover the wound or passed through a tunnel (Figure 16.2b). The reach of the flap can be extended by scoring the fascia or excising the fascia entirely to allow the muscle to gain length or width as

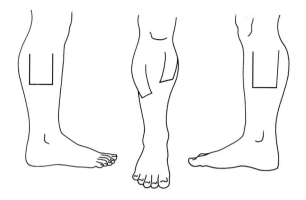

a

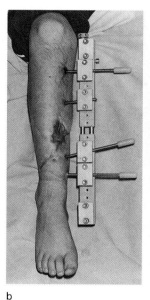

b

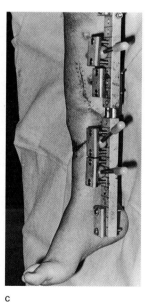

c

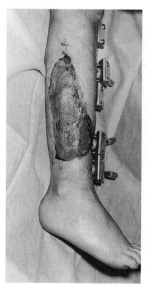

d

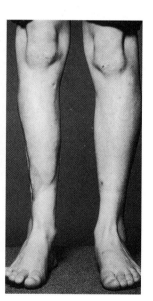

e

Figure 16.3

(a) A diagrammatic representation of the proximally based fasciocutaneous flap as described by Ponten. The flap can be raised from the medial or lateral side of the leg. (b) The use of a lateral proximally based fasciocutaneous flap is illustrated in this case. This is an adolescent boy who had a Gustilo type IIIb fracture initially treated inappropriately with split-skin grafting of a defect on the subcutaneous border of the tibia. The fracture was stabilized with a unilateral external fixator. (c) A proximally based fasciocutaneous flap was raised and used to cover the defect. (d) The donor site defect is seen on the lateral side of the leg, this being covered with split-skin graft. (e) After one year, an excellent functional result has been achieved, but cosmetic appearance of the donor site is not particularly satisfactory.

the defect dictates (Figure 16.2c). The flap is inset using multiple horizontal mattress stitches to the periphery of the defect (Figure 16.2d). The flap itself is then covered by a sheet of partial thickness skin graft which may be fenestrated.

While this flap is mainly used for soft-tissue defects around the knee and upper third of the leg the use of the medial head of the gastrocnemius for cover of soft-tissue defects in the middle third of the leg has also been reported

(Bashir 1983). In this case, the flap is distally based on communicating vessels between the two heads of the gastrocnemius. Several of these are present and the lower of them can be left as a feeding vessel. Another modification is an extension of the use of the medial head of the gastrocnemius muscle in reconstruction of the quadriceps apparatus following open injuries of the knee joint utilizing the distal tendinous part of the flap as a bridge graft (Babu et al 1994).

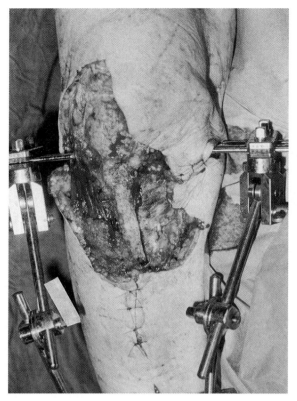

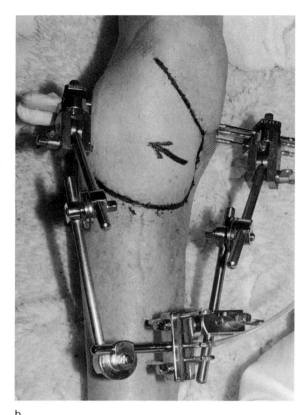

a   b

Figure 16.4

The use of a fasciocutaneous flap based on the sural artery. (a) It is difficult to cover soft-tissue defects around the knee using a conventional proximally based fasciocutaneous flap. These can be covered by raising a fasciocutaneous flap based on the sural artery. A soft-tissue defect appropriate for this type of flap is shown here. (b) The defect has been covered by the fasciocutaneous flap and an excellent cosmetic and functional result was achieved.

The proximally based fasciocutaneous flap

This is a transposition flap based on the medial or lateral aspect of the leg and is used to cover defects in the upper or middle third of the leg (Figure 16.3). A length-to-breadth ratio of about 3:1 is usually safe although higher ratios have been reported (Tolhurst et al 1983). The flap is not based on a specific septocutaneous perforator and it is therefore not safe to island it. The usual principles in designing and moving a trans-position flap are observed. The incision is made through the skin, subcutaneous tissue and fascia. The paratenon and epimysium of the donor bed are left undisturbed. Elevation is generally from distal to proximal preserving the subfascial vascular plexus on the deep surface of the flap. It is necessary to recognize and preserve the superficial peroneal nerve and, whenever possible, the sural and saphenous nerves. Their division could result in a troublesome neuroma. The subcutaneous anteromedial surface of the tibia should not be included in the planned flap donor site.

Two modifications of the original Ponten design that are particularly useful in post-traumatic reconstructions are the sural artery flap and the sliding fasciocutaneous flap. The skin bridge at the base of the standard fasciocutaneous flap can prevent adequate rotation and local deformities may be produced at the pivot point. These drawbacks, especially significant when knee cover is required, are avoided by islanding a large fasciocutaneous flap from the calf based on the sural artery (Li et al 1990). An example of the use of an islanded fasciocutaneous flap based on a sural artery is shown in Figure 16.4. Another useful modification of Ponten's flap design is the sliding fasciocutaneous flap which is based on one of the septocutaneous perforators of the lower leg. This is particularly useful for small medial ankle defects (Sinclair et al 1994).

The distally based fasciocutaneous flap

As has already been detailed there are two types of distally based fasciocutaneous flaps. The first is when an island of skin is moved from proximal to distal based on one of the three main vascular axes of the leg. An example of such a flap is the reverse pedicled anterior tibial flap which is based on septocutaneous perforators that emerge in a cleft between tibialis anterior and extensor hallucis longus and extensor digitorum longus muscles (Wee 1986, Racalde Rocha et al 1987). The anterior tibial vessels are isolated at the superior margin of the flap and transected carrying the dissection distally and incorporating the artery and its vena comitantes in the flap after elevating it from the interosseous membrane until the pivot point is reached. This is obviously a very difficult dissection and risks some damage to the motor branches in adjacent muscles as well as interrupting an important artery of the leg. The use of such a flap in the lower extremity has now largely been abandoned.

Distally based fasciocutaneous flaps based on septocutaneous perforators from the posterior tibial or peroneal arteries are easier to raise. They can be safely islanded on one perforator and its vena comitantes and they leave the main vascular axis intact. The useful perforators are those which continue in the subcutaneous tissue in a horizontal/linear fashion after an initial vertical course through the intermuscular septum and vascularize, through their multiple branches, the subdermal plexus. Flaps based on these perforators can be rotated up to 180° with the perforator as the pivot point.

Distally based peroneal island flaps

Donski and Fogestam described the first distally based fasciocutaneous flap based on the peroneal artery in a preliminary report in 1983. The technique was further refined by Valenti et al (1991) and Shalaby (1995). These flaps are based on perforators on the lateral side of the leg that arise from the peroneal artery. There are a number of laterally based perforators and the fasciocutaneous flaps that can be raised are smaller and less versatile than those based on the posterior tibial artery. They have little role in the primary management of soft-tissue defects associated with open fractures but are useful in providing soft-tissue cover for exposed lateral malleolar plates.

The distally based posterior tibial island fasciocutaneous flap

This flap has been particularly useful in reconstructing soft-tissue defects of the leg, ankle and hindfoot areas. In Edinburgh, it has become the flap of choice for such defects to the extent that free flaps are now only used for specific indications. Chapter 13 illustrates the importance of the distally based fasciocutaneous flap in orthopaedic trauma surgery but a more detailed investigation of the use of the islanded distally based fasciocutaneous flaps in the lower limb was undertaken by Erdmann et al (1994). In a five-year period, 66 distally based fasciocutaneous flaps were used of which 53 (81%) were indicated for post-traumatic soft-tissue problems. Thirty-seven (71.2%) of the flaps were used for soft-tissue defects in the lower third of the leg. A further 11 (21.2%) were used for defects in the middle third of the leg and only one (1.9%) was

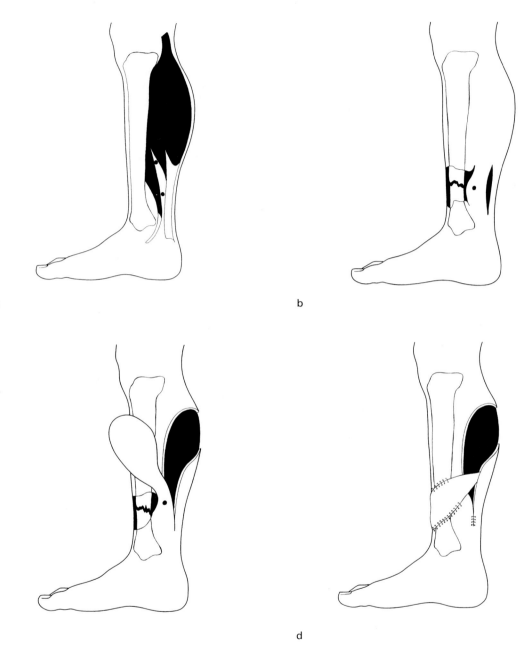

a

b

c

d

Figure 16.5

A diagrammatic representation of the operative procedure involved in raising and transposing a distally based fasciocutaneous flap. (a) Most distally based fasciocutaneous flaps are based on either the 6 mm or 12 mm perforators which are shown here. The muscles have been coloured black to illustrate their relationship to the perforators. (b) After the surgeon has decided on which perforator the flap will be based the perforator should be approached using anterior and posterior exploratory incisions. (c) The size of the desired flap is calculated and the anterior and posterior incisions extended proximally to encompass the flap which is then swung forward. (d) The flap can be islanded and moved round 180° to cover most defects in the lower leg.

used for an upper third soft-tissue defect. The remaining three (5.7%) distally based fasciocutaneous flaps were used for hindfoot defects. The commonest perforator to be used was the 12-cm perforator (Figure 16.5), this being used in 67% of the cases. The average operating time was less than two hours compared with an average of just over five hours for a free-muscle transfer and most of the surgery was carried out in the Orthopaedic Trauma Unit thereby minimizing the requirement for patient transfer. Significant flap necrosis necessitating an alternative reconstruction, usually in the form of a free-flap transfer, occurred in 7.5% of the cases. It appeared that this complication occurred mostly in patients with peripheral vascular disease or diabetes and also in patients who had had significant unrecognized degloving. There did not seem to be any correlation between major flap necrosis and the age of the patient, the specific perforator on which the flap was based or the time that had elapsed before surgery. The complication rate was considered acceptable and it was felt that the distally based fasciocutaneous flap satisfied the soft-tissue requirements for the lower third of the leg. The main criticisms of the distally based fasciocutaneous flap in this survey were twofold. The cosmetic appearance of the donor site was often unacceptable to young female patients and massive defects could not be closed by such a flap. These require free flaps. Successful use of the distally based fasciocutaneous flap relies on clinical judgement but more specifically the surgeon should be aware of the problems of local degloving and should carefully assess the state of the perforator on which the flap may be based.

Operative technique

Such is the importance of the distally based fasciocutaneous flap in the management of open fractures of the tibia that the operative technique will be described in some detail. The flap is raised with the patient in the supine position. A tourniquet should be applied to the thigh. It is helpful where possible to identify the perforators using Doppler ultrasound. These septocutaneous perforators are fairly constant, being situated about 6 and 12 cm above the tip of the medial

malleolus. The perforators are remarkably well protected within the intermuscular septum between the soleus and the flexor hallucis longus muscles. Their location is illustrated in Figure 16.5a. Experience has shown that they can only be disrupted by a very serious local injury and are in fact patent and undamaged in many Gustilo IIIb fractures.

When planning the flap, local degloving should be carefully excluded by digital palpation of the potential flap territory which is the area of skin on the medial calf between the greater and lesser saphenous veins. Usually this area escapes damage because of its protected location and the padding afforded by the underlying muscles. The flap can extend to within several centimetres of the popliteal skin crease and its width can vary from a narrow area between the greater and lesser saphenous veins to an area including most of the width of the calf. The advantage of keeping the flap within the two veins is the avoidance of damage to the accompanying cutaneous nerves, therefore minimizing the incidence of neuromata. There is no need to include any of the superficial veins in the flap and, indeed, there is a theoretical risk of increasing the venous congestion in the flap as the proximal end of any superficial vein in a distally based fasciocutaneous flap has to be ligated. The venous drainage of the flap relies on the venae comitantes which accompany the perforating arteries.

The flap can be based on either the 6 or 12 cm perforator but if the higher of the two perforators is selected a wider arc of rotation is possible. After the flap has been mapped around the appropriate vascular pedicle small anterior and posterior cuts are carried down to the deep fascia on either side of the vascular pedicle and the skin is reflected off the flexor hallucis longus anteriorly and the Achilles tendon posteriorly (Figure 16.5b). Working towards the intermuscular septum the location of the perforator is confirmed visually and hence the exact point of rotation determined. At this stage the upper limit of the flap necessary to achieve cover of a particular defect can be determined using basic plastic surgery principles. The anterior and posterior initial incisions are extended and joined at the proximal limit of the flap. Usually very few perforators are encountered above the 12 cm point and the plane is relatively avascular. The dissection is subsequently continued distally and carried through the depth of the

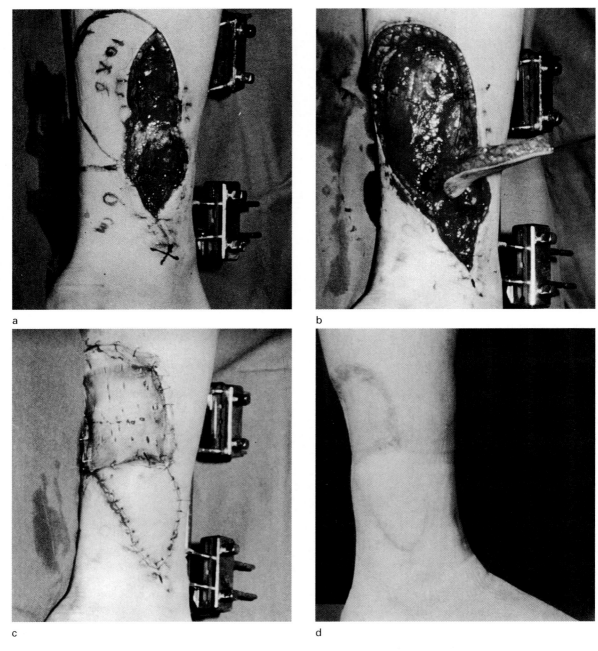

Figure 16.6

A clinical example of the use of a distally based fasciocutaneous flap. (a) The use of a distally based fasciocutaneous flap to cover a Gustilo type IIIb fracture of the distal tibia and fibula. In this case the 6 cm perforator will be used. (b) Because the flap has to be turned round through almost 180° the flap has been raised and islanded. (c) The flap is sutured into position, the donor site being covered by mesh split-skin graft. (d) After one year a satisfactory result was achieved with good patient function. However, as with the use of many distally based fasciocutaneous flaps the cosmetic appearance of the donor site leaves a little to be desired.

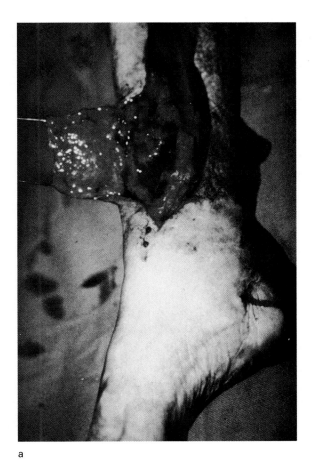

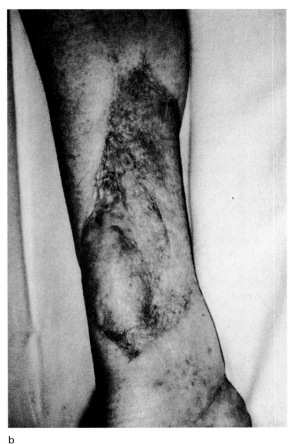

a   b

Figure 16.7

The adipofascial flap. (a) The use of an adipofascial flap in a 78-year-old lady with non-union of the lower third of the tibia. Initially the wound had been covered with split-skin grafts and this was inappropriate. After wide excision and exchange nailing had been carried out, adipofascial flap was raised and sutured into position. (b) The flap healed well as did the fracture.

intermuscular septum until the perforator is reached (Figure 16.5c). The septum distal to the site of the perforator can also be mobilized to facilitate transposition. This latter manoeuvre may not be necessary when the flap is only transposed between 30° and 45° to cover defects of the middle third of the leg. For further transposition the flap will need to be completely islanded (Figure 16.5d). This can only be achieved after careful identification of the relevant perforator and division of the skin bridge distal to it. Complete

skeletonization of the vascular pedicle is usually not necessary and is not desirable. The flap is inset over a suction drain. The part of the flap that is laid over the open fracture is usually pliable and conforms to the defect quite easily especially in the presence of a suction drain. The donor site can be grafted with a single sheet of partial thickness skin graft which can be perforated. No special flap monitoring is necessary. After wound healing and satisfactory take of the skin graft on the donor site patients may start mobilization. Obviously the amount of mobilization and weight bearing is dictated largely by the method of bone reconstruction chosen by the orthopaedic trauma surgeon as well as other factors such as the patient's age, mobilization status before the accident, extent of other injuries and general health. Support of the flap and the graft using foam compression and a tubigrip is necessary for 3–4 months to minimize flap oedema.

An illustration of the clinical use of a distally based fasciocutaneous flap is shown in Figure 16.6. This shows a Gustilo IIIb fracture of the distal third of the tibia. There is an anteromedial defect and a flap based on the 6 cm perforator has been planned (Figure 16.6a). Obviously the flap has to be swung by more than 45° and therefore it is islanded (Figure 16.6b). The flap is then placed into position with fenestrated split-skin grafts being placed on the donor site (Figure 16.6c). There were no complications and 100% 'take' of the flap was achieved. However, after one year, despite an excellent result from management of the fracture, the cosmetic appearance of the defect is perhaps less than satisfactory (Figure 16.6d). This cosmetic defect is one of the drawbacks of this type of flap. Occasionally when the soft-tissue defect is small, a modified fasciocutaneous flap without the overlying skin, the so-called 'adipofascial flap', can be used with minimal donor site defects.

The adipofascial flap

Flaps of fascia and fat have been used to provide a vascularized bed for skin grafts. They can either be based on the edge of the wound and are of the random pattern design (Lai et al 1991, 1992, Sarhadi and Quaba 1993) or designed to receive their blood supply from a recognized blood vessel, this usually being a perforator adjacent to the defect (Lin et al 1992, Tarar and Quaba 1995). The random pattern turnover adipofascial flap receives its blood supply from the narrow rim of attachment of its base adjacent to the soft-tissue defect through which vessels pass from the fascial and subcutaneous plexi (Figure 16.7). Increased vascularity of the edges of a chronic or sub-acute wound may provide additional communication channels. The flap is a quick and easy one-stage procedure and can be used to cover small or medium-sized defects in the absence of infection. It allows for some flexibility in planning and it has minimal donor site morbidity. However, it is of little use in the acute trauma situation and its use is mainly for late post-traumatic reconstruction.

In the axial pattern variety a flap is nourished by a perforator adjacent to the defect and therefore a larger flap with a narrow base can be raised. The proximity of the perforators to the tibial shaft means such a flap could be used to cover open tibial fractures, particularly in the distal third of the leg. This flap can be used for early cover of open fractures but not uncommonly partial loss of the skin grafts on the transplanted flap occurs resulting in delayed healing although this does not usually compromise the outcome of the reconstruction.

Flap cover for other open fractures

Malleolar fractures

Chapter 13 indicates the importance of plastic surgery in the management of the open ankle fractures, illustrating that almost 55% of all open ankle fractures require plastic surgery. In addition to the distally based fasciocutaneous flap, a number of reconstructive options are available including the adipofascial flap, the sliding fasciocutaneous flap and the extensor digitorum brevis muscle flap islanded on the dorsalis pedis axis (Giordano 1995).

Femoral and pelvic fractures

It is most unusual that open fractures of the femur or pelvis need flap cover although occasionally supracondylar fractures of the femur do require the use of a flap. Occasionally supracondylar fractures of the femur associated with disruption of the quadriceps mechanism need resurfacing and this could be achieved using an extended gastrocnemius or sural artery flap or an extended biceps femoris musculocutaneous flap (Quaba et al 1988). However, the size of the defect

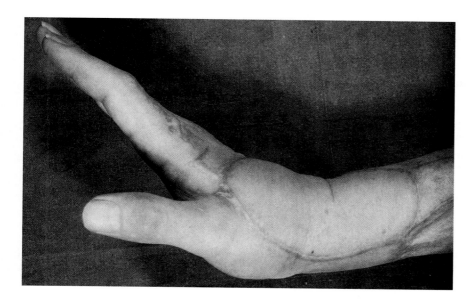

Figure 16.8

The use of a reversed forearm flap to cover a defect on the dorsal radial aspect of the hand and wrist.

in this particular injury may be such that micro-surgical tissue transfer is required.

Exposed fractures of the pelvis can be covered by a number of available regional flaps, the most useful of them being the inferiorly based rectus abdominis muscle covered by split thickness skin grafts. This flap is based on the inferior epigastric artery and is safe and easy to raise (Vergote et al 1993).

Fractures of the wrist and dorsum of hand

These can be covered using a reverse forearm flap based on the radial, ulnar or posterior interosseous arteries. An example of this type of flap is shown in Figure 16.8.

Fractures of the radius and ulna

Significant exposure of fractures of these bones is very uncommon unless the injury is very severe. In this case free-tissue transfer is more appropriate.

Fractures around the elbow

The extensor aspect of the elbow is not uncommonly damaged either as a direct result of the injury or following operative intervention. The lack of subcutaneous tissue on the extensor aspect of the elbow makes it particularly susceptible to significant soft-tissue loss. Suitable local flaps include distally based lateral or medial arm flaps based on adjacent perforators. These flaps can be completely islanded and their donor site may be closed directly. A good regional flap is a proximally based radial forearm flap and this may incorporate a tendon such as that of the brachioradialis which can be useful in restoring continuity of the triceps mechanism. The latissimus dorsi muscle flap has been used as a pedicle flap but it has to be pushed to its limit to reach the distal part of the elbow, risking significant necrosis and failure of reconstruction.

Results of the use of local flaps

There are as yet very few papers in the literature dealing with the results of the use of modern local flaps in trauma. This is perhaps understandable in that these flaps have only been in use for about ten years and surgeons have been more concerned with discovering new flaps and determining their use in the management of open fractures rather than detailing the results. The results of Erdmann et al (1994) have already been mentioned. They considered that distally based fasciocutaneous flaps were appropriate in the management of open fractures although they did stress the problems associated with graft size and cosmesis. Hallock (1989) documented the use of 41 local fasciocutaneous flaps for coverage of wounds in the lower legs. He had a 7.3% incidence of flap necrosis and felt that fasciocutaneous flaps provided a realistic option to free flaps. Keating et al (1994) documented the use of distally based fasciocutaneous flaps in the treatment of 26 open fractures of the distal third of the tibia. There were eight Gustilo type II injuries and 18 Gustilo type III fractures. Intramedullary nailing was performed in 20 cases, the remaining six fractures being managed by external fixation. Only two flaps underwent edge necrosis, both of which healed without further surgery. Bone union was achieved at an average time appropriate for the Gustilo grading of the fracture and it was felt that the combination of reamed intramedullary nails and distally based fasciocutaneous flaps was an appropriate treatment for open fractures of the distal third of the tibia.

References

Amarante J, Costa H, Reis J, Soares R (1986) A new distally based fasciocutaneous flap of the leg, *Br J Plast Surg* **39**: 338–40.

Arnold PG, Mixter RC (1983) Making the most of the gastrocnemius muscles, *Plast Reconstr Surg* **72**: 38–48.

Babu NV, Chittaranjan S, Abraham G, Bhattacharjee S, Prem H, Korula RJ (1994) Reconstruction of the quadriceps apparatus following open injuries to the knee joint using pedicled gastrocnemius musculotendinous unit as a bridge graft, *Br J Plast Surg* **47**: 190–3.

Bashir AH (1983) Inferiorly based gastrocnemius muscle flap in the treatment of war wounds of the middle and lower thirds of the leg, *Br J Plast Surg* **36**: 307–9.

Bowen J, Meares A (1974) Delayed local flaps, *Br J Plast Surg* **27**: 167–70.

Carriquiry C, Costa MA, Vasconez LO (1985) An anatomic study of the septocutaneous vessels of the leg, *Plast Reconstr Surg* **76**: 354–63.

Chatre MG, Quaba AA (1987) *Fasciocutaneous Flaps in Lower Leg Reconstructions: Experience with 100 flaps.* British Association of Plastic Surgeons Summer Meeting, Edinburgh.

Dawson RLG (1972) Complications of the cross leg flap operation, *Proc R Soc Med* **65**: 626–9.

Dibbell DG, Edstrom LE (1980) The gastrocnemius myocutaneous flap, *Clin Plast Surg* **7**: 45–50.

Donski PK, Fogdestam I (1983) Distally based fasciocutaneous flap from the sural region. A preliminary report, *Scand J Plast Reconstr Surg* **17**: 191–6.

Erdmann N, Quaba AA, Court-Brown CM (1994) *Islanded Distally Based Fasciocutaneous Flaps in the Lower Limb* (British Association of Plastic Surgeons: London).

Ger R (1970) The management of open fracture of the tibia with skin loss, *J Trauma* **10**: 112–21.

Ger R (1971) The technique of muscle transposition in the operative treatment of traumatic and ulcerative lesions of the leg, *J Trauma* **11**: 502–10.

Giordano PA (1995) Extensor digitorum brevis island flap for soft tissue coverage in the lower leg, ankle and foot, *Plast Surg Tech* **1**: 21–8.

Godina M (1986) Early microsurgical reconstruction of complex trauma of the extremities, *Plast Reconstr Surg* **78**: 285–92.

Hallock GG (1989) Local fasciocutaneous flaps for cutaneous coverage of lower extremity wounds, *J Trauma* **29**: 1240–4.

Keating JF, Court-Brown CM, Quaba AA (1994) *Open Tibial Fractures* (American Academy of Orthopaedic Surgeons: New Orleans).

Lai CS, Lin SD, Yang CC, Chou CK (1991) Adipofascial turn-over flap for reconstruction of the dorsum of the foot, *Br J Plast Surg* **44**: 170.

Lai CS, Lin SD, Chow CK (1992) Clinical application of the adipofascial turnover flap in the leg and ankle, *Ann Plast Surg* **29**: 70–5.

Li Z, Liu K, Lin Y, Li L (1990) Lateral sural cutaneous artery island flap in the treatment of soft tissue defects at the knee, *Br J Plast Surg* **43**: 546–50.

Lin SD, Lai CS, Chow CK, Tsai CW (1992) The distally based posterior tibial arterial adipofascial flap, *Br J Plast Surg* **45**: 284–7.

Masquelet AC, Beverage J, Romana C, Gerber C (1988) The lateral supra-malleolar flap, *Plast Reconstr Surg* **81**: 74–81.

McGraw JB, Dibbell DJ, Carraway JH (1977) Clinical definition of independent myocutaneous vascular territories, *Plast Reconstr Surg* **60**: 341–52.

Morris AM, Buchan AC (1978) The place of the cross leg flap in reconstructive surgery of the lower leg and foot: a review of 165 cases, *Br J Plast Surg* **31**: 138–42.

Nahai S, Mathes S (1982) *Principles of Myocutaneous Flaps* (Mosby Inc: St Louis).

Ponten B (1981) The fasciocutaneous flap. Its use in soft tissue defects of the lower leg, *Br J Plast Surg* **34**: 215–20.

Quaba AA, Davison PM (1990) The distally-based dorsal hand flap, *Br J Plast Surg* **43**: 28–39.

Quaba AA, Chapman R, Hackett MEJ (1988) Extended application of the biceps femoris musculocutaneous flap, *Plast Reconstr Surg* **81**: 91–105.

Racalde Rocha JF, Gilbert A, Masquelet A, Yousif NJ (1987) The anterior tibial artery flap: Anatomic study and clinical application, *Plast Reconstr Surg* **79**: 396–406.

Sahardi NS, Quaba AA (1993) Experience with the adipofascial turnover flap, *Br J Plast Surg* **46**: 307–13.

Shalaby HA (1995) A distally based peroneal island flap, *Br J Plast Surg* **48**: 23–6.

Sinclair JS, Gordon DJ, Small GO (1994) The sliding fasciocutaneous flap, *Br J Plast Surg* **47**: 369–71.

Song GR, Gao Y, Song Y, Yu Y, Song Y (1982) The forearm flap, *Clin Plast Surg* **9**: 21–6.

Tarar MN, Quaba AA (1995) An adipofascial turnover flap for soft tissue cover around the clavicle, *Br J Plast Surg* **48**: 161–4.

Tolhurst DE, Haeseker B, Zeeman RJ (1983) The development of the fasciocutaneous flap and the clinical application, *Plast Reconstr Surg* **71**: 597–605.

Valenti PH, Masquelet AC, Romana C, Nordin JY (1991) Technical refinement of the lateral supra-malleolar flap, *Br J Plast Surg* **44**: 459–62.

Vergote T, Revol M, Servant JM, Banzet P (1993) Use of the inferiorly based rectus abdominis flap for inguinal and perineal coverage – low pressure zone concept, *Br J Plast Surg* **46**: 168–72.

Wee JTK (1986) Reconstruction of the lower leg and foot with the reverse pedicled anterior tibial flap: Preliminary report of a new fasciocutaneous flap, *Br J Plast Surg* **39**: 327–37.

Yaremchuk MJ, Brumback RJ, Manson PN, Burgess AR, Poka A, Weiland AJ (1987) Acute and definite management of traumatic osteocutaneous defects of the lower extremity, *Plast Reconstr Surg* **80**: 1–14.

17
Free flaps

M.J. Salahuddin, J.D. Frame, A.A. Quaba and C.M. Court-Brown

Microvascular free flaps represent one of the most significant advances in the management of severe open long-bone fractures in the last 20 years. Chapter 1 illustrated the major problem facing all orthopaedic traumatologists before the era of microvascular surgery and free-flap transfer, namely what to do with the large soft-tissue defect associated with severe open long-bone fractures. The early plastic surgery techniques of tube pedicle flaps and cross-leg flaps were clearly inappropriate for the management of trauma and until the recent introduction of more sophisticated local flaps and microvascular free flaps, surgeons were forced to treat post-traumatic soft-tissue defects by repeated debridement, dressing changes and eventual split-skin grafting. Failure of this form of treatment was almost inevitable and amputation rates were high. Even when limb conservation was successful, the results were usually poor.

There have also been considerable recent advances in the use of local flaps, these being detailed in Chapter 16. There is much debate between plastic surgeons as to whether local or free flaps should be used in certain situations. However, we believe that just as orthopaedic traumatologists should be proficient in all methods of fracture stabilization so plastic surgeons who undertake the reconstruction of post-traumatic soft-tissue defects should be able to perform both local and free flaps successfully. Success will not necessarily follow a surgeon being proficient in one operation, but rather he or she should have a more flexible approach and base the decision as to which flap is appropriate on the particular characteristics of the patient and their injuries. Chapter 13 analyses the use of free flaps in the Edinburgh Orthopaedic Trauma Unit. This clearly shows the unit's preference for fasciocutaneous flaps, but this is not true of all centres and many authors have advocated the use of free-tissue transfer for the management of soft-tissue defects associated with severe open fractures (Godina 1986, Yaremchuk 1986, Melissinos and Parks 1989, Small and Mollan 1992, Campbell et al 1992).

Free-tissue transfer using microvascular techniques is now a well-established surgical procedure. Its use has expanded rapidly since 1973 when Daniel and Taylor reported the free transfer of groin skin and subcutaneous fat. The greatest proponent of microsurgical reconstruction of complex extremity trauma was undoubtedly Marko Godina of Ljubljana, Yugoslavia. He documented the results of a very aggressive policy of immediate radical debridement and early free-tissue transfer. There is no doubt that following the work of Godina and others free-tissue transfer now offers a readily available method of covering any exposed surface, reconstructing a limb and improving the cosmesis of a limb after an open fracture.

It must be understood by both plastic and orthopaedic surgeons that free-tissue transfer is only one of a number of surgical techniques which are required to treat fractures. Advances in the techniques of fracture stabilization are described elsewhere in this book, but it is also important to stress that advances in our understanding of the vascular anatomy of soft tissue and bone as well as advances in anaesthesia, microsurgical equipment and post-operative intensive care have all contributed to improved results. Increasing cooperation between plastic surgeons and orthopaedic traumatologists is vital if progress is to be maintained (Meyer and Evans 1990, BOA/BAPS Report 1993).

Free-tissue transfer to cover open fractures can be safely performed in children (Arnez and Hanel 1991), adults (Godina 1986, Melissinos and Parks 1989), the elderly (Bonawitz et al 1991) and even selected patients with diabetes (Cooley et al 1992)

and peripheral vascular disease (Shestak and Jones 1991). There is now abundant evidence that flap cover should be carried out at an early stage, with Cierny et al (1983) showing that delay beyond seven days was associated with an increase in major and minor wound healing disturbances from 20.8% to 83.3% if flap cover was delayed until after this time. More recently, surgeons have tended to perform flap cover even earlier and Godina (1986) certainly advocated waiting no more than 72 hours. Others have disagreed with Yaremchuk (1986), stating that wound closure at 7–14 days was not associated with significant morbidity. However he, like Godina, advocated a radical debridement similar to the procedure described in Chapter 5 and it may well be that if such a debridement is performed flap cover can be delayed although nowadays most surgeons would advocate covering the defect at the relook procedure or shortly thereafter.

Nowadays free-flap surgery has been refined to the point that it often takes less than four hours to perform and in all age groups it is said to have a 95% chance of success (Melissinos and Parks 1989, Salemark 1991) although in trauma cases the success rate may be lower. There is no doubt that the early coverage of exposed bone results in faster bone union, reduced infection, fewer surgical procedures, a shorter in-patient stay and less expense (Cierny et al 1983, Godina 1986, Harris et al 1987, Katsaros et al 1988, Arnez and Hanel 1991).

Early cover of an exposed fracture can of course be accomplished by both local and free flaps. As already outlined there have been major advances in both types of cover and both procedures have their proponents. Small and Mollan (1992) have summarized the traditional view of the use of the fasciocutaneous flaps in the acute phase following severe injury. They state that it is unsafe to use fasciocutaneous flaps for up to four weeks after severe limb trauma. This is said to be because of oedema and haemorrhage superficial to the deep fascia. It is felt that there is a more extensive zone of injury around the fracture than is obvious on clinical examination, and if a flap is raised, based on a traumatized vessel in this area, it may fail. There is undoubtedly some truth in this statement and great care must be taken if local flaps are to be used acutely. However, recent work by Keating et al (1994) has shown that if care is taken then good results can

be obtained by a combination of intramedullary nailing and distally based fasciocutaneous flaps.

The other stated advantage of free flaps over local flaps is that they are said to enhance bone union. This is being claimed by a number of authors (McKibben 1978, Whiteside and Lesker 1978, Small and Mollan 1992) and it is theorized that the bone actually derives a blood supply from the muscle flaps. There is actually little clinical evidence that this is the case and the apparently improved union time associated with the use of muscle flaps may well merely be a reflection of the lower infection rate associated with good flap cover.

Although these two apparent advantages of free flaps are perhaps somewhat speculative and open to debate, there are undoubtedly a number of advantages that free flaps have over local flaps.

Advantages of free flaps

Location of defect

Chapter 13 indicates that plastic surgeons are most commonly called on to cover soft-tissue defects in the lower leg, ankle and foot. This was also demonstrated by Khouri and Shaw (1989) who documented that 47% of their free flaps were performed because of soft-tissue loss in the mid-to-distal tibia with 33% being carried out for foot and ankle problems. A further 7% of their free flaps were applied to amputation stumps to lengthen the stump and thereby permit the use of a below-knee prosthesis. This concept of improving the amputation stump using free-flap techniques is an important one and is discussed further in Chapter 23. Currently local flaps have no part to play in the reconstruction of amputation stumps and while they can be used in the management of soft-tissue defects of the lower leg, ankle and hindfoot many surgeons prefer the use of free flaps in these locations.

Size of defect

Large defects can only be covered by free flaps regardless of their location in the body. Again it is likely that large defects will be more commonly encountered in open fractures of the lower limbs.

Cosmesis

The cosmetic appearance of local flaps may well be unsatisfactory principally because of the appearance of some of the skin grafted secondary defects. Thus the surgeon may select a free flap if the patient is concerned about cosmesis. Again this is particularly true of the lower limb where the use of fasciocutaneous flaps around the hindfoot and lower leg may be cosmetically unacceptable.

Degloving injuries

Degloving injuries associated with open fractures where there is either a large soft-tissue defect or exposure of the subcutaneous border of the tibia may require a free flap to facilitate soft-tissue closure. In these circumstances local flaps are either not available or are contraindicated as it is likely that the cutaneous vascular supply has been damaged and any local flap raised is almost certain to fail.

Association with bone loss

Large soft-tissue defects associated with significant bone defects can be treated by microvascular transfer of a composite soft-tissue and bone flap. The use of vascularized bone as a graft is discussed in Chapter 19.

Types of flap

Such has been the rate of progress in the development of free flaps that much of the literature written in the last ten years is already out of date. In addition, most authors have tended to publish results dealing with a mixed collection of trauma and elective reconstruction problems and it is usually impossible to ascertain which flaps were used for trauma and which were used for other reasons. Melissinos and Parks (1989) used 17 different donor sites for free-tissue transplantation in their series of 442 cases of post-trauma reconstruction, with latissimus dorsi, tensor fasciae lata and rectus abdominis flaps being the three most common. However, in their series only 249 (56.3%) of the flaps were used to treat an acute soft-tissue defect associated with a fracture and although it is clear that latissimus dorsi and tensor fasciae lata flaps were used for this purpose the authors did not specify indications for particular flaps in acute open fracture management.

Khouri and Shaw (1989) documented the use of free flaps in 260 trauma patients of whom 91% had Gustilo IIIb or IIIc open fractures, mainly situated in the lower leg, ankle or hindfoot. They used a number of different flaps but the latissimus dorsi was used in 42% of the patients. In addition a parascapular flap was used in 21% and a rectus abdominis flap in 14% of the patients. Small and Mollan (1992) also examined the use of different flaps in the management of open tibial fractures. In 70 cases of free-tissue transfer they used a latissimus dorsi flap on 31 (44.3%) occasions. The rectus abdominis flap was used 18 (35.7%) times and the radial forearm flap eight (11.4%) times. Ten of the remaining 12 flaps were combined soft-tissue and bone flaps used to treat combined soft-tissue and bone defects. Their results closely matched the distribution of free flaps used in the Edinburgh Orthopaedic Trauma Unit as detailed in Chapter 13 and it is clear that the latissimus dorsi, rectus abdominis and radial forearm flaps are the three most useful flaps in the management of open fractures. Other flaps such as the tensor fasciae lata, scapula, groin and temporoparietal fascia flaps may be used from time to time but it is likely that they will be used for specific indications and we believe it unlikely that they will enjoy widespread use in the management of soft-tissue defects associated with open fractures. Accordingly, the latissimus dorsi, rectus abdominis and radial forearm flaps will be considered in greater detail.

Latissimus dorsi free flap

The latissimus dorsi muscle can be used as either a local or free flap. The flap was initially

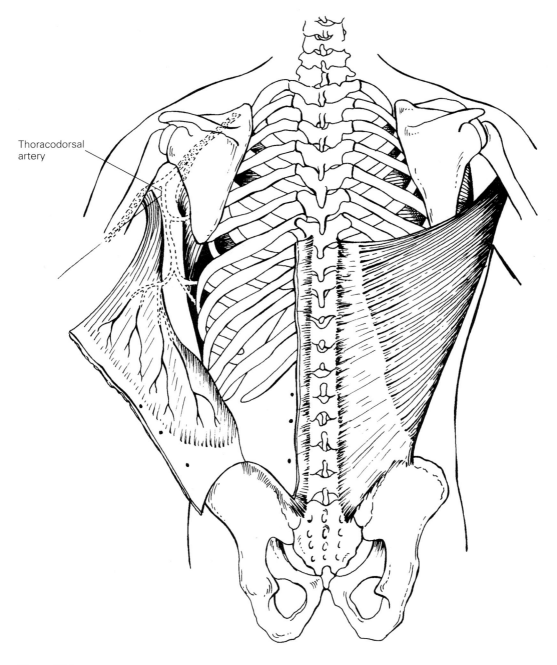

Thoracodorsal
artery

Figure 17.1

The latissimus dorsi muscle viewed from behind. On the right side, the muscle has not been mobilized and its origins and attachments are clearly seen. On the left side, the muscle has been mobilized by division of its spinal, pelvic and scapular attachments. It has been turned to show the vascular pedicle, this being the thoracodorsal artery.

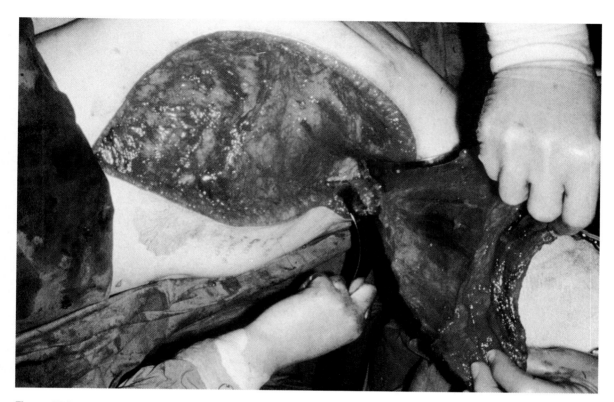

Figure 17.2

The latissimus muscle has been raised on its vascular pedicle which is clearly seen. The length of the pedicle and the size and shape of the muscle facilitate its use as a free flap.

described for reconstruction of the chest wall at the time of radical mastectomy. However, its use as a local flap has little relevance to trauma surgery. In trauma surgery, the muscle is mainly used as a motor for flexion and extension of the elbow and as a free flap for closure of large soft-tissue defects.

The latissimus dorsi muscle is a broad, thin, fan-shaped muscle with a fascial origin from the lower sixth thoracic vertebrae, the lumbar and sacral vertebrae and the posterior crest of the ileum (Figure 17.1). The anterolateral margin and the upper margin are essentially free. There is a muscular origin along the anterolateral border from the lower four ribs, this interdigitating with the external oblique muscle. There is

also a muscular origin from the tip of the scapula.

The main vascular pedicle is the thoracodorsal artery, which is a branch of the sub-scapular artery (Figure 17.1). The thoracodorsal artery is accompanied by venae comitantes and the thoracodorsal nerve. It enters the muscle on the deep surface approximately 10 cm from the insertion of the muscle into the inter-tubercular groove of the humerus. The thoracodorsal artery is usually 2–3 mm in diameter and has a pedicle as long as 10 cm. The pedicle is easily dissected, making the muscle useful for both local and free transfer.

The surgical technique is straightforward (Figure 17.2). An incision is made parallel to the anterior border of the latissimus dorsi approximately 3 cm posterior to the border. This enables the entire muscle to be dissected from its attachments and the iliac crest. Dissection is undertaken both superficial and deep to the muscle, separating it from the underlying serratus anterior. Dissection proceeds from the periphery towards the insertion of the thoracodorsal artery and its venae comitantes into the undersurface of the muscle. Care must be taken to protect the neurovascular structures but the vascular branches of the sub-scapular artery to the serratus anterior muscle are ligated and divided and subsequently the latissimus dorsi neurovascular pedicle is dissected proximally into the axilla and divided, thus providing a pedicle of sufficient length. The muscle is then positioned over the recipient site and the recipient artery and vein are dissected as close to the recipient site as possible but outside the zone of injury. The muscle is sutured into place and arterial and venous anastomosis accomplished. Usually a single artery and one or two veins are anastomosed. Vein grafts may be used if the thoracodorsal vessels will not reach the recipient vessel.

The latissimus dorsi muscle is the largest muscle in the body and obviously it can be used to cover very large defects. The use of the full muscle was, however, criticized by Godina (1987) as the large mass of muscle which overlies the proximal pedicle makes for bulky unattractive flaps. He developed the technique of tailored partial transfer of the latissimus dorsi free flap. This flap has the advantage of allowing the surgeon to design latissimus dorsi free flaps of different sizes.

The latissimus dorsi free flap can reasonably be regarded as the 'work horse' of muscle flaps. Its large size combined with Godina's modification permits different sizes of flap to be used. There are, however, a few disadvantages. A considerable amount of dissection is required and consequently seromata and haematomata may develop. The principal contraindication is in patients who have damage to the flexor and extensor muscles of the arm where the latissimus dorsi may be used to replace these muscles, although even for this problem alternative motors such as pectoralis major are available. The surgeon may also choose not to use the latissimus dorsi free flap if the patient is going to require crutches post-operatively.

One obvious potential problem is the reduction of function of the upper limb after the removal of the latissimus dorsi muscle. This was investigated by Russell et al (1986) in 24 patients. They commented that all the patients had obvious flattening of the soft tissues over the posterolateral chest wall and in 17 patients the total muscle strength of the affected shoulder was reduced. Interestingly, the authors found that the reduction affected all of the muscle groups around the shoulder. The range of motion was lessened by 0.9–44.8% in 18 patients and there was an average 6.2% disability as measured with the AMA Guide. Most patients had returned to work but eight reported shoulder weakness during routine activities. Overall, 23 patients were happy with the results of the surgery. It would therefore seem that the disability resulting from the use of this large muscle is relatively slight and is certainly acceptable when compared with the benefits to the patient of using the muscle as a free flap.

Rectus abdominis flap

The other muscle to be commonly used as a free flap following trauma is the rectus abdominis muscle. This is a long strap-like muscle which arises by a medial head from the ligaments in front of the pubic tubercle and by a lateral head from the pubic crest. The muscle widens as it passes upwards and is inserted into the anterior surface of the xiphoid process and into the fifth, sixth and seventh costal cartilages. The medial border of the muscle lies alongside the linea alba and the muscle is enclosed between the anterior and posterior layers of the rectus abdominis sheath which is formed from the aponeurosis of the internal oblique muscle. The anterior layer is joined by the aponeurosis of the external oblique muscle and passes in front of the rectus constituting the anterior wall of the sheath. The posterior layer is joined by the aponeurosis of the transversus abdominis muscle making the posterior wall of the sheath which is missing below the arcuate line. Typically three tendinous intersections are found in the muscle: one at the umbilicus, one at the xiphisternum and one between these two.

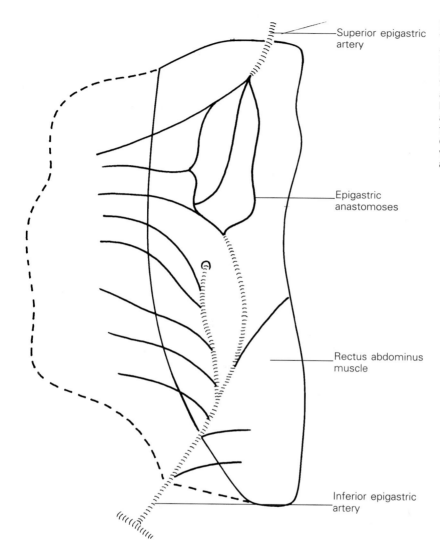

Superior epigastric artery

Epigastric anastomoses

Rectus abdominus muscle

Inferior epigastric artery

Figure 17.3

A diagrammatic view of the posterior surface of the anterior abdominal wall and vascular territories of the superior and inferior epigastric arteries. There are anastomoses between the superior epigastric and inferior epigastric arteries but the dominant artery is the inferior epigastric. This provides the vascular pedicle for the rectus abdominis free flap.

The rectus abdominis muscle is supplied by superior epigastric and inferior epigastric arteries (Figure 17.3). The superior epigastric artery averages 1.6 mm at its point of origin whereas the inferior epigastric artery measures 3.4 mm on average and has a vascular pedicle of up to 15 cm in length (Boyd et al 1984). It is therefore the inferior epigastric artery upon which the rectus abdominis free flap is based. The rectus abdominis muscle can be harvested on its pedicle quite quickly (Figure 17.4). A paramedian incision is used and the anterior rectus sheath is incised. The medial border of the muscle is identified first and the upper half of the muscle separated from the posterior sheath by finger dissection. Dissection of the lower half of the

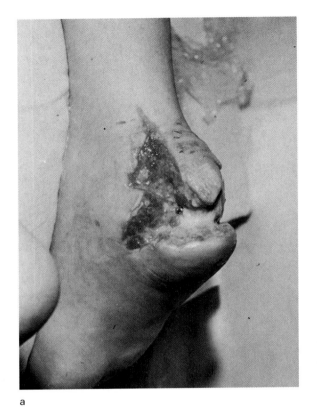

a

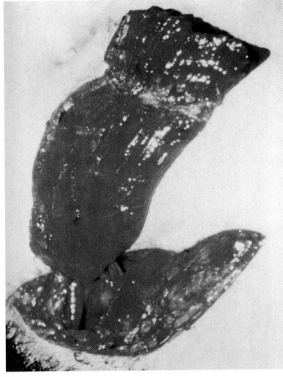

b

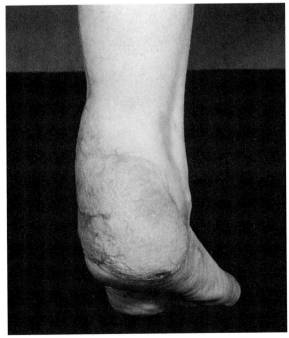

c

Figure 17.4

A rectus abdominis free flap used on a heel after an open calcaneal fracture. (a) The pre-operative heel defect. (b) The portion of rectus abdominis muscle that will be used to cover the defect. As only part of the rectus muscle will be used, a Pfannensteil incision has been used. Note the lowest tendinous intersection and the vascular pedicle. (c) An excellent result has been obtained.

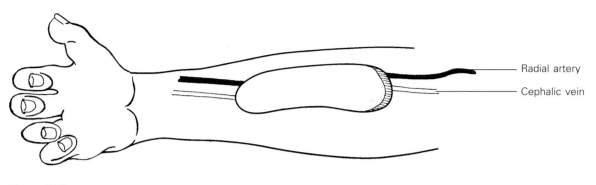

— Radial artery
— Cephalic vein

Figure 17.5

A diagrammatic representation of a radial forearm flap. It is based on the radial artery, venae comitans and occasionally the cephalic vein. It is essentially a free fasciocutaneous flap.

muscle is more difficult as peritoneal branches arise from the posterior aspect of the main artery and its venae comitantes. If these are avulsed from the main artery a tear in the side wall may ensue. The upper attachment of the muscle is divided from the chest wall and the superior epigastric pedicle ligated. The lateral border of the muscle is then filleted from its sheath and the tendinous intersections separated and each segmental neurovascular bundle ligated in turn. The inferior epigastric pedicle is dissected as far as its origin from the external iliac vessels. The rectus abdominis free flap is then transferred to the recipient site with vein grafts being used if the pedicle is not of sufficient length.

The rectus abdominis free flap was first prescribed by Pennington et al (1980). However, as with the latissimus dorsi free flap variants of the original flap have been described. Reath and Taylor (1991) have described a segmental rectus abdominis free flap particularly useful for ankle and foot reconstructions. As Chapter 13 illustrates the importance of the use of plastic surgery techniques in the management of open fractures of the ankle and foot this modification will be described.

The segmental rectus abdominis flap utilizes the inferior third to half of the muscle and is particularly useful for small defects. It is harvested through a low transverse or Pfannenstiel incision. The abdominal wall is reflected off the anterior rectus sheath and the sheath is then opened and dissected away from the underlying rectus abdominis muscle. The muscle is divided above or below the second most inferior tendinous intersection depending on the amount of muscle that is required. Usually a strip of muscle is left medially which acts to tether the remaining muscle in place, thereby preserving its function. The origin of the muscle is divided after identification of the inferior epigastric vessels. After transfer the anterior rectus sheath is repaired.

The rectus abdominis free flap has a number of advantages over latissimus dorsi flaps. It can be harvested quickly and with minimum disability to the patient. It is particularly useful in the management of traumatic defects as it can be harvested with the patient lying supine thus allowing other surgery to be carried out at the same time. Its use also allows patients to mobilize with crutches as soon as discomfort and other injuries permit. The disadvantage of the rectus abdominis flap is that central herniation may occur and great care must be exercised during the repair of the abdominal wall. A synthetic mesh may be required to strengthen the abdominal wall.

The radial forearm flap

The third most common free flap to be used in the management of open fractures is the free

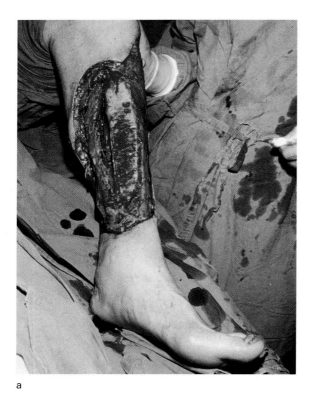

a

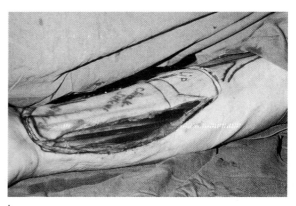

b

Figure 17.6

The use of a radial forearm flap in the late management of a Gustilo IIIa open tibial fracture which was initially treated with inappropriate soft-tissue cover. (a) The size of the soft-tissue defect after excision of the unstable skin and subcutaneous tissues. (b) The radial forearm flap is mobilized and a large flap can be taken from the forearm. (c) The final result.

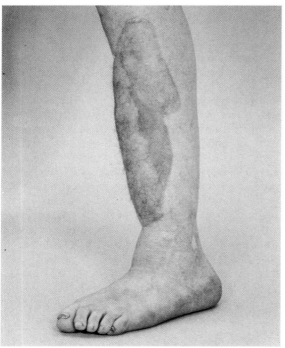

c

forearm flap. This is occasionally known as the Chinese flap because it was first described in China by Song et al (1982). The originators of the flap used it for the treatment of burn contractures in the neck but it has been applied to other areas of the body.

Forearm flaps can be based on the radial or ulnar arteries but the former is by far the most common; hence the use of the term 'radial forearm flap'. This is a free fasciocutaneous flap based on the segmental perforators from the radial artery that pass through the lateral intermuscular septum to supply the deep fascia of the forearm. Venous drainage is provided by the basilic or cephalic veins or one of their interconnecting branches (Figure 17.5). The blood vessels are large, the radial artery measuring 2–3 mm and the veins 3–4 mm. Each has a long pedicle and consistent anatomy.

The use of a radial forearm flap is illustrated in Figure 17.6. The flap is raised using a tourniquet around the arm. The required size and shape of the flap are marked on the flexor or radiodorsal surface of the forearm. The radial artery is identified at the wrist and the flap is raised by following the course of the radial artery and its venae comitantes proximally. It is important to include the fascia of the forearm in the flap to preserve the segmental perforators. The deeper branches from the radial artery to the muscles and tendon sheath are ligated.

The flap may be raised to the level of the elbow joint. The artery is usually raised throughout the entire length of the flap but it can be extended proximally or distally as the surgeon wishes. The veins of the flap are ligated distally. One of the veins of the forearm is dissected beyond the upper edge of the skin flap for an appropriate distance. Anastomosis of one of the veins is sufficient to provide drainage for the flap. Superficial branches of radial nerve should be protected to preserve sensation to the radial aspect of the hand and the fingers.

The tourniquet is then released and the viability of the flap is assessed. If there is any concern about the vascular supply to the hand, the radial artery can be clamped at its origin and at the wrist before division.

After division of the radial artery, the flap is transferred to the recipient site and the donor site in the forearm is either closed directly or with split-skin graft. The surgeon has the option of relying on the ulna artery as well as the anterior and posterior interosseous arteries to supply the hand or he or she can reconstruct the radial artery by using a reverse vein graft.

There are a number of obvious advantages to the use of the free forearm flap. The anatomy is constant and there is easy surgical access. The shape and size of the skin flap can be planned accurately to fit the recipient site. The radial artery and forearm veins are of sufficient size to allow the use of loupes instead of an operating microscope.

There have, however, been criticisms of the radial forearm flap because of the poor quality of its donor site. There are two main problems. One of these is the difficulty in using split-skin grafting on the exposed tendons of the distal forearm, delayed healing of the grafts being relatively common. Related to this is the problem of cosmesis of the forearm. Obviously this area of the body is often exposed and patients frequently complain of the cosmetic results of the radial forearm flap.

Evaluation and preparation of recipient vessels

Most free flaps are anastomosed to the anterior or posterior tibial arteries. The anterior tibial artery is difficult to expose in the upper third of the leg. It enters the leg through the upper part of the interosseous membrane, descending on the anterior surface of the membrane. In the lower part of the leg, it lies on the tibia and then on the front of the ankle joint mid-way between the two malleoli. The posterior tibial artery lies behind the soleus muscle attachment in the middle third of the leg where its exposure is quite easy and is achieved by incising through the deep fascia, reflecting the medial head of the gastrocnemius muscle and detaching the attachment of the soleus muscle from the middle third of the medial border of the tibia. This is usually carried out under tourniquet control and when completed the tourniquet is released to assess blood flow and arterial pulsation.

The vessels should be exposed outside the zone of injury, whose area is directly proportional to the magnitude of the traumatic insult. Delay in reconstruction and low grade sepsis may extend the zone of injury. Usually the relatively long pedicle of the free flaps commonly used in lower leg reconstruction allows the anastomotic site to be placed outside the zone of injury but occasionally the use of vein grafts is required. However Khouri and Shaw (1989) reported a fivefold increase in anastomotic thrombosis following the use of vein grafts.

The condition of the local vascular supply is best assessed clinically and the ideal opportunity to do this is provided by the initial debridement. More information may be obtained using angiography but this may not be possible when managing a multiply injured patient. Angiograms are particularly valuable when considering soft-tissue surgery in a severely injured leg where there have been previous attempts at reconstruction. Under these circumstances the local vascular anatomy may well have been distorted by previous surgery. Patients with a single artery supplying the distal extremity should be advised of the possibility of amputation if reconstructive efforts fail. There has been some debate about the usefulness of angiography, particularly with reference to the morbidity of the procedure.

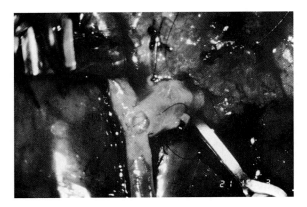

Figure 17.7

The use of an end-to-side anastomosis. This is preferable in all free-flap anastomoses and obligatory if there is only one functioning artery in the leg.

There is, however, no evidence that the dye used in angiography increases the risk of anastomotic thrombosis.

Ideally the surgery is best performed by two teams working synchronously as this can significantly reduce the operating time. One team harvests the flap while the second, more experienced, team prepares the recipient site. They will expose the recipient vessels and undertake the anastomosis. End-to-side arterial anastomoses are preferable in free-tissue transfer in both the upper and lower limbs. An example of such an anastomosis is shown in Figure 17.7. This type of anastomosis is technically more difficult to perform but is associated with a decreased incidence of spasm and post-operative thrombosis. An end-to-side anastomosis is mandatory in patients with a single artery supplying the distal extremity. It also provides a mechanism to prevent excessive flow through the free flap as the bulk of the blood flow continues through the recipient artery. One of the venae comitantes should be used as the recipient vein rather than a superficial vein, as superficial veins are thick-walled and susceptible to post-operative spasm and to thrombosis. The diameter of the venae comitantes is usually similar to that of the veins of the latissimus dorsi or rectus abdominis muscles and anastomosis is straightforward.

Cross-leg free flaps

Rarely the plastic surgeon may be faced with the necessity of carrying out a cross-leg free flap. This involves raising a standard free flap and transferring it to a recipient site, usually in the leg. The vascular pedicle is, however, anastomosed to vessels in the uninjured contralateral limb, the vessels being ligated later after the flap gains a local blood supply. This flap may be used where there is major vessel damage and the surgeon judges that a standard anastomosis will compromise the circulation to the foot. In reality, this type of flap is probably more useful in late reconstructions but it remains an option which may be considered from time to time. Documentation of this type of free flap is scanty but the problems associated with cross-leg free flaps are well documented by Hodgkinson et al (1994).

Anaesthesia

During anaesthesia, it is important to maintain the patient's body temperature. Patients should be placed on a heated water mattress and all surfaces of the body not involved in the operation should be covered with an insulated blanket. All blood and other intravenous transfusions should be warmed and the anaesthetist must be careful to regulate the patient's temperature carefully as hypothermia will induce vasospasm which is detrimental to the flap. In addition to a low body temperature, vasospasm is also produced by pain and it is therefore important to keep the patient pain-free during this prolonged operative procedure. Brachial plexus blocks are very useful for upper-limb surgery and most plastic surgeons and anaesthetists now agree that epidural anaesthesia is the most effective way for providing pain control for lower-limb surgery. This technique also provides a chemical sympathectomy at the spinal nerve root level. Scott et al (1993) compared the effect of a combination of epidural and general anaesthesia to general anaesthesia alone in patients undergoing free flaps to the lower extremities. This was a retrospective study of 35 consecutive patients over a two-year period. Sixteen patients had epidural and general anaesthesia and 19 patients had general anaesthesia. In the combined epidural/general anaesthetic group there were no flap losses and only one complication was seen. In the non-epidural group there was one flap loss and five major complications. Robins (1983) also stressed the importance of epidural anaesthesia and he recommended the maintenance of an epidural block post-operatively. He emphasized that post-operatively it is very important that the patient does not become hypoxic, hypotensive or hypothermic.

It is vital that adequate fluid and blood replacement is undertaken per-operatively. Failure to do this may precipitate vascular constriction and flap damage. It is therefore important that the anaesthetist accurately assess the haemodynamic status of the patient. It is also important that the blood viscosity is reduced to facilitate improved blood flow. It is desirable to keep the haematocrit in the region of 30–35%. This is best achieved by replacing the blood loss with either a plasma protein solution or plasma substitutes such as Dextran. Routine use of anticoagulation is not indicated but the surgeon should give consideration to the use of heparin particularly if re-exploration of a flap is being undertaken.

Post-operative flap monitoring

Even in experienced hands, up to 15% of free flaps develop post-operative complications and require further surgery. Successful revision is inversely related to the time between the onset of ischaemia and re-exploration. It has been suggested that the cutaneous vascular flow must be established within 8–12 hours but it is probable that the equivalent time for muscle reperfusion is of the order of 2 hours. It is therefore important to monitor the blood flow.

A number of methods of monitoring have been suggested. These include temperature monitors to examine the surface temperature, laser Doppler, transcutaneous oxygen, photoplethysmography and impedance plethysmography. These modalities may well have a place in the assessment of flaps but in the trauma patient, particularly those with multiple injuries, will be difficult to use. Surgeons therefore rely on clinical judgement using the same clinical criteria to assess the blood flow through a flap as they would do to assess blood flow through normal tissue. Thus in skin flaps it is important to

observe the colour, tissue turgor and capillary refill. If there is any dubiety about flap circulation the flap can be pricked with a sterile needle which should be placed well away from the pedicle and the quality of bleeding observed. In muscle flaps the surgeon should use forceps to stimulate the muscle, with active twitching providing evidence of viability. Should post-operative thrombosis occur in either artery or vein then early exploration is mandatory if the free flap is to be saved.

Post-operative care

Patients who have free flaps should be nursed post-operatively by nurses experienced in the care of free flaps. In the multiply injured patient this may not be possible because of the nature and extent of other injuries and ideally these patients should be monitored in an intensive care unit with experienced nursing staff. The body temperature should be maintained and the fluid balance watched very carefully. It is important to maintain an adequate post-operative analgesic regime as uncontrolled pain can give rise to restlessness and vascular constriction. Patient-controlled analgesia (PCA) and continuous infusion of narcotics are acceptable methods of maintaining analgesia. In addition, epidural anaesthesia can be used post-operatively.

When using free flaps for the management of open fractures it is important that orthopaedic traumatologists and plastic surgeons confer about patient and joint mobilization. This is particularly true where the units are in different hospitals. Chapter 13 has illustrated that most free flaps will be used in the lower leg, ankle and hindfoot and in this situation it is easy for the patient to develop an equinus contracture after flap cover. This may interfere with subsequent hindfoot and ankle mobilization and may even necessitate further orthopaedic surgery. This problem can be avoided by adequate cooperation between the two disciplines.

Results

The importance of flap cover in the management of open fractures is illustrated by an analysis of

Table 17.1 The aetiology of 100 cases referred for major lower-limb reconstruction in the North East Thames Regional Plastic Surgery Unit in Billericay, of whom 65 were treated by free-flap transfer. The importance of free flaps in the management of open fractures is obvious

Aetiology	Number of cases
Road traffic accident	53
Work/sport	12
Exposed plate	8
Burns	5
Osteomyelitis	4
Chronic leg ulcers	4
Miscellaneous	14

100 patients treated at the North East Thames Regional Plastic Surgery Unit in Billericay between 1987 and 1992. Table 17.1 shows the reasons for treating these 100 cases. It is obvious that most of these patients were referred follow-ing trauma either at the acute stage or secon-darily following a complication. Of these 100 cases, 14 were treated by fasciocutaneous flaps, 21 were reconstructed by muscle flaps and 65 were treated by free flaps. The results of 51 of these patients were available in full. The patients were divided into three groups based on the timing of flap cover in the manner of Godina (1986). In the early group flap cover was under-taken within 72 hours of the injury. In the delayed group flap cover was undertaken between 72 hours and three months and in the late group flap cover was delayed until more than three months had elapsed. The results are shown in Table 17.2. It is obvious that most patients fell into the delayed and late categories. It is also clear that the failures of flap cover occurred in these categories and that the bone healing time was markedly prolonged in the late group. The average duration of hospitalization and the number of procedures also increased in relation to the delay from time of injury.

Table 17.2 The results of the use of microvascular free flaps in the North East Thames Plastic Surgery Unit. The results are presented according to Godina (1986) and can be compared with those of Godina presented in Table 17.3

	Patient group (timing of surgery)		
	Early (<72 h)	Delayed (72 h–3 months)	Late (>3 months)
Patients (n)	8	21	22
Flap failures (n)	0	3	2
Post-operative infection (%)	12.5	9.5	9.1
Bone union time (months)	5	7	20
Hospitalization time (days)	28	50	145
Procedures (n)	2.2	3.7	5

Table 17.3 The results of the use of microvascular free flaps according to Godina (1986). The influence of delay is clearly seen

Parameter	Patient group (timing of surgery)		
	Early (<72 h)	Delayed (72 h–3 months)	Late (>3 months)
Patients (n)	134	167	231
Flap failures (n)	1	20	22
Post-operative infection (%)	1.5	17.5	6
Bone union time (months)	6.8	12.3	29
Hospitalization time (days)	27	130	256
Procedures (n)	1.3	4.1	7.8

Table 17.4 Sequential and cumulative information regarding post-traumatic free-flap use from Melissinos and Parks (1989)*

Parameter	Group 1	Group 2	Group 3	Group 4
Flaps (n)	98	166	178	442
Failed flaps (n)	8	4	4	16
Flap failure (%)	8.2	2.4	2.2	3.6
Re-operations (n)	25	22	18	65
Re-operation rate (%)	25.5	13.2	10.1	14.7
Operating time (hours)	8	6.2	4.5	6

*Group 1 refers to results between July 1979 and April 1982, Group 2 to the period between May 1982 and February 1985, Group 3 to the period from March 1985 to December 1987 and Group 4 to the cumulative results between July 1979 and December 1987.

The results published by Godina in 1986 are shown in Table 17.3. In his early reconstruction group there were 134 patients. In 63 of these patients the free-flap transfer was undertaken immediately after the injury, but all were done within 72 hours of the fractures. The reason for delay was usually logistic, caused by the unavailability of a microsurgeon. Godina was clear that surgery within 72 hours was acceptable and Table 17.3 illustrates the exceptional results that he gained. There was only one failure out of 134 patients and the hospitalization time was markedly less than in his delayed and late group.

In the delayed and late category, it is obvious that the morbidity is much worse. There is a higher incidence of microsurgical procedure failures and post-operative infection and the bone healing time and hospitalization time is markedly prolonged. In Godina's series there were 42 cases of free-flap failure. He showed that 14% of these were caused by arterial thrombosis with the remaining 86% being caused by venous thrombosis. The problem of venous thrombosis was also documented by Melissinos and Parks (1989) as causing 10 out of 14 flap failures involving the distal lower extremities. These authors also separated their 442 consecutive cases into three groups based on the timing of surgery. The impression is that they were able to operate rather more quickly than Godina and 328 (74.4%) of the free-tissue transfers were performed between 48 hours and 10 days after the injury. A further 46 cases (10.4%) were operated on between 10 and 60 days after the injury and the remaining 62 patients (14%) had late reconstructions performed at least 60 days after the injury.

Melissinos and Parks also documented their cumulative results between 1979 and 1987, dividing the patients into four groups based on the timing of surgery. Their results are shown in Table 17.4 and it can be seen that the cumulative results between July 1979 and December 1987 are excellent. Their average operating time had fallen to 4.5 hours with a re-operation rate of 10.1%. Their flap failure incidence had fallen to 2.2% and their conclusions were that free-flap tissue transfer is a reliable method of reconstructing post-trauma defect in all areas of the body, although as with other authors, they found that it was most useful when dealing with defects in the lower third of the legs. Table 17.4 illustrates the importance of experience when dealing with these difficult cases.

Small and Mollan reviewed the treatment of 168 open tibial fractures referred to the Northern Ireland Plastic Surgery Service over a 15-year period. Flap reconstruction was carried out in 133 (79%) of the fractures, with split-skin grafting being used for a further 22 fractures. The remaining fractures were treated by amputation. The authors made use of local flaps, cross-leg flaps and free-tissue flaps. Of the 97 local flaps, 60 were pedicled muscle flaps, with 33 fasciocutaneous flaps and four random skin flaps being used. Of the 70 free flaps, 31 involved the latissimus dorsi muscle, 18 used the rectus abdominis muscle and eight used a radial forearm flap. The remaining 13 flaps involved four different donor sites. The authors documented a 12.6% incidence of flap necrosis with a similar incidence being noted for fasciocutaneous and free flaps. Overall, however, they stated that the

Table 17.5 Comparison of free-tissue transfer in patients over and under 60 years of age (Bonawitz et al 1991). Primary flap cover is not as successful in the older group but if re-operation is performed, the eventual success rate is almost as high as in younger patients

Parameter	<60 years	≥60 years
Patients (n)	136	54
Primary cover, n (%)	116 (85.3)	37 (68.5)
Salvage surgery, n (%)	16 (11.8)	13 (24.1)
Successful, n (%)	12 (75.0)	8 (61.5)
Primary flap failure, n (%)	8 (5.9)	9 (16.7)
Eventual flap success, n (%)	131 (96.3)	50 (92.6)

fasciocutaneous flaps had a higher complication rate than free flaps and it was their view that free flaps were more useful than local flaps. It must be stressed, however, that this paper was a retrospective study over a 15-year period and the techniques of both local and free-flap transfer clearly improved over the 15 years of the survey. There is no doubt that experience with these techniques is crucial. This is illustrated by the fact that Khouri and Shaw (1989) had half the incidence of re-exploration and flap failure in their second 100 flaps compared with their first 100. These authors examined the reasons for post-operative thrombosis after free-flap transfer. They found that there was an increased incidence in Gustilo IIIc fractures, in fractures with an abnormal pre-operative angiogram, in end-to-side anastomoses and if there was a bone deficit of <4 cm. Most of their anastomotic thromboses were successfully treated by re-exploration.

With an increasing incidence of elderly in the population and the obvious association between Gustilo type IIIa fractures and the elderly pedestrian pointed out in Chapter 3, it is worthwhile examining the results of free-tissue transfer in elderly patients. Bonawitz et al (1991) examined the results of 151 patients over a 70-month period. Forty-seven of the patients were at least 60 years of age, the mean age being 69.6 years, while 25 (53.2%) of these patients were operated on because of head-and-neck tumours, and 14 (29.8%) had free flaps carried out because of wounds, 10 of the 14 being in the lower limbs. There was a high incidence of co-existing hypertension, coronary artery disease, diabetes melli-

tus, peripheral vascular disease, and tobacco and alcohol abuse in the patient groups. Again, analysis of the free-tissue donor sites showed that the latissimus dorsi muscle, scapula and radial forearm provided most of the flaps. The results of the young and older group are shown in Table 17.5 and it is clear that the elderly group had a higher incidence of further surgery than the younger group. Analysis of their data showed that they could not find a significant correlation between flap loss and conditions such as diabetes, hypertension, peripheral vascular disease, coronary artery disease, tobacco abuse, alcohol abuse, previous systemic chemotherapy or donor-site radiotherapy. They also demonstrated no beneficial effect of anticoagulation. The authors stressed that minor complications were not uncommon, but they pointed out that their eventual flap coverage rate of 92.6% confirms the feasibility of free-flap reconstruction in elderly patients and this finding is obviously important given the fact that the elderly population in all societies is rapidly increasing in size.

References

Arnez ZM, Hanel DP (1991) Free tissue transfer for reconstruction of traumatic limb injuries in children, *Microsurgery* **12**: 207–15.

Bonawitz SC, Schnarrs RH, Rosenthal AI, Rodgers GK, Newton ED (1991) Free-tissue transfer in elderly patients, *Plast Reconstr Surg* **87**: 1074–9.

Boyd JB, Taylor GI, Corlett R (1984) The vascular territories of the superior epigastric and the deep inferior epigastric systems, *Plast Reconstr Surg* **73**: 1–14.

British Orthopaedic Association, British Association of Plastic Surgeons (1993) *The Early Management of Severe Open Tibial Fractures: The Need for Combined Plastic and Orthopaedic Management* (London: BOA/BAPS).

Campbell P, McLean NR, Black MJ (1992) Free microvascular tissue transfer in Newcastle General Hospital, UK, *J R Coll Surg (Edin)* **37**: 180–2.

Cierny G, Byrd HS, Jones RE (1983) Primary versus delayed soft tissue coverage for severe open tibial fractures: a comparison of results, *Clin Orthop* **178**: 54–63.

Cooley BC, Hanel DP, Anderson RB, Foster MD, Gould JS (1992) The influence of diabetes on free flap transfer: 1. Flap survival and microvascular healing, *Ann Plast Surg* **29**: 58–64.

Daniel RK, Taylor GI (1973) Distant transfer of an island flap by microvascular anastomoses: A clinical technique, *Plast Reconstr Surg* **52**: 111–17.

Godina M (1986) Early reconstruction of complex trauma of the extremities, *Plast Reconstr Surg* **78**: 285–92.

Godina M (1987) The tailored latissimus dorsi free flap, *Plast Reconstr Surg* **80**: 304–6.

Harris GD, Nagle DJ, Lewis VL, Bauer BS (1987) Accelerating recovery after trauma with free flaps, *J Trauma* **27**: 849–55.

Hodgkinson PD, Andhoga M, Wilson GR, McLean NR (1994) Cross-leg free muscle flaps for reconstruction of open fractures of the tibia, *Injury* **25**: 637–40.

Katsaros J, Tan E, Robinson DN (1988) Cost effectiveness of free tissue transfer, *Aust NZ J Surg* **58**: 373–6.

Keating JF, Court-Brown CM, Quaba AA (1994) *Open Tibial Fractures* (American Academy of Orthopaedic Surgeons: New Orleans).

Khouri RK, Shaw WW (1989) Reconstruction of the lower extremity with microvascular free flaps: A 10-year experience with 304 consecutive cases, *J Trauma* **29**: 1086–94.

McKibben B (1978) The biology of fracture-healing in long bones, *J Bone Joint Surg (Br)* **60B**: 150–62.

Melissinos EG, Parks DH (1989) Post trauma reconstruction with free tissue transfer. Analysis of 442 consecutive cases, *J Trauma* **29**: 1095–102.

Meyer M, Evans J (1990) Joint orthopaedic and plastic surgery management of type III and IV lower limb injuries, *Br J Plast Surg* **43**: 692–4.

Pennington DC, Lai MF, Pelly AD (1980) The rectus abdominis myocutaneous free flap, *Br J Plast Surg* **33**: 277–82.

Reath DB, Taylor JW (1991) The segmental rectus abdominis free flap for foot and ankle reconstruction, *Plast Reconstr Surg* **88**: 824–8.

Robins DW (1983) The anaesthetic management of patients undergoing free flap transfer, *Br J Plast Surg* **36**: 231–4.

Russell RC, Pribaz J, Zook EG, Leighton WD, Eriksson E, Smith CJ (1986) Functional evaluation of latissimus dorsi donor site, *Plast Reconstr Surg* **78**: 336–43.

Salemark L (1991) International survey of current microvascular practices in free tissue transfer and replantation surgery, *Microsurgery* **12**: 308–11.

Scott GR, Rothkopf DM, Walton RL (1993) Efficacy of epidural anaesthesia in free flaps to the lower extremity, *Plast Reconstr Surg* **91**: 673–7.

Shestak KC, Jones NF (1991) Microsurgical free tissue transfer in elderly patients, *Plast Reconstr Surg* **88**: 259–63.

Small JO, Mollan RAB (1992) Management of the soft tissues in open tibial fractures, *Br J Plast Surg* **45**: 571–7.

Song R, Gao Y, Song Y, Yu Y, Song Y (1982) The forearm flap, *Clin Plast Surg* **9**: 21–6.

Whiteside LA, Lesker PA (1978) The effects of extraperiosteal and subperiosteal dissection: II. On fracture healing, *J Bone Joint Surg (Am)* **60A**: 26–30.

Yaremchuk MJ (1986) Acute management of severe soft tissue damage accompanying open fractures of the lower extremity, *Clin Plast Surg* **13**: 621–32.

18
Degloving injuries

C.M. Court-Brown, A.A. Quaba and J.D. Watson

'Degloving' is the term applied to the soft-tissue damage caused by traumatic avulsion of the skin and subcutaneous tissues from the underlying deep fascia. The skin contains a dermal vascular plexus which is dependent upon vessels which pierce the underlying muscles and deep fascia to enter the subcutaneous tissue. The vessels are interrupted in degloving injuries, leaving the skin dependent on blood that comes through the dermal plexus in a random fashion, and skin necrosis and death is common.

Degloving is caused by a shearing force and usually results from a rotating object with a high coefficient of friction, such as a rubber tyre, making contact with a limb (Figure 18.1). The limb is usually, but not invariably, lying on the road and incapable of being pushed away by the force of the impact. Thus commonly degloving injuries associated with underlying fractures are seen in pedestrians knocked down and run onto, or over, by motor vehicles. Usually the degloving injury is open (Figure 18.2) in that the skin has been torn by the shearing force but occasionally closed degloving injuries occur where the subcutaneous tissues have been elevated from the underlying deep fascia without a break in the skin. These may be associated with an underlying closed fracture but this situation is rare. Closed degloving injuries are beyond the scope of this book, but surgeons wishing more information about these injuries should consult the work of Hudson et al (1992).

Open degloving injuries were recognized by Slack (1952). He appreciated their relationship to tyre injuries and referred to them as 'friction injuries'. He documented skin necrosis secondary to loss of the cutaneous blood supply, delayed skin gangrene and secondary sepsis. In 12 cases, Slack noted that it was the lower leg, ankle or hindfoot that was mainly involved although he also recorded cases associated with open pelvic and open forearm fractures.

Prendiville and Lewis (1955) also documented degloving, describing the condition as a pneumatic-tyre torsion avulsion injury. Of their 50 cases, 40 involved children, but only three had upper-limb injuries. It is interesting to note that a large number of their cases presented late as surgeons at the time did not appreciate the severity of the condition. They described three distinct groups, with 66% of their patients presenting immediately or within a few weeks. A further 14% presented with granulating areas after sloughs had separated and in the remaining 20% the injury had healed with deformity. This classification is now historic, but illustrates

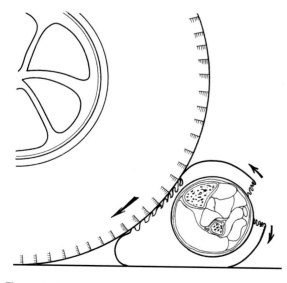

Figure 18.1

A diagram illustrating the usual cause of degloving. Such injuries are frequently caused by an automobile tyre shearing the skin and subcutaneous tissues away from the deep fascia.

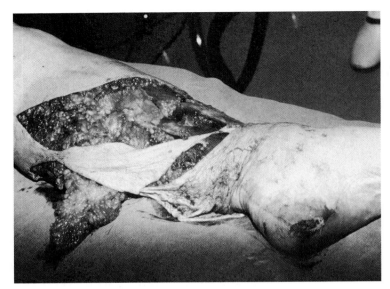

a

Figure 18.2

(a) A Gustilo type IIIb fracture in a 64-year-old pedestrian where there is clear evidence of major degloving. It is obvious that the skin in the photograph is devitalized and further inspection at the time of surgery showed there to be circumferential degloving. (b) After soft-tissue and bone debridement, there was a 7-inch bone defect and a circumferential soft-tissue defect over most of the leg. The open tibial fracture was treated by Grosse–Kempf intramedullary nail. (c) At 48 hours, the wound was re-inspected and no further debridement was required. A rectus abdominus flap was used to cover the area of tibial deficit and split-skin graft was used to cover the rectus abdominus flap and the area of degloving. Subsequently, bone grafting was performed and the fracture united.

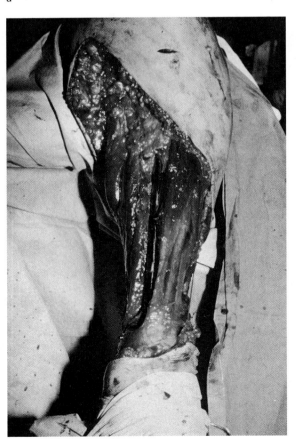

b

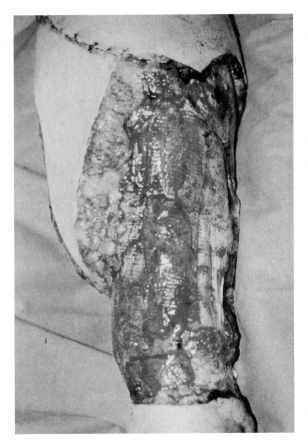

c

that the condition was not fully appreciated until recently.

Entin (1955) carried out experimental work using rats and dogs to examine the cause and treatment of degloving injuries. It was his view that three factors were important in producing degloving injuries. Firstly, there had to be a compression force between the roller and the limb; secondly, the rotating motion had to create friction and a significant torque; and lastly there was a stripping force dragging the soft tissues over the rigid bony structure of the leg. He detailed a number of factors which influenced the extent and degree of damage. These included obvious factors such as the force of compression, the speed of rotation of the rolling objects and the duration of the shearing force. However, he noted that age played a part and he suggested that younger people had more elastic tissues and had a lower incidence of degloving injuries. He also pointed out that despite the plane of cleavage in degloving injuries being outside the deep fascia there was damage to the muscles accompanied by haemorrhage and transudation from torn vessels and injured tissues. This preceded skin necrosis and secondary infection.

Clinical experience suggests that Entin's observation about the importance of age is correct. Degloving is more commonly seen in older patients presumably because of an alteration of the resistance to shearing forces secondary to changes in the composition of the subcutaneous tissues. They are also commonly seen in patients who have medical conditions such as rheumatoid arthritis where atrophy of the skin and subcutaneous tissues is a major problem.

Epidemiology

It is difficult to give accurate data about the incidence of degloving associated with fractures. There is no definition as to what constitutes significant degloving and as minor degrees of degloving are very common and frequently not associated with significant morbidity they are often not recorded by surgeons, who understandably only comment on cases of severe degloving. Circumferential degloving is uncommon but dramatic when it occurs. Kudsk et al

(1981) analysed data referring to 21 cases of degloving involving at least two thirds of the circumference of the affected area. In ten years the authors collected 21 patients aged 7–78 years. Seventeen patients were involved in road traffic accidents and 11 of the patients were pedestrians. All but two of the degloving injuries involved the lower extremities. Only three of the degloving injuries were not associated with fractures and 50% of the patients had multiple limb fractures. The authors documented a total of 38 fractures associated with degloving in the 21 patients. The commonest sites involved were the leg (31.6%), thigh (21.1%), pelvis (21.1%) and foot (13.2%). The distribution of degloving injuries was also analysed by McGrouther and Sully (1980). They excluded degloving injuries of the sole, dorsum of the foot, pre-tibial area and hand on the grounds that these injuries required individual solutions. They only looked at cases of extensive degloving but again documented a preponderance of cases in the lower limbs. They showed a similar incidence of skin loss in the thigh, knee and leg and demonstrated that the degloving injury was often circumferential. They found that 77.4% of the degloving injuries in the leg were circumferential, in addition to 63% of the thigh wounds and 58.6% of the injuries around the knee. Degloving injuries of the leg were almost six times as common as degloving injuries of the upper limbs, but most of the upper-limb degloving injuries were circumferential. McGrouther and Sully also documented a number of predisposing factors, these being age, low intelligence and high alcohol intake. They found higher rates of degloving in the young and the elderly.

In Edinburgh, the association of degloving with open fractures is not dissimilar to the results published by McGrouther and Sully (1980) and Kudsk et al (1981). However, there are some differences. Only one of the six open pelvic fractures detailed in Chapter 3 had significant degloving. The rest of the open pelvic fractures, while associated with considerable soft-tissue and bone damage, had open injuries adjacent to the vagina and rectum and did not show significant associated degloving.

Degloving was principally seen in the leg in association with open tibial fractures. The next most common location was the foot, but significant degloving was also seen in the thigh, hand

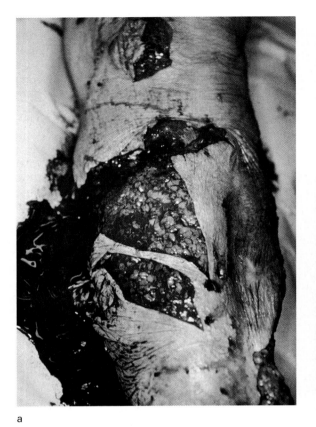

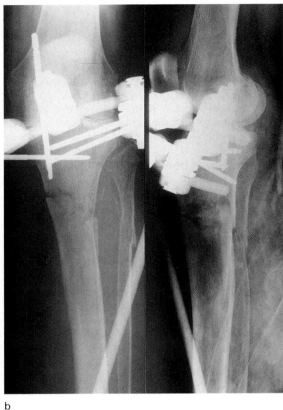

a

b

Figure 18.3

(a) Severe degloving injury in a 78-year-old pedestrian. Again, there are obvious areas of tissue degloving, but at the time of debridement, it became clear that this was a circumferential injury. There was a Gustilo IIIa proximal diaphyseal tibial fracture which was treated by a Grosse–Kempf intramedullary nail. Subsequently, the fracture site was covered by a gastrocnemius flap with split-skin grafting used for the degloved area. (b) This illustrates the relatively benign nature of the fracture compared with the severe soft-tissue injury seen in (a). This is not an uncommon combination in elderly patients.

and forearm. Degloving of the leg was frequently seen in older patients and often associated with a relatively benign Gustilo IIIa fracture pattern (Figure 18.3). This finding was, however, not invariable and a degloving component was often seen in more severe injuries (Figure 18.2). The major difference between the pure degloving injury and the mixed direct blow/degloving injury is involvement of the subcutaneous border of the tibia. The treatment of these two types of fractures is very different, with pure degloving

injuries not involving the skin overlying the subcutaneous border of the tibia being treated by split-skin grafting and fractures involving the subcutaneous border requiring flap cover.

Degloving injuries of the foot are almost invariably caused by a car or bus tyre mounting the foot and shearing off the skin and subcutaneous tissues from the dorsum (Figure 18.4). An alternative presentation is when the degloving is circumferential and the skin of the sole has also been removed (Figure 18.5). The extent of bony

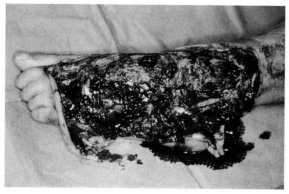

a

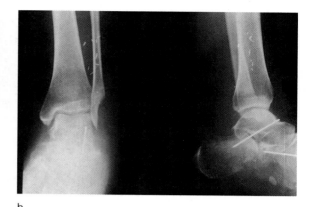

b

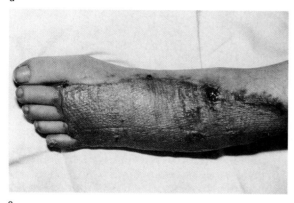

c

Figure 18.4

(a) A severe degloving injury in a 25-year-old female. Again, this was a road traffic accident and in this case a bus mounted the patient's foot. Severe degloving injury is obvious. (b) X-rays confirm severe bony injury with a fracture of the calcaneus, damage to the subtalar joint and damage to the lateral part of the mid-foot. The distal fibula was ground away by the tyre. K-wires have been used to stabilize the joints of the foot. (c) A latissimus dorsi free flap was used to cover the area. Good function was obtained.

damage in the foot is variable but not infrequently the soft-tissue injury is a major component and the fracture may be relatively minor. The variability of bony damage is illustrated in Figures 18.4 and 18.5. In the patient shown in Figure 18.4 there was considerable bony damage in addition to the obvious soft-tissue damage. There was a crush fracture of the calcaneus with damage to the mid-foot joints as well as to the bases of the fourth and fifth metatarsals. The base of the fifth metatarsal had in fact been sheared off as had most of the lateral malleolus. There was also significant tendon damage. By contrast, the patient illustrated in Figure 18.5 had very little bony injury. The foot had sustained a virtually pure circumferential degloving injury with involvement of both dorsum and sole skin. There was only an undisplaced fracture of the

base of the fifth metatarsal although the toes were damaged. There was no tendon involvement.

Degloving injuries of the thigh and forearm are very similar. Both can be closed or open and as McGrouther and Sully (1980) pointed out the area of degloving may be very extensive or even circumferential (Figure 18.6). Hand degloving injuries commonly involve the digits and classically occur in association with ring avulsion injuries. These are discussed in Chapter 10 where the classification of Carroll (1974) is presented. It can be seen that only Carroll's class IV injury involves an open phalangeal fracture and he, and other authors, suggest primary amputation as the treatment of choice.

Major degloving injuries of the palm and dorsum of the hand are relatively uncommon

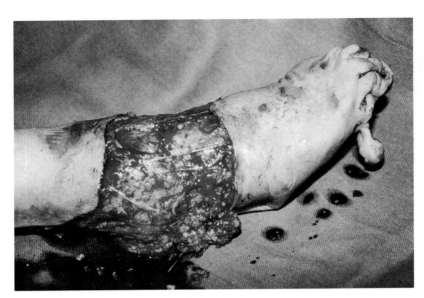

Figure 18.5

Circumferential degloving injury of the foot in a 43-year-old female pedestrian. Again the degloving injury is caused by a car tyre mounting the foot. This is a pre-operative photograph and it is clear that the foot skin has moved 6 inches distally. Clearly there was significant damage to the toes, but otherwise there was only a minor fracture to the fifth metatarsal base. The toes were amputated and the resultant soft-tissue defect treated by split-skin graft. An amputation was performed electively two years later.

except in areas with a lot of heavy industry. Figure 18.7 shows an example of such an injury. There is obvious degloving of the skin of the palm of the hand associated with damage to the thenar musculature. These are essentially severe soft-tissue injuries which may or may not have co-incidental fractures. The fractures themselves are of relatively minor importance compared with treatment of the soft tissues and because of this the reader is referred to more specific texts if further information on soft-tissue cover of the hand is desired (McCarthy and McCarthy 1990, Green 1993).

Diagnosis

The presence of degloving associated with an open fracture is usually relatively easy to determine, if the surgeon remembers to look for it! The factors that are often more difficult to determine are the extent of the degloving and the viability of the degloved skin. In small areas of degloving such as illustrated in Figure 5.5 (see page 48) it is quite possible that all of the degloved area has retained a blood supply and no resection is required. However, in larger areas

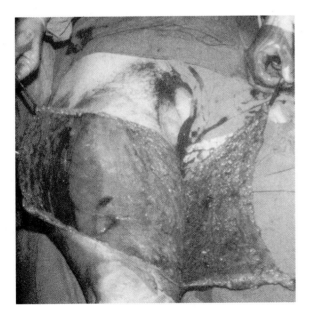

Figure 18.6

Degloving injury of the femur. The considerable extent of some thigh degloving injuries is illustrated.

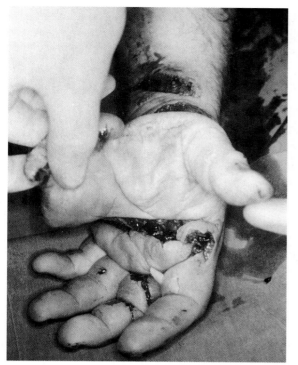

a

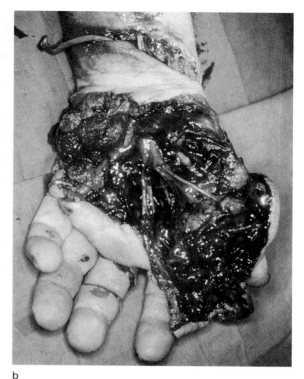

b

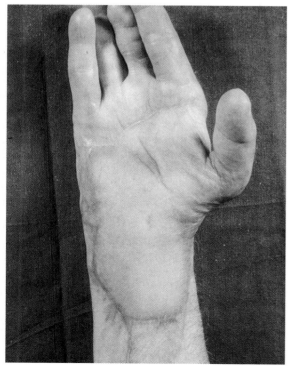

c

Figure 18.7

(a) Degloving injury of the hand. This 18-year-old man caught his hand in a milling machine, sustaining a severe degloving injury to the wrist and hand. (b) The extent of the damage to the underlying thenar musculature is seen. It is obvious that the skin bridge over the volar aspect of the wrist has also been degloved and is non-viable. (c) The results of treatment with a groin flap. This shows the fingers in full extension. The patient had full flexion of his fingers but there was impaired thumb function.

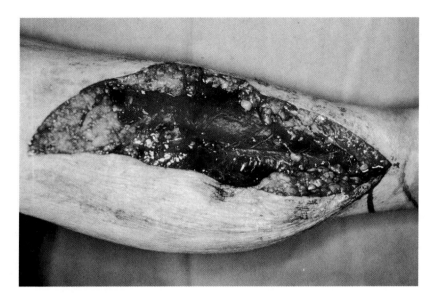

Figure 18.8

A Gustilo IIIa fracture in a 64-year-old female pedestrian. The area of skin degloving is obvious and it is clear from the picture that there is wrinkling and bunching of the degloved skin with altered colour.

of degloving, there may well be dubiety about the presence of the cutaneous blood supply, and the surgeon may find it difficult to determine the exact extent of skin resection.

Severe degloving should be considered pre-operatively in all limb injuries in pedestrians, particularly if the patient is elderly. Thus it is important to take an adequate history of the mechanism of injury. The condition should also be considered if there is a history of rheumatoid arthritis or any other autoimmune disease associated with atrophy of the skin and subcutaneous tissue. Corticosteroids, and other drugs which predispose to skin changes, may increase the incidence of degloving and thus a full history of any medications taken by the patient may be useful although in the multiply injured patient it may well not be possible to obtain.

Pre-operative inspection may alert the surgeon to the presence of degloving, particularly if it is circumferential. At worst, the skin will be hanging from the limb with the underlying muscle layer relatively undisturbed. Lesser injuries may present with wrinkling or bunching of the skin and increased pallor when compared with the normal adjacent skin. This is well shown in Figure 18.8. The skin may have lost its ability to blanch on pressure but if this test is used the

surgeon should be aware of the overall haemo-dynamic state of the patient as impaired peripheral perfusion may produce the same effect. As already detailed in Chapter 5, the presence of more than one skin wound, particularly if they are close together, should alert the surgeon to the possibility of degloving. At surgery, the surgeon should carefully explore the wound digitally to document the extent of any degloving injury. When this is done, the surgeon must be careful not to artificially enlarge the degloved area, as in elderly patients with very atrophic skin it is easy to push the skin away from the underlying deep fascia. The extent of resection of degloved skin may be difficult to determine. In practical terms the easiest way of determining the resection margin is to cut the tissue back until dermal bleeding is seen. However, there are other tests which may help the surgeon. The tourniquet test may be employed. A sphygmomanometer cuff is placed around the limb proximal to the zone of injury and inflated for some minutes. On release the distribution of reactive hyperaemia will give an idea of the extent of the normally vascularized skin. The surgeon can also employ the fluorescein test outlined in Chapter 5. This test is based on the fact that normal vascularized skin will fluoresce in ultraviolet light after the intravenous injection of fluorescein. McGrouther and Sully (1980) suggest that 1 g of 5% fluorescein be given intravenously in 200 ml of normal saline over a period of 10 minutes. After a further 10 minutes, the skin is inspected with ultraviolet light in a darkened room. If the skin shows yellow this suggests normal vascularity; a blue colour signifies skin death. Unfortunately, the middle of the spectrum, a mottled appearance, is difficult to interpret. While this test may be useful it is likely to be impractical when dealing with a seriously injured patient and the surgeon will probably elect to rely on dermal bleeding. He or she may also find other signs such as coagulation of the subcutaneous veins and damage to the subcutaneous fat to be useful when deciding on the exact margin of resection. As with all debridement procedures in cases of serious soft-tissue or bone injury, it is suggested that the surgeon should adopt the policy of re-examining the degloved area 36–48 hours after the initial surgery to re-inspect the skin and undertake further resection if this is required.

Treatment

Once the degloved skin has been excised, the surgeon must decide how to cover the soft-tissue defect. Obviously this will depend on the site of the defect and its area and the decision may be modified by the overall condition of the patient and the presence and extent of other injuries. The mainstay of treating degloving injuries is split-skin grafting. The principal message to get across to surgeons is that suturing the degloved skin is not only futile as skin death is inevitable, but it is also wasteful as the excised skin can be used as a split-skin donor site if it is harvested at the time of the initial surgery. Kudsk et al (1981) showed that reduction and closure of degloved skin was associated with 50% flap necrosis within a few days as well as a high incidence of infection. Wounds treated by packing or loose approximation had equally poor results. In contrast they showed good results using either the defatted flap applied as a full-thickness skin graft or using split-skin grafts taken from the degloved flap. Under no circumstances should the degloved skin be resutured.

The difficulty encountered in treating degloving injuries with split-skin grafting is how to take the split-skin grafts easily from the avulsed skin. The plastic surgeon faces a number of problems. The inferior surface of the degloved flap is uneven and this may interfere with taking the graft. In addition, the skin has lost its elastic property and it is often difficult to apply a pure shearing force when taking the graft. As compression of the flap is inevitable, the split-skin graft tends to have an uneven or wavy surface. To get round this problem, special dermatomes can be used. Gibson and Ross (1965) and McGrouther and Sully (1980) advocate the use of the Gibson Ross dermatome, but they suggest sticking the harvested skin onto ground glass using an adhesive made of domestic evostick diluted with ether. Goris and Nicolai (1982) suggested that surgeons cut the avulsed skin into large rectangular pieces. They then grasped the four corners of the flap rectangles with clips and stretched the skin flap over a large abdominal gauze pad on a sterile table. Two assistants pulled the four clips downwards and outwards and the authors say that large skin grafts of uniform thickness can then be cut with a conventional hand-held dermatome. They also suggested stretching the skin flaps over the patient's uninjured thigh to provide an even distribution of pressure. Zeligowski and Ziv (1987) suggested resuturing the degloved area into its original location before taking the grafts and subsequently discarding the remains of the flap. Cohen et al (1990) extended this idea and after resecting the flap they took two 0.14-inch split-skin grafts from the skin surface. They then removed the flap, turned it over and defatted it before removing a further 0.14-inch split-skin graft from the undersurface of the flap. They therefore obtained three times the quantity of split-skin graft from the flap. Once split skin has been harvested it can be stored at 4°C for about one week. Ideally the skin should be used as soon as possible but usually it can be used safely for about one week after harvesting.

As has already been noted many open fractures show a combination of degloving and direct injury. This is particularly the case in the tibia where there is often damage to the subcutaneous border of the tibia (Figure 18.2). Under these circumstances the surgeon will usually have to use a distant flap to cover the bone defect as well as split-skin grafting for the degloved area. In extensive or circumferential injuries where the subcutaneous border of the tibia is exposed, it is likely that the surgeon will employ a free rectus abdominus or latissimus dorsi flap in addition to split-skin grafting (Figure 18.2). Local flaps are rarely indicated for coverage of subcutaneus border of the tibia in degloving injuries. Usually the vascular damage associated with the degloving injury precludes the raising of a flap based on a local blood vessel. If in doubt about the potential viability of a local flap, the surgeon should use a distant flap.

Degloving injuries of the foot are similarly treated. The difference between the foot and the leg is that degloving injuries of the foot frequently expose the extensor tendons and the surgeon may well choose to use a free flap to cover the exposed tendons and areas of exposed bone. Such an approach is illustrated in Figure 18.4. Alternatively, if there is a pure degloving injury split-skin grafting can be used over the foot, but the skin is less durable and the results of split-skin grafting, particularly when used on the sole of the foot, are less satisfactory. Resurfacing the sole of the foot is a very specialized procedure. It was reviewed by Sommerlad and McGrouther (1978) who found that there was no adequate way of replacing sole skin and where possible they suggested that the skin of the sole should be preserved. In circumferential degloving injuries this will be impossible and Sommerlad and McGrouther advocate the use of local flaps. They also sensibly suggest that consideration should be given to elective below-knee amputation in cases of total loss of the sole. It is interesting to note that in the case illustrated in Figure 18.5, below-knee amputation was discussed with the patient, who rejected it. Skin grafting was used to cover the foot but even with specially adapted shoewear it proved impossible to mobilize adequately and an elective below-knee amputation was performed two years after the injury. If surgeons wish further information on replacement of the sole of the foot, it is suggested they consult an appropriate text (McCarthy and McCarthy 1990).

Treatment of degloved forearms and thighs is essentially split-skin grafting as Chapter 15 illustrates. There is virtually no requirement for flap cover in femoral fractures and the requirement for flap cover in degloving injuries of the forearm is minimal.

Outcome

Little has been documented about the results of the treatment of degloving injuries. It is important to consider the results from two points of view, namely those of cosmesis and limb function. As far as the cosmetic aspects of degloving treatment are concerned, the patient and surgeon may well have very different points of view. The surgeon may be pleased that he or she has managed to treat a difficult injury satisfactorily but the patient may well remain unhappy about the cosmetic aspect of the treatment. The results of the treatment of a degloving injury are shown in Figure 18.9. This shows the treatment of an elderly female patient who was involved in a road traffic accident as a pedestrian. On the right leg she had a Gustilo IIIa fracture with obvious degloving. Skin was removed, thinned and stored in a refrigerator. Figure 18.9a shows the appearance of the legs 48 hours after the initial surgery and by this time it is clear that the skin on the left leg has also had a major degloving injury and it was removed at the time of the re-look procedure. The right soft-tissue defect was treated by a rectus abdominus free flap and the skin taken originally from the right leg was used to treat the degloving injury on the left. Figure 18.9b shows the result. It is obvious that there is loss of contour of both legs and this is inevitable given the fact that the subcutaneous fat was missing following the degloving injury. This was noted by McGrouther and Sully (1980). They also noted that while split-skin grafting was successful in covering degloving injuries it was often associated with poor pigment match and the use of thin split-skin grafting over muscles produced a bluish discoloration. They also observed that meshed split-skin graft in the early stages was associated with marked hypertrophy and the later result was often unsatisfactory because of the persistence of the mesh pattern (Figure 18.9b).

McGrouther and Sully also observed that female patients altered their clothing patterns. Few patients, adult or children, were entirely unconcerned about the cosmetic appearance of their degloved areas.

The influence of degloving on late joint function is unknown. It could be argued that in a pure degloving injury, where the muscles are

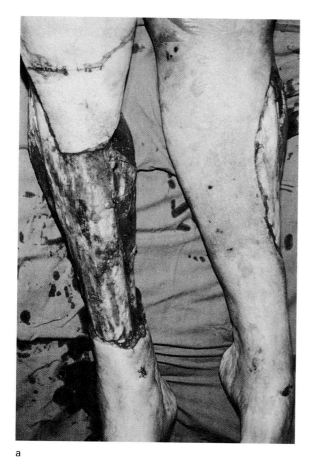
a

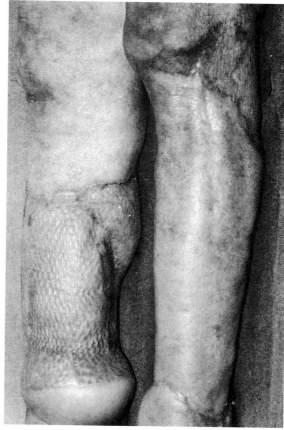
b

Figure 18.9

The late results of treatment of degloving injuries. (a) Bilateral degloving at 48 hours after injury. The degloving on the right leg was recognized immediately, but the left-side degloving was not noted by the surgeon until the time of the re-look procedure at 48 hours. Had it been the skin over the left leg, it could have been harvested and used later. (b) The cosmetic result six months after injury. The mesh pattern of the split-skin graft is clearly seen.

normal, there should be minimal loss of function in the joints adjacent to an open long-bone fracture. However, the immobilization inherent in the treatment of these extensive degloving injuries does encourage joint stiffness. It is particularly important that the plastic surgeon when treating leg degloving injuries does not allow an equinus deformity to develop in the ankle joint. McGrouther and Sully (1980) did examine function in a very basic way and noted that many of their patients walked with a limp which was usually attributed to a short leg problem. As most of the lower-limb long-bone fractures associated with the degloving injuries were managed non-operatively this is not an unexpected finding. Unfortunately no information exists on the influence of degloving on limb function in operatively managed limb fractures.

References

Carroll RE (1974) Ring injuries in the hand, *Clin Orthop* **104**: 175–82.

Cohen SR, LaRossa D, Ross AJ, Christofersen N, Low HT (1990) A trilaminar skin coverage technique for treatment of severe degloving injuries of the extremities and torso, *Plast Reconstr Surg* **86**: 780–4.

Entin MA (1955) Roller and wringer injuries. Clinical and experimental studies, *Plast Reconstr Surg* **15**: 290–311.

Goris RJ, Nicolai JPA (1982) A simple method of taking skin grafts from the avulsed flap in degloving injuries, *Br J Plast Surg* **35**: 58–9.

Green DP (ed.) (1993) *Operative Hand Surgery* (Churchill Livingstone: New York).

Hudson DA, Knottenbelt JD, Krige JE (1992) Closed degloving injuries: Results following conservative surgery, *Plast Reconstr Surg* **89**: 853–5.

Kudsk KA, Sheldon GF, Walton WL (1981) Degloving injuries of the extremities and torso, *J Trauma* **21**: 835–9.

McCarthy MC, McCarthy JG (eds) (1990) *Plastic Surgery* (W.B. Saunders: Philadelphia).

McGrouther DA, Sully L (1980) Degloving injuries of the limbs: Long-term review and management based on whole-body fluorescence, *Br J Plast Surg* **33**: 9–24.

Prendiville JB, Lewis E (1955) The pneumatic-tyre torsion avulsion injury, *Br J Surg* **42**: 582–7.

Slack CC (1952) Friction injuries following road accidents, *Br Med J* **ii**: 262–4.

Sommerlad BC, McGrouther DA (1978) Reservicing the sole: Long-term follow-up and comparison of techniques, *Br J Plast Surg* **31**: 107–11.

Zeligowski AA, Ziv I (1987) How to harvest skin graft from the avulsed flap in degloving injuries, *Ann Plast Surg* **19**: 89–90.

19
Management of bone loss

K.S. Leung

Bone loss is common in open fractures. This may happen during the initial injury or following subsequent repeated debridement of the devitalized and infected osseous tissues. As the principles of treating open fractures have become better established in the past few years, improved clinical results from the treatment of these difficult fractures have come about as a result of meticulous debridement, early revascularization and treatment of infection. Nevertheless, maintenance of the normal bone length remains a major challenge to orthopaedic trauma surgeons. Loss of bony continuity results in failure of fracture healing as well as delay in functional recovery.

To re-establish the continuity of the skeleton, bone-grafting procedures are required. There are numerous grafting techniques with different indications (Table 19.1). The success of each technique depends on the types of graft as well as the condition of the recipient sites. Three physiological goals must be attained in order to obliterate the defect and restore the normal length of bone with viable osseous tissue (Friedlaender 1987, Heiple et al 1987). The first goal is to successfully induce bone formation locally by recruiting bone-forming cells, a process known as 'osteo-induction'. The second is to provide the framework for bone deposition or 'osteoconduction'. The third, perhaps of less importance, is the provision of bone-forming cells. Different types of graft may provide one or more of these properties to varying degrees. Knowledge of the different grafting techniques aids the surgeon in choosing the most appropriate type of graft and the correct surgical approach in treating patients with bone loss after open fractures.

Timing of bone reconstruction

The importance of managing soft-tissue problems in open fractures has been well recognized in recent years. The results of the treatment of open fractures depend primarily on the management of the associated soft-tissue injuries. Adequate soft-tissue coverage and revascularization will provide the best conditions for bone-graft incorporation and subsequent fracture union. It is, therefore, vital to undertake bone grafting when these requirements are fulfilled. Cancellous bone grafting will only give good results when the recipient bed is well vascularized. It is recommended that cancellous bone grafting should not be unnecessarily delayed and it should be carried out as soon as any co-existing infection is under control and the revascularization process is complete. The necessary delay ranges from two to six weeks depending on the degree of soft-tissue injury and the type of operative procedure used to gain soft-tissue cover.

For grade I and grade II open fractures, cancellous bone grafting may be performed 2–3 weeks after soft-tissue coverage using skin grafting or

Table 19.1 Methods for reconstruction of skeletal defects in open fractures

Cancellous graft
  Posterolateral
  Papineau technique
  Allograft
Vascularized graft
  Muscle pedicle
  Vascular pedicle
  Free vascular
  Bone substitutes
Bone transport

local muscle flaps (Swartz and Mears 1986, Gustilo et al 1987, Gordon and Chiu 1988, Peat and Liggins 1990). For grade III fractures requiring major reconstruction of soft tissue using free-tissue transfer, a longer delay may be advisable for cancellous grafting, usually 4–6 weeks after the soft-tissue reconstruction (Swartz and Mears 1986, Burgess et al 1987, Caudle and Stern 1987, Johnson et al 1988b, Blick et al 1989, Melendez and Colon 1989, Fischer et al 1991). If there is to be a significant delay the technique of using antibiotic-impregnated beads as a spacer (Christian et al 1989) is particularly useful as it allows bone graft to be inserted without major dissection.

There has been a recent trend to perform free vascularized grafting at a much earlier stage, after adequate debridement. The survival of a free vascularized graft depends on the vessels and anastomosis being intact. Primary one-stage vascularized bone grafts or composite grafts have been advocated in order to reduce the duration of treatment (Byrd et al 1981, Godina 1986, Shaw 1986, Yaremchuk 1986). The disadvantage of this approach lies in the uncertainty that an adequate debridement has been performed, as often repeated debridement has to be undertaken, particularly after high-energy injury. Primary vascularized grafting necessitates major and prolonged surgery and this may not be indicated in a patient in the early stages of treatment if their condition has not been stabilized. The severity of the soft-tissue injury may also pose a challenge in achieving a successful anastomosis. It is therefore recommended that for high-energy injury with extensive soft-tissue and bone loss, a staged procedure should be used with early soft-tissue reconstruction followed by vascularized grafting at a later stage.

The method of bone transport using the Ilizarov technique is an exciting new development in the management of bone loss. Most of the current literature and clinical experience relates to bone lengthening in limb-length discrepancy and there are relatively few clinical reports of the management of established non-union with bone loss after open fracture (Paley et al 1989, Dagher and Roukoz 1991). There are even fewer clinical reports of the acute management of open fractures with bone loss using this technique. The role of the Ilizarov technique is, therefore, not fully established, and the useful-

ness and correct timing of bone transport in acute bone loss are not clear at this stage. Since some authors have shown that the presence of infection does not affect either new bone formation or fracture healing in cases of established non-union after open fractures (Pearson and Perry 1989, Golyakhovsky and Frankel 1991, Cattaneo et al 1992), it is logical to recommend that reconstruction of a bony defect using bone transport should be considered when there is satisfactory soft-tissue cover, since soft-tissue healing and revascularization are an important prerequisite in new bone formation (Ilizarov 1989, Ilizarov 1990, Moseley 1991, White and Kenwright 1991).

Cancellous grafting

Autogenous cancellous or cortico-cancellous grafts are commonly used to fill a small bony defect. These are preferred to cortical bone grafts because the more porous nature of cancellous bone is associated with easier fluid penetration, allowing more rapid revascularization and better survival of the implanted osteoblasts. This leads to a more complete and rapid incorporation of the bone graft (Hui et al 1992). The other factor which affects the incorporation of cancellous graft is the condition of the recipient bed. Regions with a good blood supply will incorporate bone graft readily (Figure 19.1). It is as important to select a suitable site for grafting as it is to achieve the correct timing.

In tibial fractures with bone loss the commonest site for bone grafting is the posterior surface of the tibia as the anteromedial surface is often injured. The posterolateral bone-graft technique in the tibia has been described by several authors (Harmon 1965, Esterhai et al 1990, Simpson et al 1990, Reckling and Rosen 1991). It is generally accepted that cancellous bone grafting will give a predictable satisfactory result with a bone defect of ≤6 cm and good soft-tissue cover (Maurer and Dillin 1987, Blick et al 1989, Meister et al 1990).

The technique is performed with the patient in the prone or lateral position. The posterior iliac crest is most suitable as the site for harvesting cancellous grafts because of the large amount of bone graft that is often required. The posterior

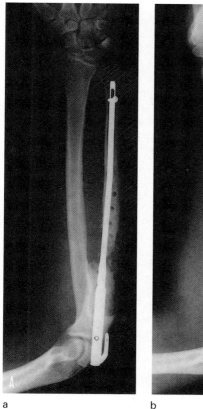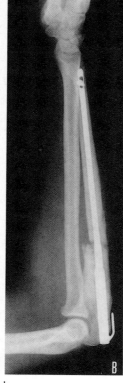

a   b

Figure 19.1

(a) Grade IIIa open fractures of ulna treated with intramedullary locked nail and massive cancellous bone graft. (b) Excellent reconstitution of the ulna after 6 months.

compartment of the leg is approached through a 10–15 cm longitudinal incision 1 cm medial to the posterolateral margin of the fibula. The gastrocnemius and soleus muscles are retracted and the flexor hallucis longus, tibialis posterior and flexor digitorum longus are elevated from bone. The posterior surface of the tibia and interosseous membrane may be exposed more easily in the normal bone proximal or distal to the fracture site. Care should be taken not to enter the anterior compartment which may be

infected. The periosteum of the posterior tibia is elevated for 5 cm on each side of the fracture. If a long segmental defect is present and the creation of a tibiofibular synostosis is planned, the corresponding length of the medial surface of the fibula should also be exposed. The bone surfaces are then decorticated and large amounts of cancellous graft are placed over the posterior surface of the tibia or across the interosseous membrane to create a tibiofibular synostosis. The deep fascia is left open, suction drains are inserted and the wound is closed. Post-operatively, the graft may be visualized radiologically using 35° internal oblique views of the tibia (An et al 1989). The advantages of the posterolateral approach include avoidance of the potentially injured anterior surface, a non-infected recipient bed which is surrounded by muscle and the ability to harvest a large amount of cancellous graft from the posterior iliac crest to place over the posterior tibial surface (Figure 19.2).

The need for a tibiofibular synostosis is still controversial. A bony bridge between the tibia and the fibula will increase skeletal stability although it has been suggested that the subsequent alteration of the biomechanics of the ankle may lead to degenerative changes (Seyfer and Lower 1989, Simpson et al 1990). Until this concern is clarified, the creation of a tibiofibular synostosis should be avoided unless there is a long segment of comminution and bone loss is best treated by cancellous grafting (Swartz and Mears 1986, Maurer and Dillin 1987).

Cancellous graft may be placed on the anterior surface of the tibia through the original wound (Figure 19.3) using the Papineau technique (Papineau 1974, Papineau et al 1976, Sachs and Shaffer 1984, Calkins et al 1987, Barquet and Masliah 1988). When using this technique, the wound must be adequately debrided and completely covered with granulation tissue induced by frequent irrigation of the bony defect with physiological saline. Cancellous graft is then laid on the granulation tissue and irrigation continued until the graft is covered with healthy granulation tissue. A second layer of graft is then inserted and the procedure is repeated until the bony defect is completely filled and bone union achieved. The skin wound is then allowed to heal by secondary intention. Although this is a technically simple method for filling a small bony

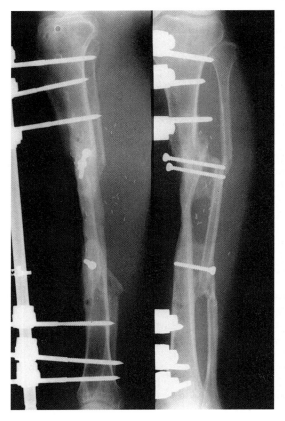

Figure 19.2

Posterolateral bone graft with fibula pro tibia operation done in grade IIIb open fractures of the tibia.

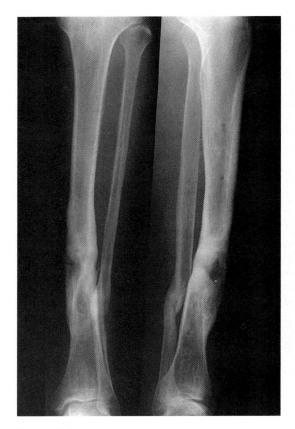

Figure 19.3

Grade IIIa open fracture of the tibia treated with Papineau technique to achieve union.

defect, it requires a considerable period for graft incorporation and wound healing to be complete. Prolonged exposure of the wound also increases the risk of infection and wound breakdown. Grafting of the anterior tibial defect may also be carried out after the revascularization process. In the tibia, the commonest method of achieving this would be with the use of local muscle flaps to fill the defect and cover the ischaemic area. Cancellous grafting can then be carried out when the wound is stable. For the proximal third of the tibia, the medial or lateral gastrocnemius muscle flap is used whilst, in the middle third, the soleal muscle flap is indicated. In the distal third, a free-muscle flap or fasciocutaneous flap is required

but if these are not possible, the Papineau technique may be used.

Cancellous bone can also be inserted percutaneously to fill in a small defect. The graft in a paste form is injected into the defect, resulting in bone formation (Ebraheim et al 1991) (Figure 19.4). Encouraging early results of the use of marrow injection have also been reported (Connolly et al 1991).

The relatively simple and safe technique of Christian et al (1989) may be applicable to a large-bone defect. The defect is filled with gentamicin beads after initial debridement and soft-tissue coverage. The gentamicin beads serve as a spacer as well as a delivery system for local

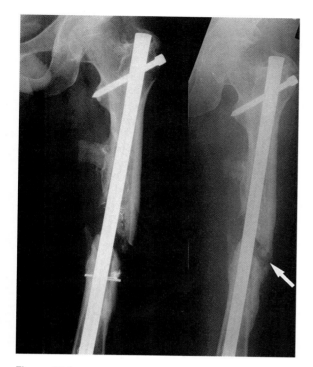

Figure 19.4

Grade IIIa open fracture of femur treated with exchange nailing and percutaneous bone grafting (arrow).

traction until callus is seen. With the current availability of locked nailing, the femoral length may be maintained without traction. This technique may be indicated in patients with open femoral fractures after control of infection in the early stage. This technique would be difficult, however, in the presence of infection and fibrosis.

The healing potential of cancellous graft may be augmented by growth factors which contribute to bone regeneration. Good results with a combination of cancellous graft and human bone morphogenetic protein have been reported in the treatment of long-segment bony defects in the tibia (Johnson et al 1988a).

Muscle pedicled graft

The treatment of major segments of bone loss with cancellous grafting often requires a prolonged period for consolidation to occur. Although there is no absolute limit for the length of defect treatable with cancellous grafting, it is generally considered that a defect of >6 cm is not suitable for cancellous grafting alone. The use of a muscle pedicled graft where the bone retains an intact muscular attachment and therefore its blood supply should be considered in this situation. With satisfactory vascularity, osteocytes remain viable and the bone retains its mechanical strength as well as the potential for incorporation (Chacha et al 1981, Chacha 1984). This technique is most commonly used in the tibia although it is equally applicable in other long-bone fractures (Braun 1983, Leung 1989a).

In the tibia, the most commonly used muscle pedicle graft is the ipsilateral fibula (McMaster and Hohl 1965, McMaster and Hohl 1975). With an intact peroneal and anterior tibial muscle attachment, the vascular supply to the fibula is from the nutrient vessels and from the rich network of musculoperiosteal vessels. This technique is applicable when the middle segment of the fibula is intact. Pre-operative angiography is required to demonstrate the patency as well as the anatomy of the tibial and peroneal vessels which may be damaged, particularly in open fractures. The fibula is exposed through a longitudinal incision and is dissected free together with a 0.5 cm cuff of the muscle

antibiotic treatment. After the soft tissues have healed, the gentamicin beads are removed and the space is filled with a massive autogenous cancellous graft. The advantage of this technique is the avoidance of major dissection during the bone-grafting operation and the elimination of scar tissue in the fracture site. Christian and co-workers reported success in eight patients with an average defect of 10 cm. This technique is also useful in areas where access to plastic and microvascular surgery is not readily available.

Chapman (1980) reported the successful treatment of three cases with large segmental defects in the femur using delayed closed intramedullary bone grafting and nailing. The cancellous graft is pushed through the proximal entry portal in the greater trochanter down to the fracture site using a plastic tube as a guide. Femoral length is then maintained with an intramedullary nail and

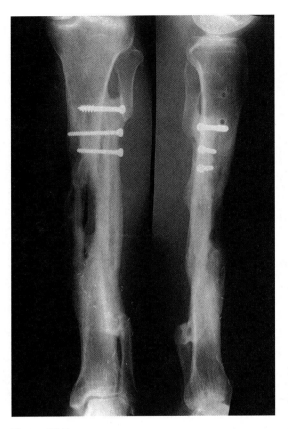

Figure 19.5

Fibula pro tibia operation in the treatment of long segment of bone loss in open tibial fracture. Note the hypertrophy of the fibula after the transposition.

attachment, thus separating the soleus and flexor hallucis longus on the posterior surface, the peroneal muscles on the lateral surface and the tibialis posterior on the medial surface from the fibula. Care must be taken to protect the peroneal vessels which pass on the medial side of the fibula. The fibula is then transected proximally and distally to give the correct length of graft required. Together with the intact peroneal vessels, the fibular graft may then be approximated to the proximal and distal ends of the tibia and stabilized with two or three screws on each side (Figure 19.5). Cancellous graft harvested from the iliac crest should then be placed around

both ends of the tibiofibular fixation to promote union. The incision may then be closed provided there is no tension; otherwise, the wound should be covered with a split skin graft. Post-operatively, it may be necessary to augment the fixation with a short leg cast. Non-weight-bearing exercises should be started as soon as possible and graduated weight-bearing may be commenced when there is evidence of union at the tibiofibular junction. With a successful vascularized fibular graft, bone union as well as fibular hypertrophy is expected (Figure 19.5).

Although this method gives predictable results and does not require microsurgical techniques, the disadvantage of losing the contribution of the intact fibula to the mechanical stability of the leg should be considered. It is, therefore, recommended that an additional stabilization procedure should be carried out at the same time. The loss of the intact fibula may also make the possibility of the creation of a tibiofibular synostosis for salvage procedures impossible (Lee et al 1990, Anderson and Green 1991).

A muscle pedicled bone graft harvested from the distal radius with an intact pronator quadratus attachment may be used to bridge a small segmental defect of the distal ulna (Figure 19.6).

Vascular pedicled graft

A common limitation of muscle pedicled grafts is the relatively short arc of rotation which restricts the area of local application. Vascular pedicled grafts may overcome this limitation and at the same time be applied without the need for microsurgery. A prerequisite for the use of such a graft is the presence of a long vascular pedicle. One available source is the vascularized pedicle iliac crest graft used to treat an ipsilateral proximal femoral-bone defect. This graft is pedicled on the deep circumflex iliac vessels (Taylor et al 1979a,b) and the arc of rotation can be as long as 10 cm (Leung 1989c). With the relatively large diameter of the artery and its venae commitante, the graft is technically easy to raise. The length of the graft may be almost half of the length of the iliac crest since the deep circumflex artery reaches the mid-point of the iliac crest before it anastomoses with the iliolumbar and superior gluteal arteries. The graft may then be trans-

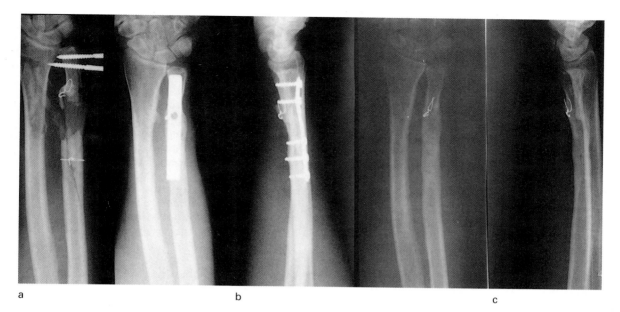

a   b   c

Figure 19.6

Muscle pedicled distal radial bone graft based on the pronatus quadratus in the treatment of open fracture of the distal ulna. (a) Immediate after operation. (b) Augmentation of fixation with plate. (c) Complete healing after 6 months with plate removed.

ferred with a pedicle of 6–10 cm which easily reaches the subtrochanteric region (Figure 19.7). An advantage of this graft is its combination of cortical and cancellous bone which provides both enhancement of graft incorporation and mechanical strength. It may also be used as a composite graft to provide both soft-tissue and skin coverage (Taylor and Watson 1978, Salibian et al 1987).

Another limited application of this technique is in the forearm where the distal radius or ulna may be used to reconstruct defects in this region, based on the pedicles of the radial and ulnar arteries, respectively (Leung 1989b).

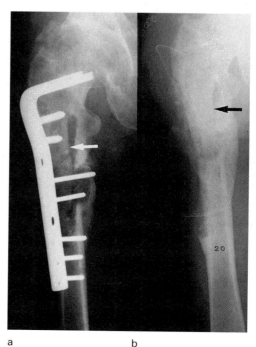

Figure 19.7

(a) Vascularized pedicled iliac crest graft (arrow) in the treatment of open fracture in the proximal femur. (b) Good consolidation after 20 months with implant removed.

a   b

Free vascularized bone graft

Free vascularized bone grafts retain their blood supply and thus the cellular components of the graft remain viable. This graft does not undergo creeping substitution and the healing of the graft to the bed is similar to fracture healing (Brunelli et al 1991). Adaptive hypertrophy is frequently observed after complete incorporation of the graft (Figure 19.8). The survival of the graft, therefore, does not depend on the conditions of the recipient bed as long as the re-established blood supply is maintained. The intact blood supply ensures an increased ability to withstand infection. These unique properties are very important in the treatment of open fractures with bone loss and, indeed, these grafts were initially designed to solve the problems of extensive bone and soft-tissue loss after open fractures (Taylor et al 1975, Taylor 1977, Weiland and Daniel 1979, Weiland 1981, Takeuchi et al 1989) as they may be transplanted as composite graft when necessary. Free vascularized bone grafting is particularly indicated in severe open fractures where there is compromise of the blood supply of the soft-tissue envelope with significant scarring, precluding the incorporation of more conventional bone grafts.

The commonest donor sites for free vascularized bone grafting are the iliac crest based on the deep circumflex iliac vessels (Figure 19.9) (Taylor 1979a,b, Leung 1989c) and the fibula based on the fibular vessels. Other donor sites include the rib (Buncke and Furnas 1977, McKee 1978, Maruyama et al 1986) based on either the anterior or posterior intercostal vessels, the lateral border of the scapula (Teot et al 1981) based on the descending branch of the circumflex scapular artery (Figure 19.10) and the distal radius based on the radial artery.

Free vascularized iliac crest graft

The iliac crest graft can provide up to 15 cm of cortico-cancellous bone (Leung 1989c). There are three main advantages to this type of graft. Firstly, a large part of the surface area is cancellous bone which allows better bone incorporation. Also, the relatively large cross-sectional area is particularly suitable for defects in the juxta-articular region and allows better end-to-end healing. Finally, the large diameter of the vessels in the pedicle makes microsurgical anastomosis easier with fewer complications. Disadvantages include the curvature of the iliac crest which may limit replacement of longer segments in long bones and the maximum length of 15 cm which may not be sufficient for large segments of bone loss.

To isolate the free vascularized iliac crest graft, the origin of the deep circumflex iliac vessels must be identified where they branch from the external iliac artery just proximal to the level of the inguinal ligament. The landmark for this origin may be found by locating the origin of the

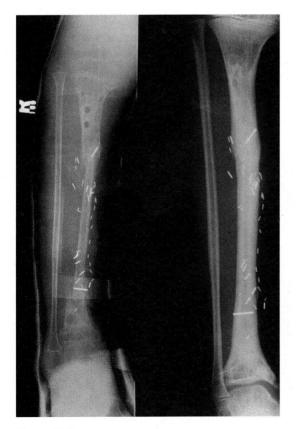

Figure 19.8

Excellent incorporation and hypertrophy of the free vascularized fibular graft in the reconstruction of long segmental bone defect in the tibia.

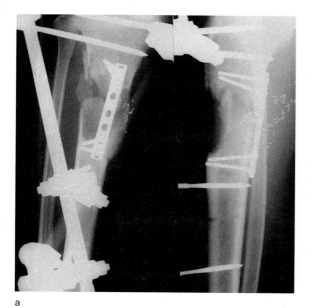

a

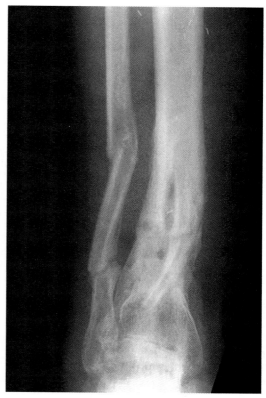

Figure 19.10

The use of the free vascularized scapular graft in the treatment of grade IIIb open fracture of the distal tibia. Consolidation 30 months after surgery.

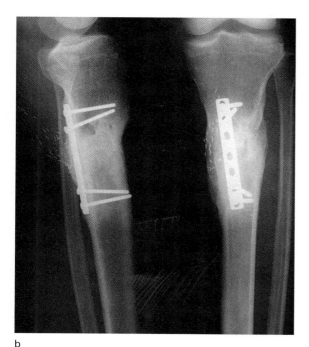

b

Figure 19.9

The use of the free vascularized iliac crest graft in the treatment of grade IIIa open fracture of the tibia. (a) Immediate after operation; (b) 24 months after operation showing good incorporation and consolidation.

inferior epigastric vessels on the lateral side of the external iliac artery (Leung 1989c). The deep circumflex iliac vessels can then be followed along their course towards the anterior superior iliac spine where they pierce the transversalis fascia and pass along the inner cortex at the iliac crest, giving out perforating branches to the bone. In order to retain these perforating branches during isolation of the graft, the three layers of the abdominal muscles attached to the crest are divided 0.5 cm superior to the iliac crest thus protecting the vessels. The external surface of the graft can then be freed by subperiosteal dissection from the tensor fascia lata and the gluteal muscle. The iliacus muscle is freed from the inner cortex of the graft and the graft can then be harvested with an osteotome on its vascular pedicle. The maximum length of the graft is 15 cm with a width of 2–5 cm. The pedicle is then transected and then anastomosis may be performed easily with double venous drainage. This graft may also be transplanted as a free composite graft. To ensure survival of the skin and soft-tissue elements, maintenance of the spatial relationship of skin to bone is important in order to prevent kinking of the musculocutaneous perforators (Salibian et al 1987). In reconstruction of small defects, a composite graft of bone and muscle is preferred to one with skin in order to avoid this complication. The surface can then be covered with split skin graft. Donor site morbidity is minimal if the abdominal muscles are carefully sutured in layers.

Free vascularized fibular graft

The fibula is mainly a cortical bone which provides excellent mechanical strength and length for large segmental bony defects (Wieland and Daniel 1979, Newington and Sykes 1991). A maximum length of 20 cm from the proximal end can be harvested. It can also be used as a composite graft with soleus muscle and skin. However, residual donor-site morbidity has been reported (Lee et al 1990, Anderson and Green 1991) mainly due to loss of motor power and knee laxity after proximal fibular osteotomy.

The free fibular graft is based on the peroneal artery which gives rise to the fibular artery as the nutrient artery. In order to ensure adequate blood supply to the bone, the periosteal branches arising from the muscular branches of the peroneal artery should be preserved by taking a cuff of the surrounding muscle. The fibula can be approached through an incision on the lateral side of the leg and the plane between peroneus longus and soleus is developed. The peroneal artery can then be identified as it enters the superomedial side of the flexor hallucis longus. With its vein, it should then be traced proximally to its origin from the posterior tibial artery. The interosseous membrane is incised leaving the posterior tibial nerve intact and the fibula is then separated from muscle anteriorly and laterally. The fibula is then divided proximally and distally

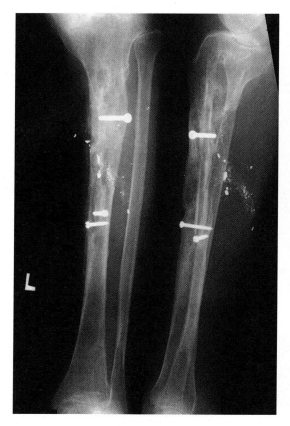

Figure 19.11

Free vascularized fibular graft in the treatment of open fracture caused by gunshot injury. The fibula is fixed with screws onto the tibia.

to give the desired length. Care should be taken to include the foramen for the nutrient artery which is located 18–22 cm from the proximal end of the fibula (Sung 1979). The donor site is then closed with a drain.

The graft may either be fixed to the recipient site with screws (Figure 19.11) or dowelled into the medullary cavity of the ends of the long bones (Figure 19.8). A successful graft will undergo adaptive hypertrophy to match the size of the recipient (Figure 19.8). In areas where early stability can be achieved or there is a large discrepancy in size between the fibula and the recipient bone, the fibular graft may be modified

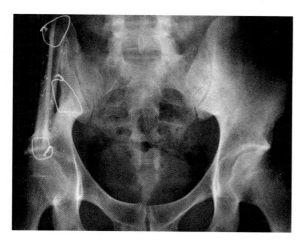

Figure 19.12

Double-barrel vascularized fibular free graft in the reconstruction of the bony defect in pelvic ring.

by an osteotomy anterolaterally just distal to the entry of the nutrient artery. The proximal part of the graft is then supplied by the periosteal and endosteal blood supply while the distal part is supplied by the periosteal vessels alone. This so-called 'double barrel' free graft (Jones et al 1988) is indicated in areas such as the pelvic ring (Figure 19.12), the distal femur and adjacent bony defects of the radius and ulna.

Rib

The rib may also be harvested as a vascularized free graft. It has two sources of blood supply: the posterior intercostal artery arising directly from the aorta and the anterior intercostal artery arising from the internal mammary artery. There is an extensive anastomosis between these two arteries and this should ensure a safe blood supply from either end. However, the rib graft does not have a wide application in restoring bony defects in open fractures, mainly owing to its relatively small diameter, its curvature and potential complications during harvesting (Brunelli et al 1991).

Distal radius

A segment of the distal radius based on the radial artery may be used as a free vascularized graft, although again the application is limited. It may be used as an osteocutaneous graft, since it has the advantage of a large radial artery for a safe anastomosis.

The experience of treating 11 cases with segmental defects after open fractures by free vascularized grafting is summarized in Table 19.2. Bony defects are due to initial comminution and repeated debridement for ensuing infection. There were three femoral fractures, five tibial fractures, two humeral fractures and one radial fracture. The average length of the bony deficit was 7.6 cm. Eight cases were treated with free vascularized iliac crest graft, and, of these, two were composite graft using skin for simultaneous soft-tissue coverage. Two cases were treated with free vascularized fibular graft and one with a free vascularized composite scapular graft for a distal tibial fracture. All the fractures finally united, with an average time to union of 2.9 months. The average length of time from injury to reconstructive surgery was 2.5 months. Functional recovery was satisfactory in all patients. In this series more than 70% of the cases were treated with bony reconstruction when infection was controlled and the soft-tissue condition was satisfactory. The results showed that complications are common when the treatment of bone loss is delayed while early reconstruction of the bony defect resulted in a smoother post-operative period and more predictable results.

Other bone-grafting techniques

The two main disadvantages of autogenous bone grafting are the limited amount available and donor-site morbidity (Keller and Triplett 1987, Chon and Krackow 1988, Kurz et al 1989, Younger and Chapman 1989). One solution to this is the use of bone substitute such as allografts and artificial bone-grafting materials. The use of the allograft has been very popular in limb salvage surgery after tumour resection and revision arthroplasty. There is a limited experience of its use in open fractures (McAndrew and

Table 19.2 Results of vascularized bone transplant in open fractures

Case	Fractures	Bony defect (cm)	Interval between injury and reconstructions (weeks)	Infection	Graft	Healing time (weeks)	Result	Complication	Fixation
1	Humerus Mid.	7	4	No	Iliac crest	8	Good	Nil	Locked nails
2	Humerus Distal	7	8	Yes	Iliac crest	10	Good	Nil	Screws and plates
3	Femur Proximal	8	6	No	Iliac crest	14	Good	Nil	AO external fixator
4	Femur Mid. shaft	8	30	Yes	Iliac crest	16	Stiff hip	Delayed union needs 20 bone grafts	Orthofix fixator
5	Femur Mid. shaft	10	12	Yes	Iliac crest	14	Stiff knee contracture of quadriceps	Pin tract infection	AO external fixator
6	Tibia Distal	6	4	Yes	Scapular composite	12	Stiff ankle	Sher's stress fracture treated with cast	Hoffmann external fixator
7	Tibia Proximal	7	6	No	Iliac crest	12	Good	Nil	AO external fixator
8	Tibia Mid. shaft	8	8	Yes	Iliac crest composite	13	Good	Superficial loss, needs skin graft	External fixator AO followed by plating
9	Tibia	7.5	7	No	Fibular	15	Good	Nil	AO external fixator
10	Tibia Mid. shaft	10	30	Yes	Iliac crest composite	15	Stiff ankle, shortening 2 cm	Prolonged wound discharge, superficial loss, haematoma, needs skin graft	AO external fixator
11	Radius Mid. shaft	5	3	No	Fibula composite	10	Good	Nil	Screws

Nelson 1989, Jaffe et al 1991). The common complications of this technique are deep infection and delay in bone union. Nevertheless, this technique is a useful option for reconstruction of large bony defects, particularly in cases with articular involvement. Complications will be minimized by eradication of infection, the use of long-term antibiotics, revascularization of the affected area with soft-tissue reconstruction and the use of rigid fixation, preferably with intramedullary locked nailing. Success has also been reported using chemical resterilization of extruded autografts (Winkle and Neustein 1987) and preservation of extruded autografts by storage in the abdominal wall (Bossi and Ronzani 1990).

Artificial bone substitute may also be used in the reconstruction of bone defects (McAndrew et al 1988, Kocialkowski et al 1990). Success has recently been reported using preformed vascularized bone graft in animal experiments (Angel and Swartz 1985, Mizumoto and Weiland 1992). Mizumoto and Weiland implanted a vascular bundle into cylindrical hydroxyapatite chambers and demonstrated a vascular connection between newly formed vessels in the pores of the chambers and the implanted vascular bundles. Further study will certainly lead to the clinical application of this artificial vascularized bone substitute.

Bone transport

Potentially one of the most exciting recent advances in orthopaedic surgery is the development of bone transport. This is a form of bone regeneration under tension stresses pioneered by Ilizarov (Ilizarov 1989, 1990, Delloye et al 1990, Moseley 1991, Green 1992, Anon 1992). He has shown that with minimal soft-tissue trauma and preservation of the endosteal circulation, bone has an unlimited potential for regeneration under continuous tension stress. He designed a distraction apparatus which allowed this biological phenomenon to be put into clinical practice. A new aspect of the Ilizarov approach included the design of circular external fixators with multiple flexible bone-holding wires and the appreciation that osteotomy

should be followed by a delay before slow distraction should proceed. This phenomenon was subsequently explored and modified by the work of DeBastiani's group. The concept of callotasis evolved from the original concept of Ilizarov (DeBastiani et al 1987, Aldegheri et al 1989, Price and Cole 1990). These authors have shown that the endosteal circulation is not as important as originally believed for the regeneration of bone under tension stress. A more important factor is the delay in distraction after osteotomy (White and Kenwright 1991) which allows distraction on newly formed callus tissue. Although different reasons are advanced for the need for delay in distraction, it is likely that re-establishment of the local blood supply and soft-tissue repair following surgery are the most important factors in the regeneration of osseous tissue. The recent finding of early suppression of osteoblastic activity after fracture (Leung 1992) also indicates that osteoblasts do not respond to mechanical stimulation in the early postosteotomy period.

It is also important to consider the site of the osteotomy which should be placed in the area with maximum potential for regeneration. This is generally in the metaphysis where there are abundant active osteoblasts. A further advantage of this site is the larger diameter of the bone in the metaphyseal region which will increase the strength of the regenerated bone. This helps to prevent fracture of the callus.

Ilizarov recommended a rate of distraction of 1 mm per day in four increments of 0.25 mm. This was much slower than previously recommended but experimental evidence has shown that many small increments in the lengthening results in better new-bone formation than a small number of large increments. Weight-bearing is also encouraged during the lengthening period as cyclical loading of the newly formed bone will improve its mechanical properties as well as the speed of new-bone formation.

The technique of callotasis allows simultaneous restoration of a bony defect, correction of limb length and deformity, improvement in the condition of the local soft tissues and the treatment of infection. This has become increasingly popular for the treatment of large-bone defects caused by open fractures (Dagher and Roukoz 1991, Tucker et al 1992).

Technique

A segment of bone is created by corticotomy or osteotomy through normal bone. This segment is transported by wires under tension and new bone forms in the gap which is created by gradual distraction. There are two basic techniques of transport (external and internal transport) which differ in their transfixion to the frame as well as the method of transport. With external bone transport, the bone segment is transfixed with transverse Kirschner wires attached to the external rings. The segment is transported by movement of the rings (Figure 19.13). This technique is indicated primarily for simultaneous bone defect, correction of deformity and limb lengthening. The advantages of external transport are the relative simplicity of ring and wire construction and the simultaneous correction of length and deformity. Its disadvantage is its inadequacy in cases with bone defects >5 cm.

Using internal bone transport, the transfixing Kirschner wires are introduced obliquely into the segment which is transported gradually to the desired position by distraction devices fixed to an immovable ring (Figure 19.14). This technique is used for bone restoration without deformity or shortening. The advantages of this technique are the possibilities of a longer distance of bone transport and less cosmetic deficit. Its disadvantages are the complexity of the construction of the frames and wires and its inability to correct deformity. It is also necessary to change the frame configuration after the transportation of the bone segment is completed since the compressive forces generated by the wires are not sufficiently strong for union to take place. There is also less control and stability of the segment during transport with the internal transport technique, although the insertion of an intramedullary wire helps to stabilize the fragment. The technique of bone transport around an intramedullary nail has been advocated (Brunner et al 1990) and this may be advantageous since an increasing number of open fractures are being treated with intramedullary implants. A combination of external and internal transport may be indicated in cases with large segment bone loss combined with deformity, soft-tissue scarring and poor local blood supply (Golyakhovsky and Frankel 1991).

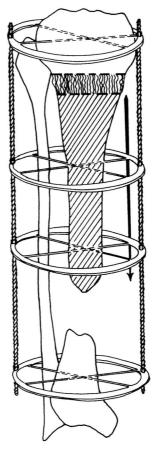

Figure 19.13

Schematic drawing of the external bone transport technique. Monofocal transport is illustrated.

Depending on the length of bone to be restored, the corticotomy or osteotomy can be performed at one level (monofocal) in which one segment of bone is transported, new-bone formation formed by distraction fills the gap and the original bone gap heals by compression (Figure 19.13). A two-level or bifocal corticotomy is indicated in large-bone loss when osteotomy is carried out in the proximal and distal fragments and the two segments of bone are brought together (Figure 19.15). Bifocal treatment shortens the duration of transport since distraction can be carried out at two levels simultaneously.

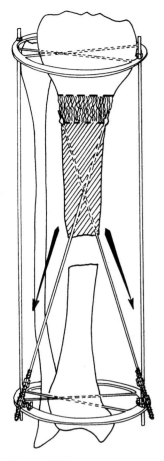

Figure 19.14

Schematic drawing of the internal bone transport technique.

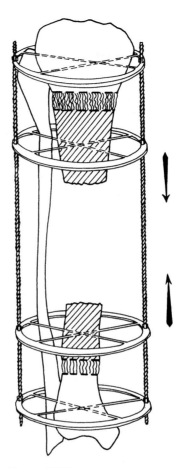

Figure 19.15

Schematic drawing of the bifocal corticotomy and bone transport.

Apart from the classic modular Ilizarov technique with a circular external fixator, the use of *monolateral tubular frames* has been reported in distraction osteogenesis (DeBastiani et al 1986, 1987). Compared with the Ilizarov fixator, the advantage of this type of fixation is its simplicity of application and the avoidance of a circular frame. The larger half-pins used in this technique are less likely to cause damage to adjacent structures during insertion. This is an advantage for the occasional user of bone transport. However, the larger half-pin causes more pain during transport and results in more scarring. A further disadvantage of the monolat-eral frame system is that the sliding component for dynamization may not be effective due to eccentric positioning and binding of the frames under axial loading (Aronson et al 1989, Fleming et al 1989, Paley et al 1990, Calhoun et al 1992).

The overall success of bone transportation depends more on an understanding of the biology of the process. Circular frames may be used in conditions where bone quality is poor and are more suitable in the lower femur and tibia. Monolateral frames may be used in good quality diaphyseal bones and in regions such as the humerus and the femur where circular

Table 19.3 Results of bone transport in open fractures

Authors	Cases (n)	Average bone loss (cm)	Infection cases n	Average delay (months)	Average time of treatment (months)	Good results Bone (n)	Functional (n)	Complications
Paley et al (1989)	25 tibiae	6.20	13	42.0	13.6	23	23	Soft-tissue obstruction, pin-tract infection
Pearson and Perry (1989)	5 tibiae	1.8–4.3 inches	5	Nil	7.7	1	Not applicable	Four needs internal fixation to achieve union
Tucker et al (1990)	7 tibiae	3.90	5	Nil	10.5	7	4	Refractures, pin-tract infection, early consolidation
Milicevic (1990)	1 tibia	14.00	1	2.0	18.0	1	1	Needs cast after removal of lengthening device
Dagher and Roukoz (1991)	9 tibiae	6.30	4	9.0	7.7	8	6	Pin-tract infection, joint contracture
Golyakhovsky and Frankel (1991)	9 tibiae, 1 femur, 1 humerus	7.80	3	15.4	12.0	10		Refractures, non-unions, residual shortening deviation
Green (1992)	17 tibiae, 1 femur	5.14	9	30.0	9.6	9	10	3.5 complications per patient, 1 amputation, 16 frame loosening, 6 bone graft, 19 wire infection
Cattaneo et al (1992)	28 tibiae	4.00	6	25.0	9 months full segment transport 2 months partial transport	22	21	3 non-unions, 3 refractures, 6 persistent infections

frames are difficult to construct and poorly tolerated. On occasion, hybrid frames may be used with a circular frame with half-pins to increase the stability in the proximal femur, or a monolateral frame with rings and tension wires in metaphyseal regions may be used. The two systems are in many ways complementary to each other (Paley et al 1990).

Since this is a relatively new technique clinical experience is limited. Most of the current literature concentrates on the management of more chronic conditions after open fractures such as the problem of established non-union with bone loss. Even less experience of this technique is reported in the English literature. Table 19.3 is a summary of the most recent reports on the treatment of bone loss after open fractures with the Ilizarov technique (Blick et al 1989, Paley et al 1989, Pearson and Perry 1989, Milicevic 1990, Tucker et al 1990, Dagher and Roukoz 1991, Golyakhovsky and Frankel 1991, Cattaneo et al 1992, Green et al 1992, Lammens and Fabry 1992). Most reports are of experience with tibial fractures requiring a long period of treatment with the fixator. The success of obtaining bone union is high and there are no problems in inducing bone regeneration with this technique, although supplementary procedures such as cancellous bone grafting and additional internal fixation are employed in some cases. Complications of the prolonged use of external fixation are common, and refracture of the fracture site and regenerated bone is also reported. Some authors recommend the application of a cast for some time after fixator removal to ensure sound consolidation of the fracture and the newly formed bone. The compliance of the patients and their psychological reaction are not considered in these reports.

Schwartsman et al (1992) and Tucker et al (1992) report the use of the Ilizarov technique in the acute management of fractures. Although their groups consist of all types of tibial fractures, their results do demonstrate that this technique is a useful part of the armamentarium for the treatment of tibial fractures. It may be particularly indicated in the acute management of high-energy injuries causing severe soft-tissue and bony damage in which a subsequent bone transport procedure may be carried out without changing the external fixator. One theoretical disadvantage of the ring fixator is the presence of the multiple Kirschner wires which may hinder soft-tissue reconstruction prior to bone transport. This may be an extra advantage in the use of the monolateral frame to give more space for soft-tissue reconstruction. Use of intramedullary locking nails in the acute treatment of open fractures has definite advantages, including a larger degree of freedom for soft-tissue reconstruction (Court-Brown et al 1990, Court-Brown et al 1991), and this makes a combination of intramedullary nailing and internal bone transport systems an attractive alternative (Brunner et al 1990). There is a need for further clinical study to document the effectiveness of these modifications of the technique.

Further study is also required to investigate methods of improving union at fracture sites. It has been demonstrated that the circular frame has good resistance to torsional and lateral bending forces but not for axial loading forces. This may be an advantage for the mineralization of newly formed bone. The alternation of compression and distraction in osteotomy sites is also a stimulus for osteoblastic activation (Paley et al 1989, Ilizarov 1989, Ilizarov 1990). With the accumulation of clinical experience it should be possible to formulate a treatment protocol for open fractures with bone loss using this new technique. The role of soft-tissue reconstruction, the timing of the start of bone transport and the use of the various types of fixator with or without internal fixation devices should be addressed. The ability of the Ilizarov technique to induce new-bone formation in large bony defects allows the surgeon to carry out extensive excision of necrotic and infected bony tissue without the fear of difficulty in subsequent reconstruction. For the future, further clinical studies should concentrate on shortening the period of application of the external fixator as well as preserving and regaining the function of injured limbs.

Conclusion

There are numerous grafting techniques available for the management of bone loss after open fractures depending on injury severity, the condition of the patient, the experience of the surgeon and the available facilities. The success of these techniques in restoring length and inducing fracture healing in clinical practice depends on a clear understanding of the biology of the various types of grafts, proper handling of the soft tissue and the early implementation of revascularization procedures in the injured area.

Acknowledgement

I wish to thank Professor P.C. Leung for allowing me to review his cases and supplying X-ray films.

References

Aldegheri R, Renzi-Brivio L, Agostini S (1989) The callotasis method of limb lengthening, *Clin Orthop* **241**: 137–45.

An HS, Ebraheim NA, Savolaine ER et al (1989) The value of internal oblique radiographs for posterolateral bone grafting of the tibia, *Clin Orthop* **238**: 209–10.

Anderson AF, Green NE (1991) Residual function deficit after partial fibulectomy for bone graft, *Clin Orthop* **267**: 137–40.

Angel MT, Swartz WM (1985) Vascularization of tricalcium phosphate, an artificial bone substitute: preliminary observation, *Microsurgery* **6**: 175–81.

Anon (1992) Orderly bone transport, *Lancet* **339**: 903–4.

Aronson J, Harrison BH, Stewart CL et al (1989) The histology of distraction osteogenesis using different external fixators, *Clin Orthop* **241**: 106–16.

Barquet A, Masliah R (1988) Large segmental necrosis of the tibia with deep infection after open fracture, *Acta Orthop Scand* **59**: 443–6.

Blick SS, Brumback RJ, Lakatos R et al (1989) Early prophylactic bone grafting of high-energy tibial fractures, *Clin Orthop* **240**: 21–41.

Bossi E, Ronzani C (1990) Preservation of detached fragments in open fractures of the limbs, *Ital J Orthop Traumatol* **16**(3): 387–95.

Braun RM (1983) Pronator pedicle bone grafting in the forearm and proximal carpal row, *J Hand Surg (Am)* **8**: 612–13.

Brunelli G, Vigasio A, Battiston B et al (1991) Free microvascular fibular versus conventional bone grafts, *Int Surg* **76**: 33–42.

Brunner U, Kessler S, Coroky J et al (1990) Defekt-behandlung langer Rohrenknochen durch Distraktion-sosteogenese (Ilizarov) und Marknagelung. Theoretische Grundlagen, tierexperimentelle Ergebnisse, klinische Relevanz, *Unfallchirurg* **93**: 244–50.

Buncke HJ, Furnas DW (1977) Free osteocutaneous flap from a rib to the tibia, *Plast Reconstr Surg* **59**: 799–804.

Burgess AR, Paka A, Brumback RJ et al (1987) Management of open grade III tibial fractures, *Orthop Clin N Am* **18**: 85–93.

Byrd HS, Cierny G, Tebbetts JB (1981) The management of open tibial fractures with associated soft tissue loss: external pin fixation with early flap coverage, *Plast Reconstr Surg* **68**: 73–82.

Calhoun JH, Li F, Ledbetter BR et al (1992) Biomechanics of the Ilizarov fixator of fracture fixation, *Clin Orthop* **280**: 16–22.

Calkins MS, Burkhalter W, Reyes F (1987) Traumatic segmental bone defects in the upper extremity. Treatment with exposed grafts of corticocancellous bone, *J Bone Joint Surg (Am)* **69**: 19–27.

Cattaneo R, Catagni M, Johnson EE et al (1992) The treatment of infected nonunions and segmental defects of the tibia by the methods of Ilizarov, *Clin Orthop* **280**: 143–52.

Caudle RJ, Stern PJ (1987) Severe open fractures of the tibia, *J Bone Joint Surg (Am)* **6**: 801–7.

Chacha PB (1984) Vascularised pedicular bone grafts, *Int Orthop* **8**: 117–38.

Chacha PB, Ahmed M, Daruwalla JS (1981) Vascular pedicle graft of the ipsilateral fibula for non-union of the tibia with a large defect. An experimental and clinical study, *J Bone Joint Surg (Br)* **63**: 244–53.

Chapman MW (1980) Closed intramedullary bone-grafting and nailing of segmental defects of the femur—a report of three cases, *J Bone Joint Surg (Am)* **62**: 1004–8.

Chon BT, Krackow KA (1988) Fracture of the iliac crest following bone grafting—a case report, *Orthopedics* **11**: 473–4.

Christian EP, Bosse MJ, Robb G (1989) Reconstruction of large diaphyseal defects, without free fibular transfer, in grade-IIIB tibial fractures, *J Bone Joint Surg (Am)* **71**: 994–1004.

Connolly JF, Guse R, Tiedeman J et al (1991) Autologous marrow injection as a substitute for operative grafting of tibial nonunions, *Clin Orthop* **266**: 259–79.

Court-Brown CM, Christie J, McQueen MM (1990) Closed intramedullary tibial nailing. Its use in closed and type I open fractures, *J Bone Joint Surg (Br)* **72**: 605–11.

Court-Brown CM, McQueen MM, Quaba AA et al (1991) Locked intramedullary nailing of open tibial fractures, *J Bone Joint Surg (Br)* **73**: 959–64.

Dagher F, Roukoz S (1991) Compound tibial fractures with bone loss treated by the Ilizarov technique, *J Bone Joint Surg (Br)* **73**: 316–321.

DeBastian G, Aldogheri R, Renzi-Brivio L et al (1986) Limb lengthening by distraction of the epiphyseal plate—a comparison of two techniques in the rabbit. *J Bone Joint Surg (Br)* **68**: 545–9.

DeBastiani G, Aldogheri R, Renzi-Brivio L et al (1987) Limb lengthening by callus distraction (callotasis), *J Pediatr Orthop* **7**: 129–34.

Delloye C, Deleforrtrie G, Coutelier L et al (1990) Bone regenerate formation in cortical bone during distraction lengthening—an experimental study, *Clin Orthop* **250**: 34–42.

Ebraheim NA, Fenton PJ, Jackson WT (1991) Percutaneous bone graft of the tibia, *J Orthop Trauma* **5**: 83–5.

Esterhai JL, Sennett B, Gelb H et al (1990) Treatment of chronic osteomyelitis complicating nonunion and segmental defects of the tibia with open cancellous bone graft, posterolateral bone graft, and soft-tissue transfer, *J Trauma* **30**: 49–54.

Fischer MD, Gustilo RB, Varecka TF (1991) The timing of flap coverage, bone-grafting, and intramedullary nailing in patients who have a fracture of the tibial shaft with extensive soft-tissue injury, *J Bone Joint Surg (Am)* **73**: 1316–22.

Fleming B, Paley D, Kristiansen T et al (1989) A biomechanical analysis of the Ilizarov external fixator, *Clin Orthop* **241**: 95–106.

Friedlaender GE (1987) Current concepts review. Bone grafts—the basic science rationale for clinical applications, *J Bone Joint Surg (Am)* **69**: 786–90.

Godina M (1986) Early microsurgical reconstruction of complex trauma of the extremities, *Plast Reconstr Surg* **78**: 285–92.

Golyakhovsky V, Frankel VH (1991) Ilizarov bone transport in large bone loss and in severe osteomyelitis, *Bull Hosp Joint Dis Orthop Inst* **51**: 63–73.

Gordon L, Chiu EJ (1988) Treatment of infected nonunions and segmental defects of the tibia with staged microvascular muscle transplantation and bone-grafting, *J Bone Joint Surg (Am)* **70**: 377–86.

Green SA (1992) Editorial comment, *Clin Orthop* **280**: 3–6.

Green SA, Jackson JM, Wall DM et al (1992) Management of segmental defects by the Ilizarov intercalary bone transport method, *Clin Orthop* **280**: 136–41.

Gustilo RB, Gruninger RP, Davis T (1987) Classification of type III (severe). Open fractures relative to treatment and results, *Orthopedics* **10**: 1781–8.

Harmon PH (1965) A simplified surgical approach to the posterior tibia for bone grafting and fibular transference, *J Bone Joint Surg (Am)* **47**: 179–90.

Heiple KG, Goldberg VM, Powell AE et al (1987) Biology of cancellous bone grafts, *Orthop Clin N Am* **18**: 179–85.

Hui J, Sher A, Leung PC (1992) Blood flow property of heterogeneous cancellous bone graft and its effect on bone regeneration. In: *Proceedings of Biomechanical Engineering Symposium, Hong Kong, April 10–11*, 104–5.

Ilizarov GA (1989) The tension–stress effect on the genesis and growth of tissues. Part I. The influence of stability of fixation and soft-tissue preservation, *Clin Orthop* **238**: 249–81.

Ilizarov GA (1990) Clinical application of the tension–stress effect for limb lengthening, *Clin Orthop* **250**: 8–25.

Jaffe KA, Morris SG, Sorrell RG et al (1991) Massive bone allografts for traumatic skeletal defects, *South Med J* **84**: 975–82.

Johnson EE, Urist MR, Finerman GAM (1988a) Repair of segmental defects of the tibia with cancellous bone grafts augmented with human bone morphogenetic protein, *Clin Orthop* **236**: 249–57.

Johnson KD, Bone LB, Scheinberg R (1988b) Severe open tibial fractures: a study protocol, *J Orthop Trauma* **2**: 175–80.

Jones NF, Swartz WM, Mears DC et al (1988) The 'double barrel' free vascularized fibular bone graft, *Plast Reconstr Surg* **81**: 378–85.

Keller EE, Triplett WW (1987) Iliac bone grafting: review of 160 consecutive cases, *J Oral Maxillofac Surg* **45**: 11–14.

Kocialkowski A, Wallace WA, Prince HG (1990) Clinical experience with a new artificial bone graft: preliminary results of a prospective study, *Injury* **21**: 142–4.

Kurz LT, Garfin SR, Booth RE (1989) Harvesting autogenous iliac bone grafts—a review of complications and techniques, *Spine* **14**: 1324–31.

Lammens J, Fabry G (1992) Reconstruction of bony defects using the Ilizarov 'bone transport' technique, *Arch Orthop Trauma Surg* **111**: 70–2.

Lee EH, Goh JC, Helm R et al (1990) Donor site morbidity following resection of the fibula, *J Bone Joint Surg (Br)* **72**: 129–31.

Leung KS (1992) Biochemistry of fracture healing and callus distraction—the measurement of bone specific alkaline phosphatase in serum and callus. In: *Symposium in Callus Distraction, International Society on Fracture Repair, Ottrott-le-Haut, France, April 22–25.*

Leung PC (1989a) *Current Trends in Bone Grafting* (Springer-Verlag: Berlin) 24–5.

Leung PC (1989b) *Current Trends in Bone Grafting* (Springer-Verlag: Berlin) 27–9.

Leung PC (1989c) *Current Trends in Bone Grafting* (Springer-Verlag: Berlin) 33–6.

Maruyama Y, Onishi K, Iwahira Y et al (1986) Free compound rib–latissimus dorsi osteomusculocutaneous flap in reconstruction of the leg, *J Reconstr Microsurg* **3**: 13–18.

aurer RC, Dillin L (1987) Multistaged surgical management of posttraumatic segmental tibial bone loss, *Clin Orthop* **216**: 162–70.

Meister K, Segal D, Whitelaw GP (1990) The role of bone grafting in the treatment of delayed unions and nonunions of the tibia, *Orthop Rev* March: 260–71.

Melendez EM, Colon C (1989) Treatment of open tibial fractures with the orthofix fixator, *Clin Orthop* **241**: 224–30.

Milicevic N (1990) Deficit (14 cm) of the tibia solved by a double sliding graft using the Ilizarov apparatus, *J Orthop Trauma* **4**: 366–9.

Mizumoto S, Weiland AJ (1992) Pre-formed vascularized bone grafts. In: *Transactions of 38th Annual Meeting, Orthopaedic Research Society, Washington, DC*, 567.

Moseley CF (1991) Leg lengthening: the historical perspective, *Orthop Clin N Am* **22**: 555–61.

McAndrew MP, Gorman PW, Lange TA (1988) Tricalcium phosphate as a bone graft substitute in trauma: preliminary report, *J Orthop Trauma* **2**: 333–9.

McAndrew MP, Nelson RL (1989) Allografting for traumatic intercalary femoral defects: a report of three cases, *J Orthop Trauma* **3**: 250–6.

McKee DM (1978) Microvascular bone transplantation, *Clin Plast Surg* **5**: 283.

McMaster PE, Hohl M (1965) Tibiofibular cross-peg grafting: a salvage procedure for complicated ununited tibial fractures, *J Bone Joint Surg (Am)* **47**: 1146.

McMaster PE, Hohl M (1975) Tibiofibular cross-peg grafting: a salvage procedure for complicated ununited tibial fractures (follow-up note), *J Bone Joint Surg (Am)* **57**: 720.

Newington DP, Sykes PJ (1991) The versatility of the free fibula flap in the management of traumatic long bone defects, *Injury* **22**: 275–81.

Paley D, Catagni MA, Argnani F et al (1989) Ilizarov treatment of tibial nonunions with bone loss, *Clin Orthop* **241**: 146–65.

Paley D, Fleming B, Catagni MA et al (1990) Mechanical evaluation of external fixators used in limb lengthening, *Clin Orthop* **250**: 50–7.

Papineau LJ (1974) Osteocutaneous resection and reconstruction in diaphyseal osteomyelitis. *Clin Orthop* **101**: 306.

Papineau LJ, Alfagerne A, Dalcourt JP et al (1976) Chronic osteomyelitis of long bones—resection and bone grafting with delayed skin closure, *J Bone Joint Surg (Br)* **58**: 138.

Pearson RL, Perry CR (1989) The Ilizarov technique in the treatment of infected tibial nonunions. *Orthop Rev* **18**: 609–13.

Peat BG, Liggins DF (1990) Microvascular soft tissue reconstruction for acute tibial fractures—late complications and the role of bone grafting, *Ann Plast Surg* **24**: 517–20.

Price CT, Cole JD (1990) Limb lengthening by callotasis for children and adolescents—early experience, *Clin Orthop* **250**: 105–11.

Reckling FW, Rosen H (1991) Treatment of infected tibial fractures: posterior vs anterior bone grafting techniques, *Orthopedics* **14**: 1025–30.

Sachs B, Shaffer M (1984) A staged Papineau protocol for chronic osteomyelitis, *Clin Orthop* **184**: 256–63.

Salibian AH, Anzel SH, Salyer WA (1987) Transfer to vascularised grafts of iliac bone to the extremities, *J Bone Joint Surg (Am)* **69**: 1319–27.

Schwartsman V, Martin SN, Ronquist RA et al (1992) Tibial fractures—the Ilizarov alternative, *Clin Orthop* **278**: 207–16.

Seyfer AE, Lower R (1989) Late results of free-muscle flaps and delayed bone grafting in the secondary treatment of open distal tibial fractures, *Plast Reconstr Surg* **83**: 77–84.

Shaw WW (1986) Acute management of severe soft tissue damage accompanying open fractures of the lower extremity: editor's discussion, *Clin Plast Surg* **13**(4): 631–2.

Simpson JM, Ebraheim NA, An HS et al (1990) Posterolateral bone graft of the tibia, *Clin Orthop* **251**: 200–6.

Sung YY (1979) The anatomical and clinical implications of the nutrient artery of the fibula, *Chin Med J (Engl)* **59**: 261–7.

Swartz WM, Mears DC (1986) Management of difficult lower extremity fractures and nonunions, *Clin Plast Surg* **13**: 633–44.

Takeuchi N, Oka Y, Arima T (1989) Clinical significance of the free vascularized bone grafts in fractures with large bone defects and non-union, *Tokai J Exp Clin Med* **14**: 35–43.

Taylor GI (1977) Microvascular free bone transfer. A clinical technique, *Orthop Clin N Am* **8**: 425–47.

Taylor GI, Watson N (1978) One-stage repair of compound leg defects with free, vascularized flaps of groin skin and iliac bone, *Plast Reconstr Surg* **61**: 494–506.

Taylor GI, Miller GDH, Ham FJ (1975) The free vascularized bone graft. A clinical extension of microvascular techniques, *Plast Reconstr Surg* **55**: 533–44.

Taylor GI, Townsend P, Corlett R (1979a) Superiority of the deep circumflex iliac vessels as the supply for free groin flaps; experimental work, *Plast Reconstr Surg* **64**: 595–604.

Taylor GI, Townsend P, Corlett R (1979b) Superiority of the deep circumflex iliac vessels as the supply for free groin flaps; clinical work, *Plast Reconstr Surg* **64**: 745–59.

Teot L, Bosse JP, Monfarrege R et al (1981) The scapular crest pedicled bone graft, *Int J Microsurg* **3**: 257.

Tucker HL, Kendra JC, Kinnebrew TE (1990) Tibial defects—reconstruction using the method of Ilizarov as an alternative, *Orthop Clin N Am* **21**: 629–37.

Tucker HL, Kendra JC, Kinnebrew TE et al (1992) Management of unstable open and closed tibial fractures using the Ilizarov method, *Clin Orthop* **280**: 125–35.

Weiland AJ (1981) Current concepts review—vascularized free bone transplants, *J Bone Joint Surg (Am)* **63**: 166–9.

Weiland AJ, Daniel RK (1979) Microvascular anastomoses for bone grafts in the treatment of massive defects in bone, *J Bone Joint Surg (Am)* **61**: 98–104.

White SH, Kenwright J (1991) The importance of delay in distraction of osteotomies, *Orthop Clin N Am* **22**: 569–79.

Winkle BAV, Neustein J (1987) Management of open fractures with sterilization of large, contaminated, extruded cortical fragments, *Clin Orthop* **223**: 275–81.

Yaremchuk MJ (1986) Acute management of severe soft tissue damage accompanying open fractures of the lower extremity, *Clin Plast Surg* **13**(4): 621–9.

Younger EM, Chapman MW (1989) Morbidity at bone graft donor sites, *J Orthop Trauma* **3**: 192–5.

20
Compartment syndromes

M.M. McQueen

An acute compartment syndrome occurs when increased pressure within a closed osteofascial compartment compromises the circulation and function of the enclosed tissues. If untreated, muscle and nerve ischaemia result, leading to disabling contractures, sensory changes and weakness.

The first description of ischaemic muscle contractures is attributed to Hamilton in 1850 by Hildebrand (1906) although the manuscript has never been found. The credit for the first full description belongs to Richard von Volkmann (1881) and in deference to this, the end stage of acute compartment syndrome is termed Volkmann's ischaemic contracture.

Volkmann described contractures caused by constrictive bandaging of the forearm and hand which he believed to be ischaemic in nature because of prolonged blockage of arterial blood. In 1888, however, Peterson cast doubt on Volkmann's reported aetiology by describing a case of ischaemic contracture occurring in the absence of bandaging. Hildebrand had been the first to suggest that raised pressure caused by an 'oedematous saturation' of muscles resulted in compression of major vessels and muscle ischaemia.

Bardenheuer (1911) gave an account of the aetiology of acute compartment syndrome which is remarkably similar to our present understanding. He noted the presence of fascial compartments, differentiated between acute ischaemia caused by 'subfascial tension' and that caused by major vessel rupture and was the first to describe fasciotomy including the detrimental effects of delay. These sound principles were echoed by Murphy in 1914 who stressed the importance of preventing ischaemic contracture by fasciotomy performed within 24–36 hours.

During the Second World War the theory of raised pressure causing muscle ischaemia was ignored and ischaemic contractures were considered to be caused by arterial spasm (Griffiths 1940, Foisie 1942, Sirbu et al 1944). Griffiths recommended excision of the affected artery and his successful results are undoubtedly due to the wide exposure required, which effectively decompressed the muscle compartments as in a fasciotomy. An unfortunate legacy of this belief persists today in the dangerously mistaken view that an acute compartment syndrome cannot exist in the presence of palpable peripheral pulses.

In the first major report on lower-limb ischaemic contractures, Seddon (1966) noted early and gross swelling in all cases, half of whom had palpable peripheral pulses. He recommended early fasciotomy for all cases. McQuillan and Nolan (1968) differentiated between ischaemia caused by major vessel disruption and 'local ischaemia' or acute compartment syndrome.

Matsen (1975) drew all these theories together and defined compartmental syndrome as a condition in which the circulation and function of tissues contained in a closed space is compromised by increased pressure within that space, with the underlying features of all compartment syndromes being the same irrespective of the aetiology of location of the condition. This is now generally accepted as the mechanism of development of the acute compartment syndrome (Matsen and Clawson 1975, Rorabeck and Macnab 1975, Whitesides et al 1975, Mubarak et al 1976, Heppenstall et al 1988, Bourne and Rorabeck 1989).

Pathogenesis

Acute compartment syndrome reduces blood flow to all the tissues in the compartment including muscle, nerve and bone. Although it is accepted that muscle blood flow is reduced, there remains considerable debate as to the mechanism of vessel shut-down. This includes proponents of a critical closing pressure with a combination of active arteriolar closure and passive capillary compression (Ashton 1975), reduction of local arteriovenous pressure (Matsen 1980) and capillary occlusion (Hargens et al 1978).

Regardless of the mechanism of vessel shutdown, the effect is to cause acute tissue ischaemia. Muscle blood flow has been studied extensively (Rorabeck et al 1972, Sheridan and Matsen 1975, Clayton et al 1977, Rorabeck and Clarke 1978, Matsen et al 1979, Reneman et al 1980, Matsen et al 1981) and there is universal agreement that increasing compartmental pressure results in decreasing muscle blood flow with an abrupt drop occurring when intracompartmental pressure reaches 60 mmHg even for a short time. Clayton and his colleagues (1977) have studied muscle blood flow clinically and found that muscle blood flow reduced as the difference between compartment pressure and diastolic pressure reduced.

The length of time for which pressure has been applied also has a significant influence on muscle ischaemia. A pressure which is tolerated over a period of a few hours may lead to significant muscle ischaemia over a longer period (Rorabeck and Clarke 1978). Other factors which reduce the tolerance of muscle to raised compartment pressure are hypotension, hypoxia, arterial occlusion and halothane anaesthesia (Matsen et al 1981).

All authors agree that loss of neuromuscular function occurs in the acute compartment syndrome although there remains debate about the level and duration of applied pressure which causes irreversible damage (Sheridan et al 1977, Matsen et al 1977, Gelberman et al 1983). Matsen and his co-authors examined the effects of raised pressure on peripheral nerve function in human subjects and noted considerable variation of pressure tolerance. Recommended pressure levels for decompression vary from 30 mmHg (Hargens et al 1979) to 55 mmHg (Gelberman et al 1983) in normotensive patients to prevent permanent neuromuscular deficit.

Bone blood flow after fracture is also affected by raised compartmental pressures. Karlstrom and his co-authors (1975) and DeLee and Stiehl (1981) noted a high incidence of delayed union or non-union in tibial fractures complicated by acute compartment syndrome. In a retrospective study (Court-Brown and McQueen 1987) a series of tibial fractures in adults complicated by acute compartment syndrome took an average of 34 weeks to unite compared to 15 weeks in a matched uncomplicated group. A recent prospective study of 25 tibial fractures complicated by acute compartment syndrome has confirmed this finding (McQueen 1995), with cases of acute compartment syndrome with sequelae taking twice as long to unite their tibial fractures as those without sequelae. Increasing the delay to fasciotomy significantly increased the union time of tibial diaphyseal fractures.

Epidemiology

There are many underlying causes of the acute compartment syndrome. The most commonly reported cause is fracture, with incidences ranging from 30% (Sheridan and Matsen 1976) to 70% (Mubarak and Carroll 1979). In a recent study of 68 acute compartment syndromes presenting to the Edinburgh Orthopaedic Trauma Unit in a 4½ year period 75% of the cases were due to fractures, half of these being tibial fractures (McQueen 1995). The proportion of cases caused by fracture varies, however, with varying patient populations.

Of the 68 cases of acute compartment syndrome there were 62 males and six females with a mean age of 32 years (range 13–83 years). The age/sex distribution (Figure 20.1) shows a unimodal distribution with a peak of young men. Four of the 68 (6%) were in open fractures.

It has previously been stated that open fractures preclude the development of acute compartment syndrome (Rorabeck and Macnab 1976) but there have now been a number of reports of acute compartment syndrome complicating open fractures mostly in tibial fractures. In 1968, McQuillan and Nolan reported nine cases of 'local ischaemia' or acute compartment syndrome in tibial fractures, three of which were open. DeLee and Stiehl (1981) had a 6% incidence of acute compartment syndrome in 104 open tibial fractures and Blick and his colleagues (1986) quote a 9.1% incidence in 198 open tibial fractures. This, however, may be

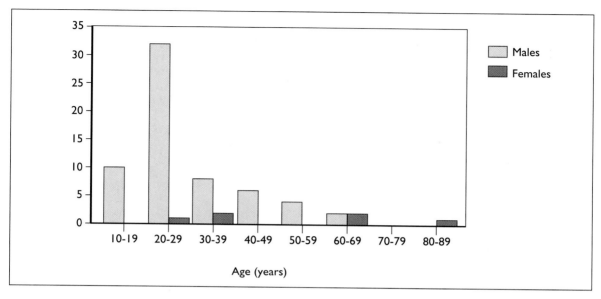

Figure 20.1

Age and sex distribution of 68 cases of acute compartment syndrome.

falsely high as their diagnoses were based on a low pressure threshold of 30 mmHg. In Edinburgh, the incidence of acute compartment syndrome in open tibial diaphyseal fractures is 1.2% (McQueen 1995) (Table 20.1).

It is difficult to assess the incidence of acute compartment syndrome in open tibial plateau or pilon fractures from the available literature as these are often included with diaphyseal fractures in reported series. Gershuni and his

Table 20.1 The incidence of acute compartment syndrome in open fractures in the Edinburgh Orthopaedic Trauma Unit, January 1988 to July 1992

Location	Open fractures (n)	Acute compartment syndromes (n)	Percentage
Femoral diaphysis	31	0	0
Distal femur	17	0	0
Tibial plateau	8	0	0
Tibial diaphysis	166	2	1.2
Tibial pilon	7	1	14.3
Ankle	25	1	4
Foot (excluding phalanges)	35	0	0
Proximal humerus	3	0	0
Humeral diaphysis	19	0	0
Distal humerus	5	0	0
Proximal forearm	14	0	0
Radial/ulnar diaphysis	24	1	4.2
Distal radius/ulna	51	0	0
Hand (excluding phalanges)	22	0	0

colleagues (1987) report a series of 32 patients with tibial fracture complicated by acute compartment syndrome of which nine were tibial plateau fractures, one of which was open. Four patients (6%) of the Edinburgh series had tibial plateau fractures and none of these was open (McQueen 1995). During the same time, one of seven open tibial pilon fractures developed acute compartment syndrome—an incidence of 14.3%. These are small numbers from which to draw conclusions but open fractures at the distal end of the tibia may be at high risk of acute compartment syndrome. Since most of the kinetic energy in these high-energy injuries is presumably absorbed at the distal end of the tibia, it may be that, unlike tibial diaphyseal fractures, the soft tissues of the leg are only minimally injured, thus preserving the limiting envelopes and in particular the interosseous membrane, allowing the development of raised compartment pressure.

In the thigh, acute compartment syndrome is recognized in association with open femoral fractures, with half of the femoral fractures in a group of patients with thigh compartment syndromes being open (Schwartz et al 1989).

In the foot, acute compartment syndrome is generally reported in association with severe crush injury often in the presence of open fractures (Ziu et al 1989, Shereff 1990) although in this site the cause of raised pressure is the severity of the soft-tissue injury rather than the open fracture. Shereff stresses that even large open wounds may be associated with a compartment syndrome and that it is wrong to assume the compartments have been decompressed by an open injury.

Only one report of an open forearm fracture being complicated by an acute compartment syndrome appears in the literature (Baumann 1973). One of seven forearm compartment syndromes in the Edinburgh series was in a Gustilo grade I open fracture of both forearm bones (McQueen 1995). During this period, there were 25 open forearm fractures. The incidence of acute compartment syndrome in open forearm fractures is therefore 4% (Table 20.1).

No other open injuries are reported as being complicated by acute compartment syndromes but there is no reason to believe they do not occur. Other open injuries are much less common than those in the tibia and femur so cases complicated by acute compartment syndrome are rare (Table 20.1).

It is clear that an open wound does not prevent the development of an acute compartment syndrome, but it is debatable whether the size of the wound has any influence on intracompartmental pressure. This is only documented in open tibial fractures. DeLee and Stiehl (1981) reported six grade II open injuries complicated by acute compartment syndromes while Blick and his co-authors found that 64% of their grade III open tibial fractures had acute compartment syndrome albeit with a very low-pressure threshold for decompression. Woll and Duwelius (1992) reported on 31 segmental tibial fractures, 80% of which were open fractures, mainly grade II and grade III injuries; 48% of their cases required fasciotomy. Of 25 tibial fractures complicated by acute compartment syndrome, McQueen (1995) reports two open fractures, one grade I and one grade II. Despite treating over 200 open tibial fractures in the last six years, with continuous compartment monitoring being performed routinely, no grade III open tibial fractures have been complicated by acute compartment syndrome in this period in Edinburgh. It is probable that the more extensive the wound, the better protected the compartment is against raised pressure, but compartments which are not open are still at high risk of acute compartment syndrome.

Clinical diagnosis

The clinical symptoms and signs of acute compartment syndrome are those of muscle and nerve ischaemia. The commonest and most reliable symptom is pain which is out of proportion to the clinical situation (Eaton and Green 1975, DeLee and Stiehl 1981, Bourne and Rorabeck 1989). Rollins and his co-authors (1981) found pain to be present in 83% of their patients requiring fasciotomy, while in the Edinburgh series 95% of conscious patients had significant pain (McQueen 1995). However, pain can be an unreliable symptom as it can be very variable in degree (Whitesides et al 1975, Eaton and Green 1975, Matsen and Krugmire 1978). Acute compartment syndrome may be painless either in association with nerve injury (Holden 1979, Wright et al 1989) or in its early stages (McQueen et al 1990). In the deep posterior compartment syndrome, pain may be minimal (Matsen and Clawson 1975, Matsen and Krugmire 1978) while pain is not a useful symptom in the unconscious patient. Pain is normally increased by passive stretching of the affected muscle group but this may often be confused by muscle injury which will cause similar findings.

Sensory symptoms and signs are usually the first indication of nerve ischaemia with paraesthesia or anaesthesia in the territory of the nerves running through the affected compartments (Matsen and Krugmire 1978, Bourne and Rorabeck 1989). Sensory deficit is reported in 42–100% of cases (Rollins et al 1981, DeLee and Stiehl 1981, Rorabeck 1984). In the Edinburgh series, 30% had sensory deficits prior to fasciotomy.

Progression of nerve ischaemia causes paralysis of muscles which is reported in varying frequency in different series. It is generally believed that motor deficit is a late finding and is associated with irreversible damage to muscle and nerve (Willis and Rorabeck 1990); 15% of patients had developed motor weakness at the time of fasciotomy in the Edinburgh series. There was a statistically significant increase in permanent sequelae in these patients (McQueen 1995).

A potentially disastrous error in the clinical diagnosis of the acute compartment syndrome is to underestimate the severity of the condition because peripheral pulses are present. Compartment pressure is only rarely high enough to occlude a major vessel and the acute compartment syndrome often occurs with pressure lower than the diastolic pressure (Whitesides et al 1975, Mubarak 1983, Bourne and Rorabeck 1989, Symes 1991, McQueen 1995). The only exception to this is in associated arterial injury where the absent pulse is due to arterial damage rather than high compartment pressure. Distal ischaemia and absent pulses are an indication for arteriography.

Swelling or tenseness is a common sign of acute compartment syndrome provided it is possible to palpate the compartment. However, in cases where the leg is encased in plasters or dressings or where there is marked peripheral oedema this sign may be difficult to elicit.

The early diagnosis of the acute compartment syndrome is of paramount importance. Delay in diagnosis is often due to either inexperience and insufficient awareness of the condition or to an indefinite and confusing clinical presentation with unreliable clinical signs. Delay in treatment can lead to catastrophic consequences including contracture, infection and occasionally amputation and is cited as the single most important cause of failure (McQuillan and Nolan 1968, Matsen and Clawson 1975, DeLee and Stiehl 1981, Rorabeck 1984, McQueen 1995).

Anatomy of the limb compartments

A knowledge of the anatomy of limb compartments is essential in order to assess and treat acute compartment syndromes wherever they may arise.

Thigh

The thigh is divided into two compartments, both of which are bounded by the fascia lata and separated by the lateral and medial intermuscular septa (Figure 20.2).

The anterior compartment contains the quadriceps muscles and sartorius along with the femoral nerve supplying them. The femoral nerve eventually becomes the saphenous nerve, supplying sensation to the medial part of the leg and foot. Thus an acute compartment syndrome in the anterior compartment of the thigh will cause pain on passive knee flexion, quadriceps weakness and hypoaesthesiae over the medial leg and foot.

The posterior thigh compartment contains the hamstring and adductor muscles with the sciatic and obdurator nerves. Thus, with an acute compartment syndrome there will be pain on passive knee extension and weakness of knee flexion. It is extremely rare to see sensory changes from sciatic or obturator involvement but this presumably occurs in severe cases.

Leg

There are four compartments in the leg— anterior, lateral, superficial posterior and deep posterior (Figure 20.3).

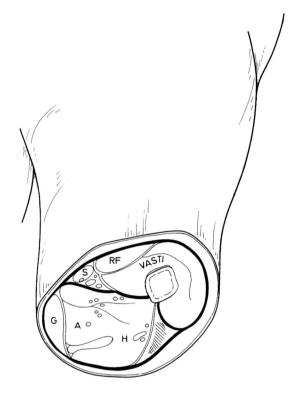

Figure 20.2

The two compartments of the thigh: anterior (S, sartorius; RF, rectus femoris) and posterior (G, gracilis; A, adductor muscles; H, hamstrings).

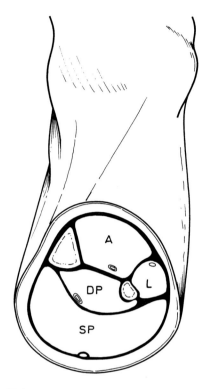

Figure 20.3

The four compartments of the leg: anterior (A); lateral (L); deep posterior (DP); and superficial posterior (SP).

The *anterior compartment* is bound anteriorly by skin and fascia, laterally by the anterior intermuscular septum, posteriorly by the fibula and interosseous membrane and medially by the tibia. It contains the dorsiflexors of the foot (tibialis anterior, extensor digitorum longus, extensor hallucis longus, peroneus tertius), the anterior tibial nerve (deep peroneal nerve) and the anterior tibial artery. Thus an acute anterior compartment syndrome will cause pain on stretching the extensors, passive flexion of the toes or ankle and numbness in the first web space whose sensation is supplied by the anterior tibial nerve. Progression of the compartment syndrome causes paralysis of the foot and toe dorsiflexors.

The *lateral compartment* is bounded laterally by skin and fascia, posteriorly by the posterior intermuscular septum, medially by the fibula and anteriorly by the anterior intermuscular septum. It contains the peroneus longus and brevis and the superficial peroneal nerve. An acute compartment syndrome affecting the lateral compartment causes pain on passive stretching of the peronei by passive inversion of the foot and sensory change on the dorsum of the foot which is supplied by the superficial peroneal nerve. Weakness of the peronei is generally a later sign. Theoretically, numbness may occur in the first web space as the deep peroneal nerve passes through the lateral compartment before entering the anterior compartment.

distally in the leg by skin and fascia. It contains tibialis posterior, flexor hallucis longus and flexor digitorum longus along with the tibial nerves. Acute compartment syndrome in this compartment causes pain on passive extension of the toes and ankle or eversion of the foot which stretches tibialis posterior. Numbness may be found on the sole of the foot and in later stages weakness of toe flexion, plantar flexion and inversion of the foot may be found.

Foot

The foot contains four compartments—medial, lateral, central and interosseous (Figure 20.4). The *medial compartment* lies on the plantar surface of the first metatarsal and contains the intrinsic muscles of the great toe. The *lateral compartment* lies in a similar relationship to the fifth metatarsal and contains the flexor and abductor digiti minimi. The *central compartment* lies on the plantar surface of the metatarsals and contains adductor hallucis, the tendons of the long toe flexor and flexor digitorum brevis. The *interosseous compartment* lies dorsal to all of the other three between the metatarsals and as well as the interosseous muscles it contains the digital nerves.

The clinical diagnosis of acute foot compartment syndrome is suspected in the presence of severe swelling but differentiating the affected compartment is extremely difficult because of the normally limited function of the toes. Sensation in the toes, nevertheless, should be evaluated.

Arm

There are two compartments in the arm—anterior and posterior (Figure 20.5). The *anterior compartment* is bounded by the humerus posteriorly, the lateral and medial intermuscular septa and the brachial fascia anterior. It contains the biceps, brachialis and coracobrachialis muscles along with the median, ulnar, musculocutaneous, lateral antebrachial cutaneous nerve and the radial nerve in the distal third. Thus, in acute compartment syndrome, elbow extension would

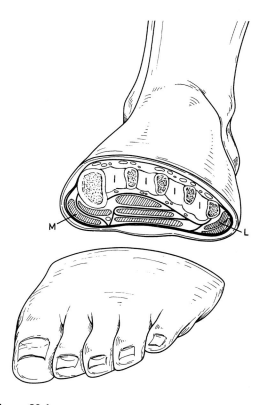

Figure 20.4

The four compartments of the foot: medial (M); lateral (L); central and interosseus.

The *superficial posterior compartment* is bounded anteriorly by the intermuscular septum between the superficial and deep compartments and posteriorly by skin and fascia. It contains the soleus, gastrocnemius and plantaris muscles and the sural nerve. Thus the signs of acute compartment syndrome affecting the superficial posterior compartment are pain on passive dorsiflexion of the ankle, numbness on the dorsolateral aspect of the foot and weakness of ankle plantar flexion.

The *deep posterior compartment* is limited anteriorly by the tibia and interosseous membrane, laterally by the fibula, posteriorly by the intermuscular septum separating it from the superficial posterior compartment and medially

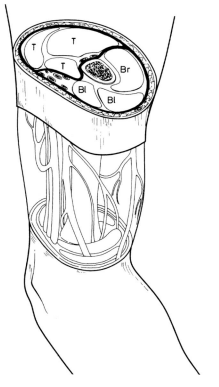

Figure 20.5

The two compartments of the arm: anterior (Bl, biceps; Br, brachialis) and posterior (T, triceps).

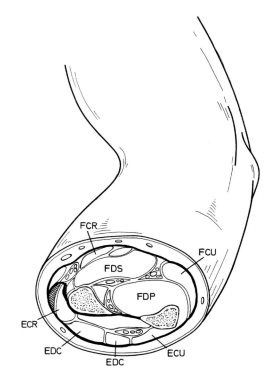

Figure 20.6

The two compartments of the forearm: volar (FCR, flexor carpi radialis; FDS, flexor digitorum superficialis; FCU, flexor carpi ulnaris; FDP, flexor digitorum profundus) and dorsal (ECR, extensor carpi radialis; EDC, extensor digitorum communis; ECU, extensor carpi ulnaris).

be painful, with weakness of elbow flexion and sensory changes in the median and ulnar distributions as well as over the lateral volar part of the distal forearm. In severe cases, there will be paresis in the muscles innervated by the median, ulnar and radial nerves.

The *posterior compartment* has the same boundaries as the anterior but lies posterior to the humerus. It contains the triceps muscle, the radial nerve and the ulnar nerve distally. An acute compartment syndrome here causes pain on passive elbow flexion, weakness of elbow extension and sensory changes on the dorsum of the hand and in the ulnar distribution. As the condition progresses there may be weakness in radial and ulnar innervated muscles.

Forearm

The forearm contains a volar and a dorsal compartment (Figure 20.6). The *volar compartment* has the ulna, radius and interosseous membrane as its posterior limit and the deep or antebrachial fascia as its anterior limit. It contains the two wrist flexors, the deep and superficial finger flexors as well as the two pronators, teres and quadratus. The median and ulnar nerves both run through the compartment. Thus, volar forearm compartment syndrome causes weakness of finger flexion often with flexor spasm, pain on passive extension of the fingers, and a loss of sensation on the palmar surface and ulnar dorsal surface of the hand with intrinsic muscle weakness.

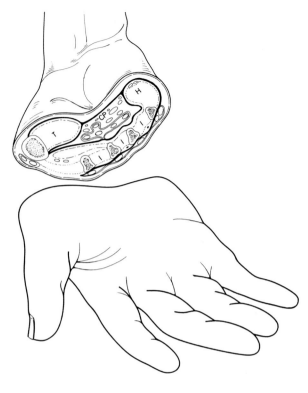

Figure 20.7

The four compartments of the hand: thenar (T); hypothenar (H); central (CP); and interosseous (I).

The *dorsal compartment* of the forearm lies dorsal to the radius, ulna and interosseous membrane and is surrounded posteriorly by the antebrachial fascia. It is split into two sections, with the mobile border of brachioradialis and the radiocarpal extensors making one and the finger extensors, extensor carpi ulnaris, thumb extensors and abductor pollicis longus making the second. Passive wrist or finger flexion causes pain and there may be weakness of wrist and finger extension.

Hand

The hand has four compartments—central, hypothenar, thenar and interosseous (Figure

20.7). The *central compartment* is surrounded by the palmar fascia anteriorly, the thenar and hypothenar septa laterally and medially and the interosseous fascia posteriorly. It contains the flexor tendons of the fingers and the digital arteries and nerves. The *hypothenar compartment* is bounded by the hypothenar (or palmar) fascia, the hypothenar septum and the fifth metacarpal and contains the hypothenar muscles—abductor, flexor and opponeus digiti minimi. The *thenar compartment* is contained by the thenar (or palmar) fascia, the thenar septum and the first metacarpal. It contains the thenar muscles—abductor and flexor pollicis brevis and opponens pollicis. The *interosseous compartments* are bound anteriorly and posteriorly by the interosseous fascia and laterally by the metacarpals. They are separate compartments and must each be decompressed individually.

Monitoring intracompartmental pressures

Because of the unreliability of the clinical diagnosis of the acute compartment syndrome, methods of measuring pressure within the muscle compartment have been developed. The first method reported was the needle manometer method (Whitesides et al 1975) but this technique has been criticized by several authors because of the potential for falsely high readings caused by injection of saline (Mubarak et al 1976), the impossibility of continuous pressure readings (Reneman 1968) and the awkwardness of observing an air–fluid meniscus and a manometer simultaneously, with possible interobserver error (Matsen et al 1976).

Matsen et al (1976) described a continuous infusion method of monitoring pressure which relies on measurement of the pressure required to infuse fluid slowly into the muscle compartment. Matsen and his colleagues concluded that the method is simple to use and accurate to within 2 mmHg. The main disadvantages are a slow response time and the risk of aggravating swelling by continuous infusion (Rorabeck et al 1981).

The wick catheter technique (Mubarak et al 1976) depends on braided Dexon wicks which protrude from the end of an epidural catheter

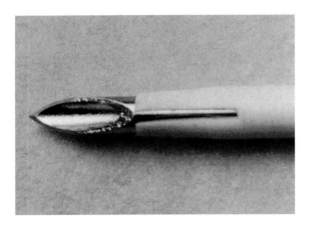

Figure 20.8

A slit catheter.

and provide an extensive contact area preventing obstruction of the catheter tip. Mubarak and his co-authors found the method to be accurate and reproducible and to allow continuous long-term measurement. A possible disadvantage of this technique is the risk of leaving part of the catheter *in situ*.

The slit catheter technique (Rorabeck et al 1981) depends on slits being cut at the tip of a catheter, resulting in a large surface area preventing occlusion by muscle. A continuous infusion is therefore not required but a disadvantage of this technique is its susceptibility to the presence of an air bubble at the tip of the catheter, reducing catheter response to changes in intracompartmental pressure (Mubarak 1983).

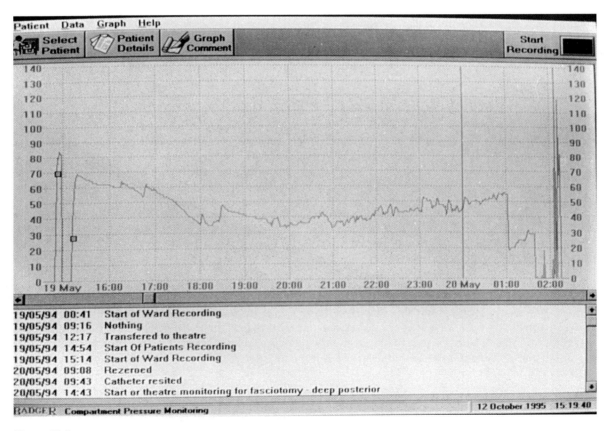

Figure 20.9

Computerized compartment pressure recording system as used in the Edinburgh Orthopaedic Trauma Unit.

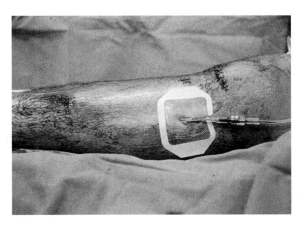

Figure 20.10

Catheter inserted into the anterior compartment of the leg.

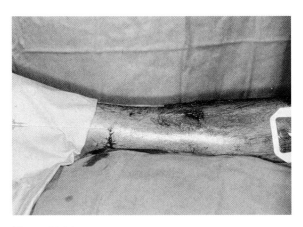

Figure 20.11

A deep posterior compartment catheter inserted from distal to proximal.

It is possible to set up a compartment monitoring system with equipment which is readily available in the operating theatre. The assistance of an interested anaesthetist is invaluable as the equipment is used on a daily basis by anaesthetic departments. A slit catheter is simple to manufacture by using a 20 gauge 6-inch central venous pressure catheter and cutting two slits in its tip (Figure 20.8). This is then inserted into the appropriate compartment and the trocar withdrawn. A small amount of sterile saline is used to fill the catheter, which is then connected to an external dome transducer via a length of saline-filled manometer tubing. The transducer is connected to a pressure monitor and zeroed to atmospheric pressure, ensuring that the transducer is placed at the same level as the catheter tip. Care must be taken to exclude air bubbles from the system, as otherwise falsely low pressure levels will be recorded. The patency of the system should be confirmed by squeezing the calf, which should elicit an immediate rise in compartment pressure. If this does not occur the system should be disconnected and refilled with saline. Saline should not be injected through the catheter as this will result in a rise in compartment pressure. It is important that there should be a continuous record of the compartment

pressures and this is achieved in Edinburgh by a computerized recording system (Figure 20.9).

It is possible to place the catheter in any of the four leg compartments without difficulty. In practice, the anterior compartment is most often monitored although in severe open fractures the catheter is probably best placed in the compartments least compounded. The catheter is introduced from an entry point approximately 7.5 cm distal to the tibial tuberosity and 2.5 cm lateral to the subcutaneous border of the tibia (Figure 20.10). As in all compartments, a characteristic 'give' is felt as the trocar penetrates the tough fascial layer after which it should be advanced so that the catheter lies at approximately the level of the fracture. This ensures that the highest possible compartment pressure will be measured (Heckmann et al 1994).

The lateral compartment and superficial posterior compartments are both superficial and easily entered either lateral to the fibula for the lateral compartment or in the mid-line posteriorly for the superficial posterior compartment.

The deep posterior compartment is entered distally in the leg where it becomes superficial on the medial border of the distal tibia. The surgeon stands at the patient's feet and the trocar is inserted alongside the subcutaneous border of the distal tibia (Figure 20.11). The trocar is then 'walked' along the posteromedial edge of the tibia until it no longer makes contact with bone at which point the tip should be lying well within the muscle compartment.

Catheters can be placed without difficulty in the other muscle compartments in both upper and lower limbs. The multiple hand or foot compartments make monitoring difficult and it is probably best to monitor the interosseous compartments, which are easily entered dorsally between the metacarpals or the metatarsals.

Tissue pressure thresholds for decompression

There is considerable debate about the pressure level over which muscle compartments should be decompressed. Whitesides and his co-authors (1975) stress the importance of relating the tissue pressure to the systemic blood pressure and stated that ischaemia begins when the tissue pressure rises to within 10–30 mmHg of the diastolic pressure. This statement was supported by Heckmann and his co-authors (1993) who studied the effect of varying differences between the compartment pressure and the diastolic pressure (Δp) on canine muscle and concluded that a Δp of 10–20 mmHg was an indication for fasciotomy. Other authors have quoted critical tissue pressures of 30 mmHg (Mubarak et al 1978, Hargens et al 1989), 40 mmHg (Matsen et al 1976, Koman et al 1981, McDermott et al 1984, Schwartz et al 1989) and 45 mmHg (Matsen et al 1980). Some of this variation may be explained by differing techniques and some by failure to take the patient's blood pressure into account. It is recognized that there is considerable variation in the individual's tolerance of increased tissue pressure (Mubarak et al 1978, Matsen et al 1980) and that the use of a single absolute pressure as an indication for fasciotomy may result in unnecessary decompressions (Blick et al 1986).

A series of 116 patients with tibial diaphyseal fractures underwent continuous compartment monitoring in the Edinburgh Orthopaedic Trauma Unit (McQueen 1995). Continuous pressure monitoring of the anterior compartment was carried out for at least 24 hours using the slit catheter method. Review was carried out at an average of 15 months after injury to document the incidence of late contracture.

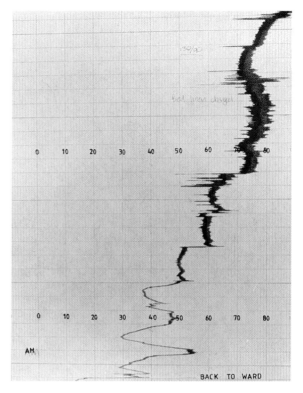

Figure 20.12

Postoperative compartment pressure in a 19-year-old male with a Tscherne grade I tibial diaphyseal fracture complicated by acute compartment syndrome.

There were three acute compartment syndromes with Δ levels of 15 mmHg, 10 mmHg and 15 mmHg, respectively. The third patient illustrates the use of continuous compartment pressure monitoring. He was a 19-year-old male with a Tscherne grade I (Oestern and Tscherne 1984) tibial diaphyseal fracture sustained whilst playing football. Six hours after injury the wound was excised, the fracture was reduced and stabilized with an intramedullary nail and compartment monitoring was commenced. His compartment pressure immediately postoperatively was 45 mmHg (Δp 45 mmHg) (Figure 20.12). The patient was symptom-free after recovery from anaesthetic. Over the following 12 hours the pressure rose to 75 mmHg (Δp 15 mmHg) (Figure 20.12) and the patient developed some stretch pain. Fasciotomy was performed and the surgical findings confirmed the diagnosis. Recovery was uneventful and no sequelae of the acute compartment syndrome were found 13 months after injury. This case illustrates that compartment monitoring allows the early diagnosis of compartment syndrome.

In the group of 116 patients, a Δp of <30 mmHg was taken as an indication for decompression. Fifty-three patients had compartment pressures of >30 mmHg and 30 of these had pressures >40 mmHg in the first 12 hours after injury but only one had a Δp <30 mmHg and he had a fasciotomy.

During the second 12 hours after injury, 28 patients had pressures >30 mmHg and seven had pressures >40 mmHg. Two patients had Δp levels of <30 mmHg and underwent fasciotomy. None of the patients with a Δp of >30 mmHg had any sequelae of the acute compartment syndrome at final review. Had a compartment pressure of 30 mmHg been the threshold for decompression, 50 patients would have had an unnecessary fasciotomy. Even if a higher threshold of 40 mmHg were used, 27 patients would have had an unnecessary decompression.

Decompression of involved compartments should be performed if the Δp level drops to <30 mmHg. It is safe to observe relatively high compartment pressures provided there is the protection of a Δp level of >30 mmHg. Continuous monitoring is essential until the Δp is steadily rising and the compartment pressure is dropping, as there may be a lag period between injury and the onset of muscle ischaemia.

Indications for pressure monitoring

Currently accepted indications for pressure monitoring are the unconscious patient (Whitesides et al 1975, Mubarak et al 1978, Matsen et al 1980, Hargens et al 1989), in patients difficult to assess such as young children (Whitesides et al 1975, Willis and Rorabeck 1990), in patients with equivocal symptoms and signs especially in the presence of concomitant nerve injury (Gelberman et al 1981, Wright et al 1989) and in patients with multiple injury (Bourne and Rorabeck 1989). Compartment monitoring has also been recommended to assess the adequacy of decompres-

sive fasciotomy (Mubarak et al 1978) and in patients 'at risk' of compartment syndrome. Some authors (Viegas et al 1988) consider that pressure monitoring should not replace clinical assessment despite stating that clinical findings are well known to be unreliable while others (Rollins et al 1981) feel that the usefulness of pressure monitoring is limited because most surgeons would find pressure monitoring cumbersome and the need for fasciotomy is readily apparent clinically. Despite this statement, this series had five patients with complications of acute compartment syndrome caused by delay in decompression.

Of 25 tibial fractures complicated by acute compartment syndrome presenting to the Edinburgh Orthopaedic Trauma Unit over a 4½-year period 13 patients underwent early continuous compartment monitoring and 12 either had no monitoring performed or had a single pressure measurement carried out immediately before fasciotomy to confirm the clinical diagnosis. The choice was dictated by surgeon preference. The severity of injury was not statistically different on comparing the two groups.

At review, almost one year after injury, the monitored group demonstrated no complications of acute compartment syndrome. In contrast, in the non-monitored group, there were 10 patients with complications of acute compartment syndrome. There was an associated dramatic reduction in delay to fasciotomy in the monitored group. This clearly demonstrates the effectiveness of compartment pressure monitoring in tibial fractures. Compartment monitoring heightens awareness amongst medical and nursing staff of the possibility of the syndrome developing and acts as an 'early warning system' for cases of impending compartment syndrome. These factors combine to reduce delay and to reduce the long-term sequelae.

Ideally, all tibial fractures should undergo compartment pressure monitoring and this is currently part of the routine management of tibial fractures in Edinburgh. It is recognized, however, that compartment monitoring may be a limited resource in some centres and in these circumstances, patients most at risk should be monitored. Identified 'at-risk' groups are younger tibial fractures, high-energy forearm and femoral fractures and patients on anticoagulants (McQueen 1995). Open fractures do not reduce the risk of acute compartment syndrome and are considered to be at increased risk by some authors (Blick et al 1986) as are segmental tibial fractures (Woll and Duwelius 1992). Open tibial pilon fractures have a high incidence of compartment syndrome as has the successfully revascularized grade IIIc open fracture because of the possible development of postischaemic swelling.

Management

The only reliable method of treating an established acute compartment syndrome is surgical decompression by incision of overlying fascia or fasciotomy. No other method has been documented which is either sufficiently reliable or rapid in reducing compartment pressures.

Impending acute compartment syndromes may on occasions be aborted by release of external limiting envelopes such as dressings or plaster casts. Volkmann (1881) was the first to note that tight bandaging could cause paralysis and contractures in the hands. Garfin and his colleagues (1981) demonstrated a 65% reduction in intracompartmental pressure by splitting and spreading a cast in experimentally elevated compartment pressures and a further 10% reduction by splitting the underlying dressings. The split and spread cast has also been shown to be the only method of casting which can expand to accommodate increasing swelling in a limb (Younger et al 1990). In most cases, however, splitting of a cast or dressings will not prevent progression from impending to established acute compartment syndrome and fasciotomy is required.

In the leg several techniques are available but whichever is employed all authors agree that exposure of all four compartments is necessary (Kelly and Whitesides 1967, Ernst and Kaufer 1971, Gaspard and Kohl 1975, Mubarak and Owen 1977, Rollins et al 1981, Rorabeck 1984). The double incision four compartment fasciotomy (Mubarak and Owen 1977) is one of the most commonly used techniques in clinical practice. The anterior and lateral compartments are approached through a longitudinal incision placed just anteriorly to the fibular shaft. The anterior intermuscular septum is identified as a thin white line underlying the skin incision and

the skin is retracted anteriorly to allow a longitudinal incision in the fascia which should be placed halfway between the septum and the lateral border of the tibia and should extend the whole length of the compartment. The skin is then retracted posteriorly and a longitudinal fasciotomy made in line with the fibular shaft, taking care not to injure the superficial peroneal nerve which pierces the fascia and lies superficial to it in the distal third of the leg.

A second incision is then made longitudinally and approximately 2.5 cm medial to the medial border of the tibia. The superficial posterior compartment is easily accessible in the proximal two-thirds of the leg and the overlying fascia is incised. The deep posterior compartment is superficial in the distal third immediately posterior to the tibia and is readily accessible. Care must be taken, however, to protect the saphenous vein and nerve which run just behind the tibia. Generous skin incisions are important as skin has been reported to act as a limiting boundary for acute compartment syndromes (Gaspard and Kohl 1975, Cohen et al 1991) and for this reason closed fasciotomy is absolutely contraindicated in the acute compartment syndrome.

Fasciotomy of all four compartments through a single incision has been described (Kelly and Whitesides 1967, Ernst and Kaufer 1971, Nghiem and Boland 1980, Cooper 1992) and has the advantage of improving the appearance of the leg in the long term. Excision of the fibula was advocated initially to expose all four compartments (Kelly and Whitesides 1967, Ernst and Kaufer 1971) but this is unnecessarily destructive, risks damage to the common peroneal nerve and removes any potentially stabilizing influence of the fibula on a tibial fracture.

Single-incision fasciotomy of all four compartments without fibulectomy is performed through a lateral incision which allows easy access to the anterior and lateral compartments. Anterior retraction of the peroneal muscles then allows exposure of the posterior intermuscular septum overlying the superficial posterior compartment. The deep posterior compartment is entered by an incision immediately posterior to the posterolateral border of the fibula.

Double-incision fasciotomy is faster and since the fascial incisions are all superficial is probably safer than single-incision methods although both appear to be equally effective at reducing compartment pressures (Mubarak and Owen 1977, Vitale et al 1988).

In the thigh, the surgical approach is over the involved compartment and fascial division is simple. In the foot the approach must be tailored to the involved compartment which makes a sound knowledge of the anatomy essential. The most commonly involved compartments are the interosseous compartments which are approached through longitudinal dorsal incisions.

As in the thigh, arm compartments are approached by longitudinal incisions over the compartments through which fasciotomy is performed. In the forearm, the most common area requiring decompression is the volar compartment. This should be performed through a long incision from the antecubital fossa and extended across the wrist crease in order to decompress the carpal tunnel. Raised pressure in the dorsal compartment is frequently relieved after volar fasciotomy but if any doubt remains a dorsal fasciotomy should be carried out through a straight dorsal incision.

Whichever technique is employed or compartment decompressed, a clear and complete view of the whole compartment should be obtained. This may necessitate a slight variation in the approach to adapt the incision to incorporate the open wound. In the leg there is no indication to decompress fewer than four muscle compartments.

The principles of treatment thereafter are the same as the primary treatment of the open fracture itself—muscle viability must be assessed, necrotic muscle should be excised and the wounds left open as closure would restore a potentially limiting envelope. At 24–48 hours later, the leg should be inspected for any further muscle necrosis, following which the technique of skin closure or coverage will be dictated by a combination of the site of the open wound and the fasciotomy. Methods of delayed primary closure by gradual approximation using a shoelace technique have been reported (Harris 1993, Berman et al 1994) but are not appropriate in the presence of skin and soft-tissue loss with an open fracture. In practice, the type of closure is probably determined by the nature of the open wound.

It is now accepted practice that fractures should be stabilized by internal or external fixation when complicated by acute compartment syndrome and fasciotomy (Gelberman 1981, Rorabeck 1984, Gershuni et al 1987). No conflict arises in the management of open fractures with acute compartment syndrome as this principle applies to both. Stabilization facilitates wound care and allows early mobilization of surrounding joints thereby reducing the development of fibrosis and joint stiffness.

References

Ashton H (1975) The effect of increased tissue pressure on blood flow, *Clin Orthop* **113**: 15–26.

Bardenheuer L (1911) Die Aneang und Behandlung der ischaemische Muskellähmungen und Kontrakturen, *Samml Klin Vortrage* **122**: 437.

Baumann E (1973) Mutilation of hand and arm with Volkmann's ischaemic contracture following a compound Monteggia fracture treated by circular plaster cast, *Therap Umschau* **30**: 877–80.

Berman SS, Schilling JD, McIntyre KE, Hunter GC, Bernhard VM (1994) Shoelace technique for delayed primary closure of fasciotomies, *Am J Surg* **167**: 435–6.

Blick SS, Brumback RJ, Poka A, Burgess AR, Ebraheim NA (1986) Compartment syndrome in open tibial fractures, *J Bone Joint Surg* **68A**: 1348–53.

Bourne RB, Rorabeck CH (1989) Compartment syndromes of the lower leg, *Clin Orthop* **240**: 97–104.

Clayton JM, Hayes AC, Barnes RW (1977) Tissue pressure and perfusion in the compartment syndrome, *J Surg Res* **22**: 333–9.

Cohen MS, Garfin SR, Hargens AR, Mubarak SJ (1991) Acute compartment syndrome. Effect of dermotomy on fascial decompression in the leg, *J Bone Joint Surg* **73B**: 287–90.

Cooper GG (1992) A method of single incision four-compartment fasciotomy of the leg, *Eur J Vasc Surg* **6**: 659–61.

Court-Brown CM, McQueen MM (1987) Compartment syndrome delays tibial union, *Acta Orthop Scand* **58**: 249–52.

DeLee JC, Stiehl JB (1981) Open tibia fracture with compartment syndrome, *Clin Orthop* **160**: 175–84.

Eaton RG, Green WT (1975) A volar compartment syndrome of the forearm, *Clin Orthop* **113**: 58–64.

Ernst CB, Kaufer H (1971) Fibulectomy—fasciotomy. An important adjunct in the management of lower extremity arterial trauma, *J Trauma* **11**: 365–80.

Foisie PS (1942) Volkmann's ischemic contracture, *N Engl J Med* **226**: 671–9.

Garfin SR, Mubarak SJ, Evans KL, Hargens AR, Akeson WH (1981) Quantification of intracompartmental pressure and volume under plaster casts, *J Bone Joint Surg* **63A**: 449–53.

Gaspard DJ, Kohl RD (1975) Compartmental syndromes in which the skin is the limiting boundary, *Clin Orthop* **113**: 65–8.

Gelberman RH (1981) Upper extremity compartment syndromes: treatment. In: Mubarak SJ, Hargens AR, eds, *Compartment Syndromes and Volkmann's Contracture* (WB Saunders: Philadelphia).

Gelberman RH, Garfin SR, Hergenroeder PT, Mubarak SJ, Menon J (1981) Compartment syndromes of the forearm: diagnosis and treatment, *Clin Orthop* **161**: 252–61.

Gelberman RH, Szabo RM, Williamson RV, Hargens AR, Yaru NC, Minteer-Convery MA (1983) Tissue pressure threshold for peripheral nerve viability, *Clin Orthop* **178**: 285–91.

Gershuni DH, Mubarak SJ, Yani NC, Lee YF (1987) Fracture of the tibia complicated by acute compartment syndrome, *Clin Orthop* **217**: 221–7.

Griffiths DL (1940) Volkmann's ischaemic contracture, *Br J Surg* **28**: 239–60.

Hargens AR, Akeson WH, Mubarak SJ, Owen CA, Evans KL, Garetto LP, Gonslaves MR, Schmidt DA (1978) Fluid balance within the canine anterolateral compartment and its relationship to compartment syndromes, *J Bone Joint Surg* **60A**: 499–505.

Hargens AR, Romine JS, Sipe JC, Evans KL, Mubarak SJ, Akeson WH (1979) Peripheral nerve conduction block by high muscle compartment pressure, *J Bone Joint Surg* **61A**: 192–200.

Hargens AR, Akeson WH, Mubarak SJ, Owen CA, Gershuni DH, Garfin SR, Lieber RL, Danzig LA, Botte MJ, Gelberman RH (1989) Kappa Delta Award Paper. Tissue fluid pressures: from basic research tools to clinical applications, *J Orthop Res* **7**: 902–9.

Harris I (1993) Gradual closure of fasciotomy wounds using a vessel loop shoelace, *Injury* **24**: 565–6.

Heckmann MM, Whitesides TE, Grewe SR, Judd RL, Miller M, Lawrence JH (1993) Histologic determination of the ischaemic threshold of muscle in the canine compartment syndrome model, *J Orthop Trauma* **7**: 199–210.

Heckmann MM, Whitesides TE, Grewe SR, Rooks MD (1994) Compartment pressure in association with closed tibial fractures, *J Bone Joint Surg* **76A**: 1285–92.

Heppenstall RB, Sapega AA, Scott R, Shenton D, Park YS, Maris J, Chance B (1988) The compartment syndrome. An experimental and clinical study of muscular energy metabolism using phosphorus nuclear magnetic resonance spectroscopy, *Clin Orthop* **226**: 138–55.

Hildebrand O (1906) Die Lehre von den ischaemischen Muskellähmungen und Kontrakturen, *Zeitschr Chir* **108**: 44–201.

Holden CEA (1979) The pathology and prevention of Volkmann's ischaemic contracture, *J Bone Joint Surg* **61B**: 296–300.

Karlstrom G, Lonnerholm T, Olerud S (1975) Cavus deformity of the foot after fracture of the tibial shaft, *J Bone Joint Surg* **57A**: 893–900.

Kelly RP, Whitesides TE (1967) Transfibular route for fasciotomy of the leg, *J Bone Joint Surg* **49A**: 1022–3.

Koman LA, Hardaker WT Jr, Goldner JL (1981) Wick catheter in evaluating and treating compartment syndrome, *South Med J* **73**: 303–9.

McDermott AGP, Marble AE, Yabsley RH (1984) Monitoring acute compartment pressures with the STIC catheter, *Clin Orthop* **190**: 192–8.

McQueen MM (1995) Acute compartment syndrome: its effect on bone blood flow and bone union, MD Thesis, University of Edinburgh.

McQueen MM, Christie J, Court-Brown CM (1990) Compartment pressures after intramedullary nailing of the tibia, *J Bone Joint Surg* **72B**: 395–7.

McQuillan WM, Nolan B (1968) Ischaemia complicating injury, *J Bone Joint Surg* **50B**: 482–92.

Matsen FA (1975) Compartmental syndrome. A unified concept, *Clin Orthop* **113**: 8–14.

Matsen FA (1980) *Compartmental Syndromes* (Grune and Stratton: New York).

Matsen FA, Clawson DK (1975) The deep posterior compartmental syndrome of the leg, *J Bone Joint Surg* **57A**: 34–9.

Matsen FA, Krugmire RB (1978) Compartmental syndromes, *Surg Gynecol Obstet* **147**: 943–9.

Matsen FA, Mayo KY, Sheridan GW, Krugmire RB (1976) Monitoring of intramuscular pressure, *Surgery* **79**: 702–9.

Matsen FA, Mayo KA, Krugmire RB, Sheridan GW, Kraft GH (1977) A model compartment syndrome in man with particular reference to the quantification of nerve function, *J Bone Joint Surg* **59A**: 648–53.

Matsen FA, King RV, Krugmire RB, Mowery CA, Roche T (1979) Physiological effects of increased tissue pressure, *Int Orthop* **3**: 237–44.

Matsen FA, Winquist RA, Krugmire RB (1980) Diagnosis and management of compartment syndromes, *J Bone Joint Surg* **62A**: 286–91.

Matsen FA, Wyss CR, King RV, Barnes D, Simmons CW (1981) Factors affecting the tolerance of muscle circulation and function for increased tissue pressure, *Clin Orthop* **155**: 224–30.

Mubarak SJ (1983) A practical approach to compartmental syndrome. Part II. Diagnosis, *AAOS Instr Course Lect* **32**: 92–102.

Mubarak SJ, Owen CA (1977) Double-incision fasciotomy of the leg for decompression in compartment syndromes, *J Bone Joint Surg* **59A**: 184–7.

Mubarak SJ, Carroll NC (1979) Volkmann's contracture in children: aetiology and prevention, *J Bone Joint Surg* **61B**: 285–93.

Mubarak SJ, Hargens AR, Owen CA, Garetto LP, Akeson WH (1976) The wick catheter technique for measurement of intramuscular pressure. A new research and clinical tool, *J Bone Joint Surg* **58A**: 1016–20.

Mubarak SJ, Owen CA, Hargens AR, Garetto LP, Akeson WH (1978) Acute compartment syndromes. Diagnosis and treatment with the aid of the wick catheter, *J Bone Joint Surg* **60A**: 1091–5.

Murphy JB (1914) Myositis, *JAMA* **63**(15): 1249–55.

Nghiem DD, Boland JP (1980) Four-compartment fasciotomy of the lower extremity without fibulectomy: a new approach, *Am Surg* **46**: 414–17.

Oestern H-J, Tscherne H (1984) Pathophysiology and classification of soft tissue injuries associated with fractures. In: Tscherne H, Gotzen L, eds, *Fractures with Soft Tissue Injuries* (Springer-Verlag: Berlin) 1–9.

Reneman RS (1968) *The Anterior and the Lateral Compartment Syndrome of the Leg* (Moutin: Paris).

Reneman RS, Slaaf DW, Lindbom L, Tangelder GJ, Arfors KE (1980) Muscle blood flow disturbances produced by simultaneously elevated venous and total muscle tissue pressure, *Microvasc Res* **20**: 307–18.

Rollins DL, Bernhard VM, Towne JB (1981) Fasciotomy: an appraisal of controversial issues, *Arch Surg* **116**: 1474–81.

Rorabeck CH (1984) The treatment of compartment syndromes of the leg, *J Bone Joint Surg* **66B**: 93–7.

Rorabeck CH, Macnab I (1975) The pathophysiology of the anterior tibial compartmental syndrome, *Clin Orthop* **113**: 52–7.

Rorabeck CH, Macnab I (1976) Anterior tibial compartment syndrome complicating fractures of the shaft of the tibia, *J Bone Joint Surg* **58A**: 549–50.

Rorabeck CH, Clarke KM (1978) The pathophysiology of the anterior tibial compartment syndrome. An experimental investigation, *J Trauma* **18**(5): 299–304.

Rorabeck CH, Macnab I, Waddell JP (1972) Anterior tibial compartment syndrome: a clinical and experimental review, *Can J Surg* **15**: 249–56.

Rorabeck CH, Castle GSP, Hardie R, Logan J (1981) Compartmental pressure measurements: an experimental investigation using the slit catheter, *J Trauma* **21**: 446–9.

Schwartz JT, Brumback RJ, Lakatos R, Poka A, Bathon GH, Burgess AR (1989) Acute compartment syndrome of the thigh, *J Bone Joint Surg* **71A**: 392–400.

Seddon HJ (1966) Volkmann's ischaemia in the lower limb, *J Bone Joint Surg* **48B**: 627–36.

Shereff MJ (1990) Compartment syndromes of the foot, *AAOS Instr Course Lect* **39**: 127—32.

Sheridan GW, Matsen FA (1975) An animal model of the compartmental syndrome, *Clin Orthop* **113**: 36–42.

Sheridan GW, Matsen FA (1976) Fasciotomy in the treatment of the acute compartment syndrome, *J Bone Joint Surg* **58A**: 112–15.

Sheridan GW, Matsen FA, Krugmire RB (1977) Further investigations on the pathophysiology of the compartmental syndrome, *Clin Orthop* **123**: 266–70.

Sirbu AB, Murphy MJ, White AS (1944) Soft tissue complications of fracture of the leg, *Calif West Med* **60**: 53–5.

Symes J (1991) Compartment syndrome, *Can J Surg* **34**: 307–8.

Viegas SF, Rimoldi R, Scarborough M, Ballantyne GM (1988) Acute compartment syndrome in the thigh: a case report and a review of the literature, *Clin Orthop* **234**: 232–4.

Vitale GC, Richardson JD, George SM, Miller FB (1988) Fasciotomy for severe, blunt and penetrating trauma of the extremity, *Surg Gynecol Obstet* **166**: 397–401.

Volkmann R (1881) Die ischaemischen Muskellähmungen und Kontrakturen, *Centrabl Chir* 51–801.

Whitesides TE, Haney TC, Morimoto K, Harada H (1975) Tissue pressure measurements as a determinant for the need of fasciotomy, *Clin Orthop* **113**: 43–51.

Willis RB, Rorabeck CH (1990) Treatment of compartment syndrome in children, *Orthop Clin N Am* **21**: 401–12.

Woll TS, Duwelius PJ (1992) The segmental tibial fracture, *Clin Orthop* **281**: 204–7.

Wright JG, Bogoch ER, Hastings DE (1989) The 'occult' compartment syndrome, *J Trauma* **29**: 133–4.

Younger ASE, Curran P, McQueen MM (1990) Backslabs and plaster casts: which will best accommodate increasing intracompartmental pressures? *Injury* **21**: 178–81.

Ziu I, Mosheiff R, Zeligowski A, Lilbergal M, Lowe J, Segal D (1989) Crush injuries of the foot with compartment syndrome: immediate one-stage management, *Foot Ankle* **9**: 185–9.

21
Post-traumatic osteomyelitis

C.R. Perry

Osteomyelitis means inflammation, secondary to bacterial infection, of bone and marrow. Post-traumatic osteomyelitis denotes that the infected area has been previously traumatized. It is a serious clinical problem which results in significant disability. The severity of the problem is compounded by the fact that many of the patients are relatively young and in the peak of their productive years. In this chapter we will review the pathogenesis of osteomyelitis, describe a classification scheme designed to guide our management and to give us an approximate prognosis, and finally describe the specific techniques used to manage osteomyelitis.

Pathogenesis

Osteomyelitis is a unique infectious process in that it remains localized and frequently becomes chronic. Other infectious diseases, such as pneumonia or endocarditis, either kill the patient or are themselves eradicated by the patient's defence mechanisms. A knowledge of the pathogenesis of osteomyelitis leads us in understanding the interplay between host defence mechanisms and the invasive growth of virulent bacteria, helping us, as orthopaedic surgeons, to optimize host defences and to neutralize those factors which aid bacterial growth.

The initial event in the pathogenesis of post-traumatic osteomyelitis is the introduction of bacteria into a fracture. This may occur either at the time of injury, through a break in the skin, or at surgery when the fracture has been surgically exposed in order to reduce and stabilize it. Haematogenous inoculation of closed fractures has been described; however, this is an extremely rare occurrence. The size of the inoculum (i.e. the number of organisms intro-

duced into the fracture) is important as it determines whether an infection will develop and the rate of onset of signs and symptoms. There is a threshold number of bacteria which must be in the inoculum for infection to develop. If there are less than this number, the bacteria will be eradicated by the host. Bacteria reproduce by binary fission, so the size of the inoculum also affects the rate of onset of infection. The clinical implications at this stage are that we can diminish the incidence of osteomyelitis in two ways: (1) administer antibiotics directed specifically at the organisms to which the patient is likely to be exposed; and (2) decrease the number of bacteria in the wound by debridement of contaminated tissue.

Following an open fracture, cultures of the wound are obtained, and antibiotics are administered. The antibiotic must be an effective anti-staphylococcal agent (e.g. the second-generation cephalosporin cephalexin), as *Staphylococcus aureus* is the most common cause of post-traumatic osteomyelitis. Gram-negative organisms are becoming increasingly common pathogens and therefore some investigators recommend the routine addition of an antibiotic effective against Gram-negative organisms (e.g. the aminoglycoside gentamicin). Certainly this should be done if the wound is grossly contaminated.

To reduce the size of the inoculum, wounds are washed out in the emergency room. Macroscopic foreign bodies are removed and a sterile dressing is applied. It is important to prevent inoculation of the wound with nosocomial organisms (e.g. methicillin-resistant *Staphylococcus aureus*), as these are extremely virulent and invasive.

Once bacteria have been introduced into the area surrounding the fracture, they find an environment which in many respects is ideal for their growth and reproduction. This environment contains nutrients which the bacteria ingest and surfaces to which bacteria can adhere and form colonies. To a great extent it is isolated from the host defence mechanisms, i.e. white blood cells, antibodies and antibiotics. The clinical implications are that the incidence of infection can be decreased by debriding the wound of haematoma, foreign bodies and avascular soft tissue and bone.

As the bacteria grow and multiply they release substances which induce migration of polymorphonuclear leukocytes (PMNs) into the area. This process of induced migration is chemotaxis. The chemotactants (i.e. factors which cause chemotaxis) are initially released by bacteria; later, other chemotactants are generated by the host via the complement cascade and macrophages stimulated by specific antigens. Chemotaxis is depressed in patients with rheumatoid arthritis, correlating with a possible increased incidence of infection in these patients. The PMNs adhere to bacteria and begin to phagocytose them. This process is aided by opsonins or molecules which attach to the bacteria. Opsonins are produced by the complement system and by antibodies. As the infectious process continues, the host defence systems are honed by activating lymphocytes specifically to the antigens found on and in the bacteria. This is a complex system which involves processing of the specific antigens by macrophages. Activated lymphocytes produce specific antibodies or become cytotoxic clones (T-cells). The clinical implications are that the competence of the immune system is dependent upon the overall state of health of the patient. When nutritional imbalances are corrected, the immune system becomes more effective.

As the host defences become more active and more effective at killing bacteria, the bacteria adapt and become more resistant. They form colonies on surfaces. These fixed bacteria are more resistant to phagocytosis and the action of antibiotics than free-floating bacteria. This is primarily on the basis of glycocalyx, a mucopolysaccharide produced by the bacteria. The glycocalyx coats the bacteria, preventing penetration by leukocytes and antibiotics.

The bacteria develop resistance to many of the antibiotics. Resistance is either on the basis of preventing penetration of the antibiotic into the bacteria, or on the basis of enzymes that inactivate the antibiotic. At this stage the patient has chronic osteomyelitis.

Classification

Post-traumatic osteomyelitis is classified as *acute* or *chronic*. Chronic osteomyelitis is further classified according to the extent of involvement and the immunocompetency of the host.

Acute osteomyelitis

We arbitrarily define osteomyelitis as being acute if it has been symptomatic for less than four weeks. After four weeks of symptoms, we define it as chronic. A less arbitrary and more accurate definition is that osteomyelitis is acute as long as the predominant histological and clinical picture is that of acute infection. When chronic inflammation and the secondary changes due to dysvascularity and scarring begin, the disease is defined as chronic. Even this definition is unclear, because chronic osteomyelitis is frequently complicated by acute flare-ups.

Chronic osteomyelitis

The diagnosis of chronic osteomyelitis is based on the presence of chronic drainage from sinuses, or ulcers. There is always a history of acute osteomyelitis. The patient is seldom systemically ill. The diagnosis is confirmed by growing organisms in culture from material obtained from the area in question. An acute 'flare-up' as indicated by pain, swelling, cellulitis and abscess formation may be superimposed on chronic osteomyelitis.

Cierny et al (1985) classify chronic osteomyelitis into 12 groups. These groups have implications regarding management and prognosis, but they do not necessarily imply the origin or pathophysiology of the infection. This classification system is based upon the location and extent of involvement of the bone and the physiological status of the patient. Location and extent of involvement is classified into four groups: (1) *superficial*, in which only the outer surface of the cortex is involved; (2) *medullary*, in which the medullary canal is involved; (3) *localized*, in which a full-thickness area of cortex is involved; and (4) *diffuse*, in which there is segmental involvement. The physiological status of the patient is classified into three groups: an *A host* is a patient who mounts a normal response to infection; a *B host* is one who cannot mount a normal response either because of local compromise, or because of systemic compromise; a *C host* is a patient for whom treatment is worse than the effects of the disease. This is usually because the disease is minimally symptomatic, or because the required therapy is so extensive that its risk outweighs that of the infection. The management implications of this classification system are that more extensive involvement requires more extensive resection and reconstruction, B hosts should be changed to A hosts prior to therapy and C hosts should not be treated. The prognostic factors are that more extensive involvement and compromise of the host carry a poor prognosis.

Management

It is essential that the patient realizes the severity of the problem before treatment is initiated. In many cases despite our best efforts, the infection will persist. In other cases, the patient and surgeon focus on the infection, not realizing that even if the infection were eradicated, the extremity would be useless because of other injuries or deficits. Some patients have so little disability associated with the infection, or will require such extensive and numerous surgeries, that treatment is not warranted.

There are five basic tools with which we manage post-traumatic osteomyelitis:

1. Debridement of necrotic tissue and foreign bodies.
2. Stabilization of associated fractures or non-unions.
3. Soft-tissue coverage of exposed bone or fractures.
4. Management of dead space.
5. Effective antibiotic administration.

Debridement

Debridement of necrotic tissue and foreign material is the starting point in the management of post-traumatic osteomyelitis. Necrotic bone and foreign material provide surfaces to which bacteria adhere, increasing their resistance to antibiotics, humoral factors (e.g. antibodies and complement) and white blood cells. This has two clinical implications:

1. It may be very difficult to control the progression of an infection complicated by the presence of necrotic tissue and foreign bodies. Cellulitis, osteolysis, purulent drainage and pain may result in permanent loss of function and necessitate complex reconstructive procedures.
2. Adherent bacteria may remain dormant, and there may be no clinical signs of infection for years until a stimulus activates the bacteria, they begin to replicate and the infection becomes clinically evident. Therefore, in cases in which the infection is progressing uncontrollably, or in which cure or permanent suppression of the infection is the goal, all necrotic soft tissue, bone and foreign material must be surgically debrided.

Carrying the principle of surgical debridement to the extreme may lead to the removal of viable tissue and implants which are vital to the function of a limb or are providing necessary stability. This may result in loss of function or even amputation. The central problem is to identify tissue which is necrotic, and implants which are not serving a constructive purpose.

Soft tissue

Necrotic soft tissue is easily recognized. It does not bleed when cut, and differs in appearance from surrounding viable tissue. Necrotic muscle will not contract when stimulated by electrocautery or pinching with a forceps. Haematoma is considered to be necrotic and is removed by irrigation and curettage.

The viability of tendons and ligaments is difficult to assess, and unnecessary debridement is associated with significant loss of function. This problem is most frequently encountered with infections involving the patellar ligament and Achilles' tendon. One way to approach this problem is with a staged procedure. At the first operation, all fragmented tissue is removed. Tendon or ligament which appears structurally intact is left undisturbed. The wound is kept moist with wet dressings which are changed daily. Further fragmentation of tendon or ligament necessitates a second debridement. If the tendon or ligament remains intact, and granulation tissue forms on its surface, it is viable and is covered with a free or local soft-tissue transfer.

Sinus tracts consist of viable tissue, but harbour large numbers of bacteria. They are excised if their excision will not result in a more difficult reconstructive procedure. When they are left in situ, they involute spontaneously as the infection is brought under control.

Bone

The surgical exposure for debridement of necrotic bone is tailored to each case. The approach must be extensive enough to expose all suspect areas and yet it must be designed to minimize devitalization of tissue which has been compromised by previous surgery. Usually it is best to use previous incisions when debriding post-traumatic osteomyelitis.

During the surgical exposure and debridement care is taken to minimize further devitalization of bone. The vascular supply of diaphyseal bone is via periosteal vessels and nutrient arteries in the medullary canal. The metaphysis is also supplied by metaphyseal vessels which perforate the cortex of the metaphysis. It is important to minimize damage to these sources of vascularity. Therefore the technique of 'sub-periosteal exposure' is seldom utilized. Retractors which result in soft-tissue stripping (e.g. Hohman, Bennet, and Criego retractors) are avoided as they may damage the periosteum, or strip it from the underlying bone. Sequential reaming of a medullary canal destroys the medullary vessels and is therefore avoided in most cases. The one instance in which we routinely use reaming is following removal of an infected intramedullary nail. The alternative is to unroof the medullary canal in order to adequately debride it. This is reserved for cases in which there is persistent

infection following nail removal and reaming. In these cases, the surgical procedure can usually be limited to one portion of the bone (e.g. proximal middle or distal third) and is not as extensive as it would be if done as a primary procedure. The combination of periosteal stripping and reaming of the medullary canal must be avoided as it will result in segmental devitalization of the cortex.

Viable bone is identified by active 'pin-point' bleeding from osteons. Bleeding can only be seen if a tourniquet is not being used. High-speed burrs or osteotomes are used to remove necrotic bone. The use of high-speed burrs minimizes the risk of fracture; however, the burr will cause thermal necrosis if not constantly irrigated. The use of osteotomes increases the chance of fracturing a bone already attenuated by debridement, but there is no risk of thermal necrosis. The bone is irrigated throughout the debridement to clear its surface of blood and debris so that the pin-point bleeders can be identified. It may be difficult to determine whether dysvascular bone and scar should be removed. We tend to err on the side of debridement at the cost of requiring more extensive secondary procedures for closure and management of dead space. As with soft-tissue debridement, the presence of granulation 4–7 days after the initial debridement indicates a healthy vascularized wound.

Foreign bodies

The foreign body encountered most frequently in post-traumatic osteomyelitis is an internal fixation device. The concept is to leave the device in situ until the fracture or non-union has healed, as long as it is providing stability. After the fracture or non-union has healed, the device is removed and the wound debrided of necrotic tissue (Figures 21.1–21.3). If an implant is not stabilizing a fracture or non-union because it has loosened, it is removed. Radiographic signs of loosening are broken screws, plates or nails, the 'windshield wiper' sign and a change in alignment seen on stress radiographs. Occasionally an implant is left in situ because the exposure necessary to remove the implant is so extensive that less harm is done by leaving the implant in place (e.g. a broken screw in the femoral head).

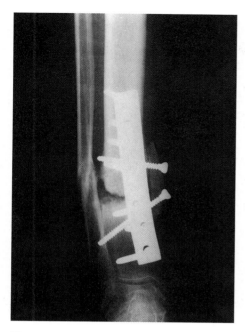

Figure 21.1

Radiograph of a distal tibia fracture which has been stabilized three months previously with a broad dynamic
compression plate. In addition to the plate, there is a cortical fragment of bone bridging the fracture fastened to the
medial side of the tibia with screws. Post-operatively, the
patient developed a wound slough, and presented with a
draining wound and exposed hardware, but minimal cellulitis. Alignment is marginally acceptable with medial translation of the distal fragment and 2–4° of valgus. There are
no signs of loosening of fixation. An electrical stimulator
was added, non-weight-bearing was continued, dressing
changes were continued and antibiotics were not started.

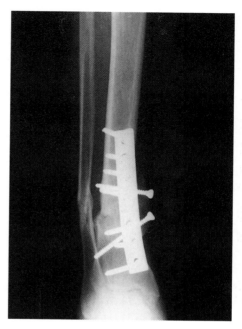

Figure 21.2

Three months later the fracture has consolidated (see
Figure 21.1). There is still exposed hardware and active
drainage.

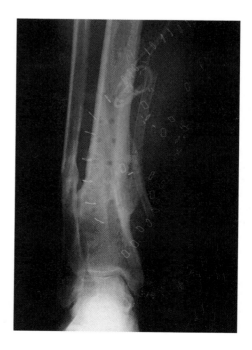

Figure 21.3

The plate and screws have been removed and necrotic
bone has been removed (see Figure 21.2). A free-tissue
transfer has been performed, and the tissue has been
contoured to fill the dead space. Six weeks of local antibiotics were administered with an antibiotic pump. The
patient has done well with no further signs of infection.

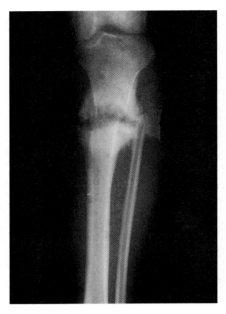

Figure 21.4

Anteroposterior radiograph of an infected hypertrophic non-union of the proximal tibia resulting from an open fracture.

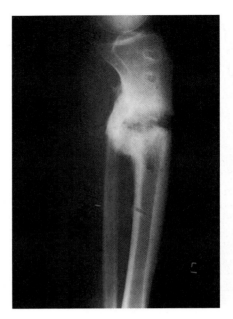

Figure 21.5

Lateral radiograph of the same patient as in Figure 21.4.

Stabilization of associated fractures and non-unions

Motion, or instability, through infected fractures and non-unions seems to exacerbate the symptoms of infection, and to make it more difficult to suppress the infection. When the wound has been thoroughly debrided of necrotic tissue and implants, re-establishment of stability begins. This may entail nothing more than plating or nailing a non-union, or it may entail an extremely complex procedure, such as a free fibular transfer. In general, the greater the bony defect, the more difficult the reconstruction. This section is divided in two parts. The first covers techniques used to re-establish bony continuity in the absence of a segmental defect, e.g. a hypertrophic non-union. The second deals with re-establishment of bony continuity in the presence of a segmental defect.

Absence of a segmental defect

There are three ways to achieve stability: (1) external fixation; (2) plates; and (3) intramedullary nails. In addition to stabilizing the fracture or non-union, we must also consider how to stimulate the fracture or non-union to heal. In general, hypertrophic non-unions only require stability as a stimulus to consolidate. Fractures and atrophic non-unions may have to be stimulated by bone grafting or dynamic axial compression via an external fixator.

The advantage of **external fixation** in the management of infected fractures and non-unions is that stabilization is achieved without placing a foreign body into an infected wound. An additional advantage is realized with dynamic external fixators. These fixators can be used to compress or distract fractures and non-unions, and therefore can be used not only for stabilization, but also to achieve bony consolidation (Figures 21.4–21.8). Previously, the use of

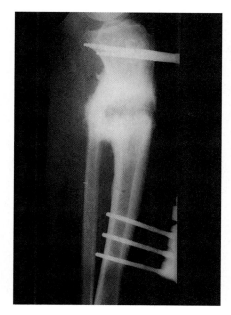

Figure 21.6

A lateral radiograph following debridement and application of a dynamic external fixator. As expected, minimal necrotic tissue was found at debridement. Systemic antibiotics were started, and the patient cyclically compressed and distracted the non-union with the external fixator.

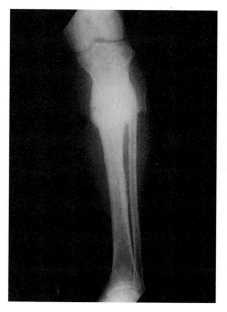

Figure 21.7

Anteroposterior radiograph six months after fixator application and two months after removal, indicate that the non-union has consolidated. There are no signs of infection.

external fixation was limited to fractures and non-unions of the diaphysis. Small wire circular frame external fixators have expanded the indications to peri-articular and even intra-articular fractures and non-unions. The disadvantages of external fixation are that patient acceptance is frequently limited, and that the pin tracts may become infected.

The key to the successful application of an external fixator is the location of the pins and the technique with which the pins are inserted into the bone. The pins should be located in healthy bone, away from the site of the infection. To minimize the risk of injury to nerves and arteries during pin insertion, pins are inserted via 'safe zones', or areas in which there are no major nerves or arteries. When it is not feasible to insert a pin via a safe zone, nerves or arteries at risk are exposed surgically and retracted out of harm's way. Surgical exposure of a neurovascular structure at risk is most frequently necessary when applying a lateral fixator to the humerus

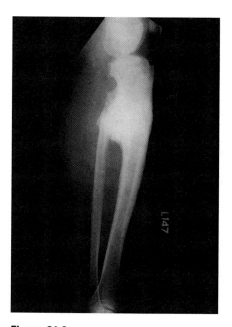

Figure 21.8

Lateral radiograph of the same patient as in Figure 21.7.

(radial nerve) or a dorsal fixator to the distal radius (superficial radial nerve). Ideally, the pins should not violate muscles or tendons. Therefore, when applying the fixator to the tibia, half-pins are inserted from the anteromedial side of the tibia. In cases in which a pin must be inserted through a muscle, the pin is inserted when the muscle is stretched to its maximum length (e.g. when inserting a lateral frame on the femur, the vastus lateralis is stretched by flexing the knee; when inserting a pin through the peroneal muscles, the ankle is dorsi-flexed and the foot supinated; and when inserting a pin through the anterior tibial muscle, the ankle is plantar flexed).

When the optimum location has been determined, the pin is inserted into the bone. It is important to cause as little tissue necrosis as possible when inserting the pin. Therefore skin and soft tissue overlying the bone is incised down to the bone. The bone is predrilled to minimize heat necrosis of the bone. Tissue-protecting sleeves are utilized during the drilling and insertion of the pins. At the conclusion of the procedure, all pin sites are examined to determine whether any of the pins are exerting tension on the overlying soft tissue. If they are, releases are performed by incising the soft tissue, or the pins are removed and replaced.

Weight-bearing, and the length of time that the fixator is maintained, is tailored to each case. Follow-up care is designed to prolong the life of the fixator by minimizing pin-tract complications. The patient is instructed to keep the pin sites scrupulously clean. Cotton swabs are used to remove debris from around the pins twice a day. Rinsing the fixator in clean tap water once a day is encouraged. When pin sites become inflamed, there are four possible courses of action: (1) release the pin sites using local anaesthesia and a scalpel; (2) prescribe whirlpool therapy to insure cleanliness and re-emphasize the importance of pin care; (3) administer broad-spectrum oral antibiotics; and (4), as a last resort, remove the pins. In cases in which the pins are removed because of inflammation, the pin site should be managed as a focus of osteomyelitis.

The use of **plates** to re-establish bony continuity has two advantages: (1) fixation is rigid and therefore surrounding joints can be mobilized; and (2) malalignment associated with the non-union can be accurately corrected. The disad-

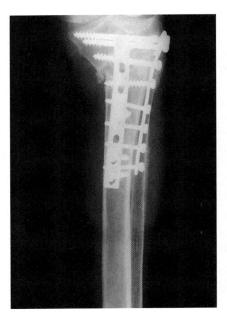

Figure 21.9

Radiograph indicating a proximal tibia fracture stabilized in unacceptable varus angulation. Pain, increasing angulation and a persistent radiolucent line all pointed to the diagnosis of non-union. There was active drainage but no soft-tissue loss.

vantages of using plates to re-establish bony continuity in the presence of infection are: the possibility of exacerbation of infection due to the extensive dissection necessary to position the plate; the plate is a foreign body and may become a source of persistent infection; and the plate is load-bearing, so there is a high incidence of failure of fixation. Plate osteosynthesis is a particularly good way to manage peri-articular and intra-articular non-unions. Juxta-articular fragments of bone are frequently best held in place with buttress plates and interfragmentary screws (Figures 21.8 and 21.9).

The technique of plate osteosynthesis of infected non-unions is broken down into three stages: (1) surgical exposure; (2) correction of associated deformity; and (3) application of the plate.

The surgical exposure is the key to success. The exposure is designed to minimize the chance of tissue necrosis in an area of soft tissue that is frequently at increased risk because of prior surgical procedures and the presence of infection. Therefore, the skin incision is through scars from previous incisions; flaps are not raised unless absolutely necessary. If a flap is raised, it is thick, if possible consisting of skin subcutaneous tissue and periosteum. In cases in which there is a hypertrophic non-union, the flap can also include bone.

When adequate exposure of the non-union has been achieved, any associated malalignment is corrected. This is most frequently accomplished by 'taking down' the non-union, i.e. the removal and lysis of fibrous tissue between the unhealed bone ends. Occasionally, a malaligned non-union is left *in situ*, and a corrective osteotomy is performed proximally or distally. This technique is useful in the management of hypertrophic peri-articular non-unions in which there is limited room for fixation. The osteotomy is located so that the non-union is between it and the joint, allowing the hypertrophic bone about the non-union to be used as a point of fixation. In the specific case of a malaligned tibial non-union, the fibula must be osteotomized if it has healed, prior to correcting the malalignment of the tibia. The fibular osteotomy is performed through a second incision if necessary. The fibular osteotomy is located at least 5 cm distal to the head of the fibula (to avoid injury of the common peroneal nerve) and 3 cm proximal to the ankle joint (to avoid destabilizing the ankle joint). Locating the fibular osteotomy at the level of the non-union facilitates correction of malalignment, but may eliminate the possibility of other procedures, such as posterior lateral bone graft and Huntington fibular transfer, in the future.

Plate application is straightforward. In general, larger plates are used for the osteosynthesis of infected non-unions than for fresh fractures. Cancellous and cortical screws are utilized according to the judgment of the surgeon.

Use of **intramedullary nails** is an ideal method of treatment of non-unions and fractures. It allows compression across the non-union or fracture with weight-bearing, maintains alignment and has a low incidence of implant failure. Locking the nail extends the indications from non-unions and fractures of the diaphysis to non-unions and fractures of the metaphysis. However, the procedure is not fool-proof and intra-operative mishaps are common particularly in the management of non-unions. The most clinically significant complication that can occur when intramedullary nailing is used in the management of infected non-unions and fractures is the conversion of a focal osteomyelitis to intramedullary osteomyelitis. In our experience, this occurs in about 10% of cases. Usually this complication is successfully managed with suppression of the infection until the non-union or fracture heals. The nail is then removed, the medullary canal debrided and antibiotics are administered.

In the intramedullary nailing of tibial non-unions, the non-unions or fractures associated with significant deformity are nailed with the patient on a radiolucent table as opposed to a fracture table. This facilitates manipulation of the tibia at the expense of making distal locking more difficult. The patellar tendon is split and the tibial cortex beneath it is perforated. A bead-tipped guide wire is inserted and if possible driven across the non-union or fracture site. If it is not possible to cross the non-union site, the proximal tibia is reamed, and a trochar tipped guide wire is inserted down the medullary canal and driven across the non-union while being monitored fluoroscopically. In the case of significant deformity that cannot be corrected even after reaming the tibia, the fibula may have to be osteotomized, or a percutaneous lysis of the non-union of the tibia may have to be performed. The nail is always locked proximally to prevent backing out at the knee. If the non-union or fracture is axially or rotationally unstable, the nail is locked statically.

Post-operatively, the patient is carefully followed for abscess formation. Systemic antibiotics are continued for a minimum of three weeks. Weight-bearing is tailored to each case. After the non-union or fracture has consolidated, routine removal of the nail followed by six weeks of systemic antibiotics is recommended. The author has seen several cases of activation of latent infections with retained implants.

Presence of a segmental defect

Remarkable advances have been made in the techniques used to reconstruct segmental defects. At the present, management is a modification or combination of three basic techniques: (1) cancellous bone grafting; (2) vascularized bone-segment transfer; and (3) distraction osteogenesis using external fixation. These techniques share in common a prolonged period of disability and numerous surgical procedures. It is important to remember that amputation may be the optimal management in terms of duration of disability and eventual function of the extremity. This is particularly applicable in young patients with involvement of the tibia.

There are three techniques which use **cancellous grafting**: the Papineau procedure; the closed Papineau procedure (closed cancellous bone grafting); and posterolateral bone grafting. The success of these techniques is dependent upon the osteo-inductive capacity of autogenous cancellous bone. When using these techniques, it is extremely important to use only cancellous bone as cortical bone will become a sequestrum.

The technique of radical surgical debridement and delayed open cancellous bone grafting was described by Papineau in the 1970s. The advantages of the *Papineau technique* are its simplicity and reproducibility. Disadvantages are: extended hospitalization; the large amount of autogenous cancellous bone required; numerous surgical procedures; and the prolonged period of disability while the graft incorporates. Certain conditions militate against the use of open cancellous grafting. Stable fixation of the affected bone is mandatory and, therefore, segmental defects which cannot be adequately stabilized should be avoided. Also, the granulation bed into which the bone graft is placed must be vascular for graft incorporation. Therefore, this method is not always applicable to chronically infected segmental defects in which the granulation bed is typically dysvascular. A modification of open cancellous grafting has been described. Following a radical debridement, the wound is closed. The dead space is filled with polymethylmethacrylate (PMMA)-antibiotic beads, which serve to deliver antibiotics locally and to maintain a potential dead space. After the wound has stabilized, the beads are removed and autogenous cancellous graft is inserted into the defect. This 'closed cancellous bone grafting' has the advantage of better soft-tissue coverage of bone, and requires less strenuous post-operative care than open cancellous grafting. It has the disadvantage of usually requiring a lengthy technically

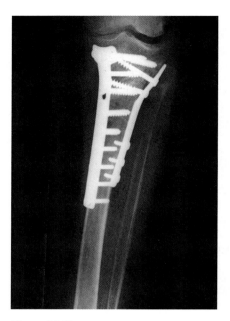

Figure 21.10

The non-union has been replated and angulation corrected (see Figure 21.9). Necrotic bone and the previous implants have been debrided. Autogenous cancellous graft containing vancomycin was placed in the non-union. A primary closure was performed. Systemic antibiotics were administered for six weeks.

difficult procedure (free soft-tissue transfer) (Figures 21.9–21.12). Alternatively, the technique of posterior lateral bone grafting does not require free soft-tissue transfer. In this technique, the non-union or segmental defect is approached via a posterior lateral exposure. Cancellous graft is placed in the non-union site or in the segmental gap. Because the bed into which the cancellous graft is placed is very vascular, the graft usually incorporates. In addition, this approach avoids compromised soft tissue anteriorly. Disadvantages of this technique include its limited usefulness in the proximal and distal tibia and the difficulty of performing an adequate debridement, as the surgical approach does not provide adequate exposure for this task.

The first stage in the Papineau procedure is radical debridement and stabilization of the bone ends. All devitalized and compromised soft tissue and bone are removed. The margins of the

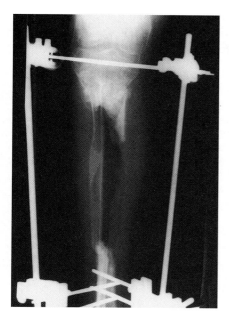

Figure 21.11

Radiograph of a tibia indicating a large segmental defect following debridement of post-traumatic osteomyelitis. An external fixator stabilizes the tibia. A primary closure over PMMA-antibiotic beads was performed.

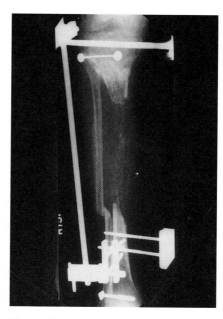

Figure 21.12

Three weeks later the beads were removed (see Figure 21.11), and cancellous graft from both iliac crests was placed in the defect. In addition, the proximal and distal tibiofibular joints were fused. The graft contained vancomycin. Systemic antibiotics were administered and were continued for a total of eight weeks.

wound must be well vascularized and granulate readily. Stabilization is most frequently accomplished with an external fixator. The wound is left open and dressing changes are performed daily until there is a healthy bed of granulation tissue. The defect is then filled with fragments of autogenous cancellous bone from the iliac crest, and the wound is left open. Cortical bone is carefully excluded from the graft because it has minimal osteo-inductive potential and because it will become a sequestrum. The first dressing change is at two days, and thereafter at daily intervals. Initially, the appearance of the wound filled with necrotic cancellous graft is disturbing. However, granulation tissue grows slowly around and through the bone graft. A split thickness skin graft is applied once a layer of granulating tissue covers the graft. Systemic antibiotics are administered until the skin graft is performed.

In follow-up, pin care is essential as the external fixator must remain in place until consolidation of the graft has occurred. Usually the patient is hospitalized for his dressing changes. Systemic antibiotics are continued until the split thickness skin graft has been applied. Weight-bearing is not allowed until removal of the external fixator. The external fixator should be removed only when the defect is healed clinically and radiographically.

The *closed-bone grafting technique* is similar to the Papineau technique in that it entails autogenous cancellous grafting of a bony defect. It differs from the Papineau technique in that the site to be grafted must have adequate soft-tissue coverage. The first stage is radical debridement, closure of the soft-tissue defect with well-perfused flaps and stabilization of the bone fragments. Closure is most frequently accomplished with a local rotational muscle flap (gastrocnemius or soleus) or a free flap. Dead space beneath the flap is maintained with PMMA-antibiotic beads. In the second stage, after the wound has healed and the flap has stabilized, the beads are removed and the dead space is filled with autogenous cancellous graft. Removal of the beads should be as atraumatic as possible. One edge of the flap is carefully lifted, exposing the beads, which are removed. The bed of granulation tissue lining the dead space is gently irrigated of haematoma and the cancellous graft is placed into the defect. Prior to insertion, antibiotics are mixed with the bone graft (i.e. 1 g of vancomycin, 1 g of a second-generation cephalosporin, or 1.2 g of tobramycin). The wound is closed.

In the immediate post-operative period, the patient is examined daily for abscess formation. Antibiotics are continued three weeks from insertion of the bone graft. When the patient is discharged, he or she is followed at intervals based on the surgeon's clinical judgment. Weight-bearing is not allowed until the graft is consolidated.

In *posterolateral bone grafting*, the patient is positioned prone. A cancellous graft is harvested from the posterior iliac crest. This wound is then closed and covered.

A longitudinal incision is made parallel with, and 1 cm posterior to, the posterior border of the fibula. The interval between the triceps surae and the peroneals is developed. The peroneals are retracted anteriorly and the gastrocnemius and soleus posteriorly, exposing the fibula. The dissection is carried around the posterior surface of the fibula to the interosseous membrane. Here the posterior tibialis is stripped from the interosseous membrane and posterior surface of the tibia. The posterior tibial artery and nerve are between the posterior tibial muscle and the flexor hallucis distally and the soleus proximally. Therefore, these structures are not at risk if the posterior tibialis is identified and elevated from its origin subperiosteally. The cortex of the tibia is decorticated with an osteotome, and the autogenous bone graft is placed in the non-union site. Bone can also be placed on the interosseous membrane, bridging the space between the fibula and the tibia. The wound is closed over a drain. In cases which are actively infected, stabilization is best achieved with an external fixator. Casting, plating and intramedullary nailing have

also been described as methods of stabilization.

In the immediate post-operative period, the patient is carefully monitored for signs of abscess formation. These signs include increasing pain, swelling and drainage. If these signs are present, the graft site is debrided emergently. In cases which are actively infected, systemic antibiotics are initiated at the time of surgery and are continued for a minimum of three weeks. In cases with a quiescent infection, the antibiotics may be discontinued when the patient is discharged from the hospital (usually at 4–7 days). Weight-bearing is tailored to each patient.

Vascularized bone transfer differs from reconstruction with autogenous cancellous grafts or allografts in that the segment of transferred tissue is living. Theoretically, living tissue is more resistant to infection and will heal more quickly to the bone ends. In reality, healing of the graft to the bone ends is not reliable and frequently supplemental autogenous cancellous grafting is required.

There are two techniques of vascularized bone transfer. The first was described by Huntington in 1905. The *Huntington technique* involves fixation of the ipsilateral fibula to the ends of the tibia. Disadvantages of the Huntington procedure are: prolonged immobilization and non-weight-bearing is necessary to protect the synostosis; an intact fibula is sacrificed; hypertrophy of the fibula is necessary to achieve a good functional result; and, segmental tibial defects with a very short proximal or distal segment are difficult to treat with this method. There has not been an extensive experience with this technique reported in the literature. The two largest series reviewed a total of 12 cases. Union was achieved in all of these cases. Posterolateral bone grafting is a modification of Huntington fibular transfer. In this technique bone graft is placed between the tibia and fibula producing a synostosis. The fibula is not centralized. In our experience this is not an adequate technique in the management of tibial segmental defects. We have found that the eccentrically loaded fibula is not strong enough to withstand weight-bearing. For this reason we reserve posterolateral bone grafting for patients with simple non-unions.

In the Huntington technique, a virgin area of the tibia proximal to the segmental defect is chosen and, through an anterior incision, a notch is made in the lateral cortex of the tibia. Similarly, the distal tibia is notched for acceptance of the fibular graft. Posterolateral incisions are used to expose the fibula at the level of the synostosis. A transverse osteotomy of the proximal fibula is completed just proximal to the notch in the tibia. The transverse osteotomy of the distal fibula is made at a level just distal to the distal tibial notch. Using both incisions, the fibula is wedged into the recipient notch sites, locking the fibula into place. The fibula is fixed to the tibia with screws and the synostosis is reinforced with cancellous grafts.

Alternatively, the procedure can be performed in two stages as originally described by Huntington. The proximal tibiofibular synostosis comprises the first stage. Following union at the proximal synostosis site, the distal synostosis is performed.

In follow-up, a non-weight-bearing long leg cast is applied until the synostosis sites are united, usually 3–4 months. If the procedure was performed in stages, a second immobilization period of 3–4 months is necessary. Once union has occurred, both proximally and distally, partial weight-bearing in a short leg walking cast is maintained for approximately 2–3 months while the fibula hypertrophies. Full weight-bearing in a protective brace is allowed.

The second technique is *free vascularized transfer*. This technique involves the mobilization of a segment of bone with its vascular pedicle. The vascular pedicle is anastomosed to nearby arteries and veins at the site of the defect. A defect of 2½ inches is the minimum indication. The disadvantages of free vascularized bone grafts include: donor-site morbidity; the extensive and difficult surgical procedure; and the protracted period of non-weight-bearing necessary to protect the synostosis sites. The technique of free vascularized fibula transfer will not be described.

The success of **distraction osteogenesis** is dependent upon osteogenesis which occurs during distraction of an osteotomy site. To accomplish this, the cortex of the involved bone is cut circumferentially at a site distant to the segmental defect, and the resulting free segment of bone is distracted and transported slowly within its periosteal sleeve through the segmental defect to the non-union docking site. Stimulated by this distraction, regenerate bone forms in the osteotomy site. It is this *de novo* formation of bone which make this technique unique.

A Russian, Gavriel Ilizarov, is credited with originating distraction osteogenesis. As experience with distraction osteogenesis in the management of post-traumatic defects has accumulated in Western Europe and North America, it has been possible to make several generalizations. The production of regenerate bone during the technique of distraction osteogenesis is a reliable phenomenon. Major complications are common and include psychological intolerance of the frame and failure to obtain union of the transported segment at the 'docking site'. Minor complications such as pin breakage, pin-tract infection, joint stiffness and premature consolidation of the regenerate bone are also common, but their occurrence does not preclude a good result. Finally, the lowest incidence of complications occurs when the technique is used for tibial defects.

The advantages of this procedure are that large autogenous bone grafts are unnecessary and early weight-bearing is encouraged. In addition, angiogenesis of small vessels may be stimulated, thus increasing local blood flow. The disadvantages include: the need for exceptional patient compliance and tolerance; frame application is a technically difficult procedure with an extended learning curve; and finally, patients must be followed closely and the frame adjusted frequently (Figures 21.13–21.20).

In distraction osteogenesis, patient selection and education are extremely important. A history of mental disorders or substance abuse is a contraindication to this technique. The ideal patient is motivated and stoic. The patient must understand what the technique entails and the necessity of his cooperation for success.

The first stage of the surgical procedure is application of the external fixator to the extremity. The frame configuration is based on preoperative planning and varies for virtually every case. External fixation is achieved using one of two basic types of fixators, either a half-pin monolateral frame or a small wire circular fixator. The half-pin monolateral frame is used when no angular correction is required (i.e. simple unipolar lengthening). The half-pin monolateral frame is less bulky than equivalent small wire circular frames, and has a lower profile which is better tolerated by the patient.

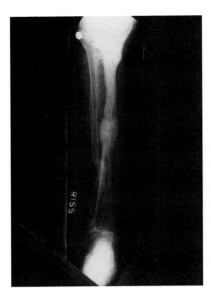

Figure 21.13

At 18 months from the original debridement (see Figure 21.12), the graft has incorporated. There has been a fracture in the mid-portion of the graft. This fracture has healed with no ill effects.

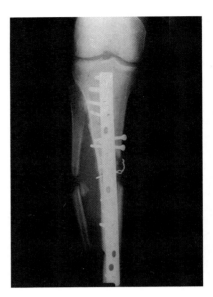

Figure 21.15

Radiograph of a tibia fracture stabilized with a broad compression plate. Clinically, the entire plate was exposed and there was obvious active infection.

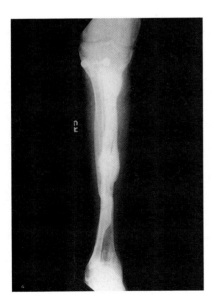

Figure 21.14

At five years from the original debridement, the patient presented with cellulitis and pain which responded to oral antibiotics (see Figure 21.13). The tibia is solidly healed.

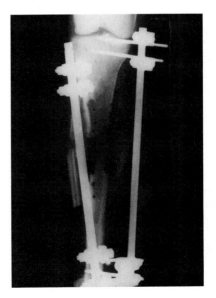

Figure 21.16

Following debridement an external fixator was applied and a free-tissue transfer was performed (see Figure 21.15). The tissue was contoured to fill the dead space. Systemic antibiotics were initiated.

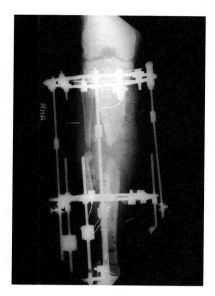

Figure 21.17

Four weeks following debridement and three weeks following the free-tissue transfer, a small wire external fixator has been applied and a corticotomy performed at the distal metaphysis (see Figure 21.16).

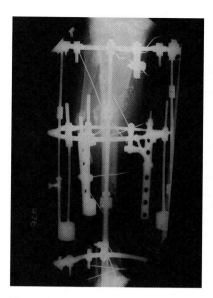

Figure 21.19

At the conclusion of transport, olive wires have been added to compress the docking site (see Figure 21.18). This did not result in consolidation.

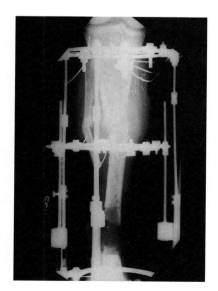

Figure 21.18

The segment is being transported proximally (see Figure 21.17). The patient underwent four additional operative procedures to replace broken wires and correct malalignment. Equinas deformity of the ankle was a constant concern during transport.

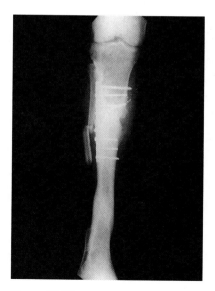

Figure 21.20

Three years after plating and bone grafting of the docking site, the tibia is solidly healed (see Figure 21.19). The patient subsequently developed a flare-up, which responded to removal of the plate and four weeks of systemic antibiotics.

The small wire circular frames are utilized in cases in which there is angular deformity which requires correction. Pin placement is chosen to minimize the chance of neurovascular damage. When a monolateral half-frame is utilized, this is fairly simple; the full pins used with small wire circular frames make avoidance of these structures more difficult.

The second stage of the procedure is osteotomy. The cortex of the involved bone is cut circumferentially with as little damage to the periosteum and medullary contents as possible. Because only the cortex is cut this osteotomy is more specifically called a corticotomy. The corticotomy is usually performed in the metaphyseal region of the involved bone. In the tibia a longitudinal incision is made over the crest of the tibia, exposing the periosteum. The periosteum is incised and carefully elevated. A one-quarter inch osteotome is used to cut medial and lateral cortices. Every effort is made to protect the medullary contents and the periosteum. The corticotomy is completed through the posterior cortex of the tibia by twisting the osteotome or by loosening the frame and using it to gently twist the tibia. The free segment of bone produced by the corticotomy is connected to the frame by half-pins or wires, and transported into the segmental defect within its periosteal sleeve. The transported segment of bone is moved at a rate of 0.5–1 mm per day in 0.25 mm increments. The rate and rhythm of distraction can be varied according to the patient's profile (e.g. age, nutritional status and clinical response). Several variations of this technique have been described. Two corticotomies can be performed in the same bone: one distal and one proximal to the segmental non-union. With two transported segments of bone, the period of treatment can be shortened. Another variation involves acute shortening of the leg with apposition of the non-union fragments. Leg lengthening is then performed using distraction osteogenesis. The non-union can be compressed during the lengthening and consolidation stages.

The surgical procedure is technically demanding but straightforward. The follow-up is extremely challenging and frequently frustrating. Patients are usually discharged 1–4 days following frame application and corticotomy. Pin care is extremely important as the frame will be in place for months. At 7–14 days after corticotomy, distraction is begun at the corticotomy site at a rate of 1 mm a day. The patient is followed weekly for at least one month and then biweekly. At each follow-up, radiographs are obtained to evaluate distraction, regenerate bone formation and frame position. If distraction is not occurring, the corticotomy may have to be redone. Regenerate bone should appear about four weeks following the corticotomy. If it has not appeared by six weeks, distraction should be stopped or temporarily reversed. The patient is carefully monitored for pin-tract infections, weight-bearing status and development of joint contractures. Pin tract infections are treated with systemic or local antibiotics, whirlpool and, if necessary, by changing the pins. If weight-bearing decreases or contractures develop, the rate of distraction is slowed and rigorous physical therapy initiated. If the contractures do not resolve, surgical releases may have to be performed. In our experience all patients treated with this method have significant pain and require analgesics during therapy. External fixation is maintained until the regenerate bone begins to consolidate. Dynamization of the frame may accelerate this process. Typically, the external fixator is maintained for a total period roughly equal to three times the distraction period. After removal of the frame, cast immobilization and partial weight-bearing is maintained until corticalization of the regenerate bone occurs.

Soft-tissue coverage

In many cases, debrided wounds can be closed primarily. In cases in which primary closure is not possible, local or free soft-tissue transfer is used to achieve coverage. These soft-tissue transfers also function to increase the local vascularity and to fill dead space created by the debridement. The issue of local vascularity is important. Frequently, the area to be covered is hypovascular, and soft-tissue flaps which are parasitic (e.g. cross-leg flaps or split thickness skin graft) or which have precarious intrinsic circulation (e.g. fasciocutaneous flaps) are associated with a high incidence of failure. The three types of closure which are most useful in the management of bone and joint infections are:

primary closure; local muscle transfer; and free soft-tissue transfer. Free soft-tissue transfer will not be described.

Primary closure

Primary closure denotes approximating the wound edges with sutures. Primary closure of an infected wound runs counter to historical surgical principles. The risk of closure is that an infected cavity is created and develops into an abscess. Today, administration of antibiotics specifically directed at the pathogenic organisms, management of dead space with spacers or autogenous bone graft, and adequate transcutaneous suction drainage, make primary closure of selected infected wounds an excellent method of coverage. Primary closure is done only when the infection is under control, and only when it can be accomplished with minimal tension on the surrounding soft tissue.

Dead space must be occupied with beads or bone graft prior to closure. Large-bore suction drains are left in all wounds unless they are so superficial that adequate drainage will occur through the suture line. In general, buried sutures are avoided when at all possible. Instances in which this is not possible are: when not using buried sutures, will result in dead space between the sides of the wound; when not closing deep tissues, results in tension being put on the skin edges; when not closing deep tissues, results in later disability or loss of function (e.g. the medial retinaculum must be closed after draining an infected total knee or the patella will dislocate laterally). Vertical mattress sutures are used to close the skin because they minimize the amount of subcutaneous dead space. Wire, monofilament proline or monofilament nylon are used as they cause minimal inflammation.

The patient is followed up very carefully in the peri-operative period, for signs of an abscess. These signs are swelling, pain, temperature spikes and cellulitis. If there is any doubt, skin sutures are removed over the most suspicious area and the wound is probed. In cases in which buried sutures have been utilized, the wound must be explored in the operating room. If an abscess has accumulated, all sutures are removed, and the wound is debrided and packed open.

If all goes well and an abscess does not develop, the drains are removed after drainage has decreased to <30 cc per day. If the drainage does not decrease to this level, the drains are left in place for 3–4 weeks. This allows enough time for the incision to heal and a sinus tract to develop around the drainage tubes. This minimizes the chance of drainage occurring through the surgical incision, and the scar becoming inverted and macerated. Antibiotics are continued for a minimum of three weeks following primary closure to protect the skin and soft tissue.

Local muscle transfer

The principle of local muscle transfer is to dissect free a muscle, or portion of a muscle, from surrounding tissue, while preserving its vascular pedicle. The end result is a muscle which can be transferred on its vascular pedicle and rotated to cover a neighbouring defect. The advantage of local muscle transfer is that, unlike free soft-tissue transfer, the procedure is simple, and does not require any special expertise or equipment. The disadvantage of local muscle transfer is that the number and types of transfers are limited, and therefore not all areas can be adequately covered. The distal tibia is an example of an area which cannot be adequately covered with a local muscle transfer. Using local transfers successfully requires a knowledge of the vascular supply of the muscle to be transferred, and an understanding of which transfer should be used in a given situation. The two muscles most frequently transferred are the medial head of the gastrocnemius and the medial soleus. The **medial gastrocnemius muscle** is the most useful of all the local tissue transfers and can be rotated to cover defects from the patella to the junction of the proximal and middle thirds of the tibia. The vascular supply of the medial gastrocnemius is from the sural artery, and enters the undersurface (anatomically, the anterior surface) of the muscle in the popliteal fossae.

The patient is supine with the entire leg and foot prepped and draped free. A tourniquet is used. The skin incision is parallel and 1 cm posterior to the posterior medial border of the tibia. It extends from the level of the distal pole of the patella to the junction of the distal and middle third of the tibia. The gastrocnemius is easily freed from the overlying subcutaneous tissue with blunt dissection. The interval between the soleus and the gastrocnemius is identified and these two muscles are separated in the proximal third of the calf. The tendon of the plantaris muscle is found between the gastrocnemius and soleus and confirms that the correct interval has been entered. The raphe of the gastrocnemius is identified approximately in the coronal midline of the muscle. It is easier to identify the raphe proximally, where the medial and lateral heads merge, than distally near their insertion on the Achilles' tendon. The raphe is gently separated with a scissors and blunt dissection, from proximally to distally. At the musculotendinous junction, the medial half of the Achilles' tendon is divided. A suture is passed through the distal tip of the flap and is used for retraction. The dissection of the raphe is now carried proximally as needed to increase the arc of rotation. As the dissection proceeds proximally, adequate exposure is mandatory to visualize and protect the sural artery. The dissection can be carried to the origin of the medial gastrocnemius from the medial femoral condyle. The tourniquet is deflated and haemostasis is achieved. The flap is rotated to cover the defect. If more coverage is needed, the fascia on the undersurface of the muscle can be incised in line with its fibres at 1 cm intervals to increase the width of the transfer. Horizontal mattress sutures are used to hold the gastrocnemius in the desired location. A split thickness skin graft is applied, and the skin incision is closed over a drain. A bulky dressing is applied to the extremity.

In follow-up care, the drain is removed and the dressing is changed according to the surgeon's preference. In the immediate post-operative period, the patient must be carefully examined daily for signs and symptoms of an abscess developing beneath the flap. The leg is kept elevated for 2–4 weeks after surgery. At 2–4 weeks, active range of motion of the ankle and knee is begun. The mattress sutures holding the flap in place are left in for a minimum of four weeks to prevent delayed retraction of the flap.

The **soleus muscle** transfer is the most useful local tissue transfer for defects of the middle third of the tibia. Its usefulness is somewhat limited by its vascular supply, which is segmental in the proximal third of the muscle and

primarily from the posterior tibial artery. In addition, because the soleus blends gradually with the Achilles' tendon, as opposed to the medial head of the gastrocnemius which has a more discrete insertion, the dissection of the muscle distally from the tendon is difficult. The soleus can be transferred medially or laterally; however, the medial transfer is much more useful, as the lateral transfer is hindered by the fibula. Indications for lateral transfer include patients with a lateral tibial defect, with a mid-third tibial defect with destruction of the medial side of the soleus and in whom the fibula has been resected.

The positioning of the patient is as described for a medial gastrocnemius transfer. The skin incision extends from below the level of the knee joint to the ankle and is 1 cm posterior to the posterior medial border of the tibia. The plane between the soleus and gastrocnemius is identified and opened. The plantaris tendon is found in this intermuscular interval. Anteriorly, the interval between the soleus and the muscles of the deep posterior compartment is identified, confirmed by the presence of the posterior tibial artery and opened. The soleus is dissected off the Achilles' tendon. Sutures are placed in the distal end of the muscle and are used for retraction of the muscle. The dissection is carried as far proximally as needed. As the dissection proceeds proximally, vascular pedicles to the muscle from the posterior tibial artery are identified. One, or at most two, of these pedicles can be ligated to increase the arc of rotation of the soleus. Suture ligation, as opposed to electrocautery, is necessary because of the proximity of the posterior tibial artery. If only the medial half of the soleus is required, the muscle is split in line with its fibres, and the lateral half is left *in situ*. The muscle is rotated to the desired position and the wounds are closed as described for the medial gastrocnemius transfer.

Follow-up care is identical to that described for a medial gastrocnemius transfer.

Dead-space management

Dead space is defined as the space left in a wound after it has been closed. In the surgery of post-traumatic osteomyelitis, dead space is frequently created by the debridement of necrotic tissue and the removal of implants. Post-operatively, this space quickly fills with exudate and haematoma. If bacteria are present, the exudate and haematoma provide nutrients and an environment ideal for replication. The problem is compounded by the fact that penetration of this large haematoma by antibiotics and humoral elements (e.g. antibodies and complement) and cellular elements (e.g. polymorphonuclear leukocytes) of the immune system is limited. For these reasons, dead space must be managed. Methods of dead-space management are: not closing the wound, in essence externalizing the defect; modifying wound closure to fill the dead space (e.g. closure with a local or free-tissue transfer); or occupying the space with something (i.e. bone graft, beads, or an absorbable spacer) that prevents the accumulation of haematoma.

Externalization of infected wounds

Externalization, or saucerization, of infected wounds is a classic method of management which was in use long before the advent of antibiotics. The concept was that, by leaving debrided wounds open widely, through excision of overhanging soft tissue and bone, the wound would drain freely, abscesses would not form, and cellulitis would slowly resolve. When saucerization alone was used to manage war wounds, the defect was covered with a split thickness skin graft after the infection had been controlled. The technique of saucerization in a less radical form (i.e. packing a wound open) is still useful as a salvage procedure, or to temporize and delay definitive management of the wound. This technique keeps us out of trouble in the occasional instance when we find that debridement has resulted in a greater defect than anticipated. The initial step of a Papineau procedure, in essence, is externalization of an infected wound.

This technique is limited to areas in which it will result in an acceptable loss of function, such as the diaphysis of the tibia or femur. Saucerization of peri-articular infections is performed only as a last resort because it results in ankylosis of the joint. Infections involving the proximal femur and hip are seldom managed by saucerization,

because the excision of overlying soft tissue necessary to open the wound widely results in unacceptable loss of function.

When it is elected to manage an infected wound by externalization, it is critical that an adequate debridement be performed. All overlying bone and soft tissue is excised. This may result in a segmental defect of the bone which requires stabilization with an external fixator. Casting and then windowing the cast to obtain exposure of the wound is not recommended as the cast quickly becomes soiled with wound drainage. The wound is packed loosely with gauze soaked in a topical antibiotic.

Dressing changes start no later than the second post-operative day, and then at daily intervals. The type of dressing is according to the surgeon's preference. Reconstruction of the defect can be undertaken when the wound has started to granulate, and can range in complexity from something as simple as filling the defect with autogenous cancellous bone (Papineau procedure) to distraction osteogenesis or free-tissue transfer.

Tissue transfer

Free- or local soft-tissue transfers are utilized not only to close wounds and cover exposed bone and joints, but also to fill dead space with healthy well vascularized tissue.

The technique and follow-up care of soft tissue transfers has been described in Chapters 15–17. When using transferred tissue to fill dead space, it is critical that no dead space be left under the transfer. It may be necessary to contour the bed and even the tissue to be transferred in order to create a better fit. The transferred tissue is carefully positioned to fill any bony or soft-tissue defects, and is firmly sutured in place in order to prevent its retraction as it heals. Suction drains are left under the transferred tissue to prevent fluid accumulation in the potential space between it and the bed.

Occupying dead space

The third method of managing dead space is to occupy it with something that will prevent it from filling with haematoma. This can be accomplished with bone graft, methylmethacrylate beads or an absorbable spacer.

Cancellous graft in the management of dead space

Autogenous cancellous bone graft is frequently used to fill dead space, the primary limitation being the amount of graft that can be easily obtained. It is important to use only cancellous bone and to exclude all cortical bone. Cancellous bone is more osteo-inductive and is readily absorbed, so it will not become a sequestrum. When antibiotics are mixed with the graft, it also serves as an antibiotic delivery system, and osteo-induction is not suppressed (Lindsey 1933).

Sources of readily available cancellous bone are the iliac crest, in particular the posterior crest, and the distal femur. More graft can be obtained from the iliac crest than from the distal femur, but there is significant post-operative pain following an iliac crest graft. The advantages of obtaining a graft from the distal femur are that it is a simple operative exposure, and there is minimal post-operative pain.

In the **iliac crest bone graft**, if a large amount of graft is required, the patient is positioned on his or her side or prone. If graft is only to be taken from the anterior one third of the crest, the patient is positioned supine, with a bolster under the operated side. The skin incision is at the brim of the iliac crest and is carried down to the crest itself. The muscles which attach to the superior aspect of the crest (i.e. the internal and external obliques and the erector spinae) are left undisturbed. The periosteum overlying the outer lip of the iliac crest is incised and the gluteus maximus is stripped from the outer table of the ilium using a large periosteal elevator. When stripping the gluteus, it is useful to remember that the majority of the cancellous bone is located just under the brim of the ilium, and that the ilium quickly becomes very thin distally, so it is not necessary to strip the muscles off more than the proximal 3 cm of the ilium. The exception to this is posteriorly where the ilium is very thick and there is a large amount of graft along the entire length of the sacro-iliac joint. The superior gluteal artery and nerve exit the sciatic notch posteriorly and run anteriorly. To avoid injury to these structures,

the exposure of the ilium must be subperiosteal. An osteotome is used to cut the outer cortex of the ilium along its brim. This cut can be extended as far anteriorly as the anterior superior iliac spine and as far posteriorly as the posterior superior iliac spine. Two vertical cuts are now made at the anterior and posterior ends of the horizontal cut. The outer cortex of the ilium is peeled back by undercutting it with a broad osteotome. Cancellous bone is harvested from under the crest with curettes and gouges. If the inner cortex of the ilium is inadvertently windowed, the iliacus muscle protects the intrapelvic structures from injury. When all the required cancellous bone has been harvested, the raw bony surfaces are covered with a haemostatic agent, and the outer table of the ilium is pushed back into place. The gluteus maximus is sutured back to periosteum and fascia of the crest of the ilium, holding the outer table reduced. A suction drain is left in the wound. There are no restrictions post-operatively.

In **distal femoral bone graft**, the patient is positioned supine on the operating table, with a tourniquet around the upper thigh. After the leg has been exsanguinated, and the tourniquet inflated, a midlateral skin incision is made over the lateral femoral condyle. The skin incision extends from the knee joint proximally for 4 cm. The fascia lata is divided in line with its fibres, exposing the periosteum of the lateral femoral condyle. The periosteum is incised and elevated. A half-inch osteotome is used to window the cortex 2 cm proximal to the distal articular surface of the femur. Curettes are used to harvest the graft. The wound is closed in layers without leaving a drain.

Toe touch-weight-bearing is maintained for one month. Active and passive range of motion of the knee is encouraged post-operatively.

Methylmethacrylate beads

Methylmethacrylate beads serve three purposes. They fill dead space, preventing it being filled with serum and blood. They maintain dead space, making it easier to bone graft or perform a revision arthroplasty and they deliver antibiotics to the surrounding cavity. When using beads to manage dead space, it is vital to remember that they are temporary. In most cases they must be removed and the dead space occupied with a tissue transfer or a bone graft.

Beads are made by mixing powdered antibiotics with polymethylmethacrylate (PMMA) polymer. Prior to adding the liquid monomer, the antibiotic must be well dispersed in the polymer, or the rate of elution will be unpredictable. The antibiotic and powdered cement are stirred until there is no doubt that they are well mixed; alternatively, a small amount of a sterile powdered dye can be added. When the powdered dye is well dispersed, the antibiotic is also assumed to be dispersed. Virtually any powdered antibiotic can be added to cement. Commonly used antibiotics and amounts per 40 g pack of cement are cephazolin 1 or 2 g, vancomycin 1 or 2 g (vancomycin presents a problem because it forms aggregates which must be powdered prior to mixing) and tobramycin 1.2–3.6 g. As the volume of antibiotic is increased per given amount of cement, the time or polymerization of the cement increases. After the polymer and the antibiotic have been mixed, the liquid monomer is added. When the PMMA-antibiotic composite has reached the stage that it is workable, and does not adhere to surgical gloves, it is rolled into small balls and strung on heavy non-absorbable suture. After polymerization is completed, and the composite has cooled, the beads are implanted in the defect. Care is taken to fill the defect as completely as possible, leaving the minimum amount of dead space unoccupied. Following implantation of beads, the wound must be closed to prevent the emergence of bacterial strains resistant to the antibiotic in the beads.

Systemic antibiotics are initiated during bead implantation and continued a minimum of three weeks. The author rationalizes administration of antibiotics during bead implantation as being necessary because the beads do not occupy all the dead space. Theoretically, we would like antibiotics to be in the haematoma surrounding the beads. Continued administration of antibiotics systemically is necessary because the local levels of antibiotic due to elution of antibiotic from the beads falls very quickly.

The timing of bead removal is determined by the rate and amount of antibiotic elution and the fact that the beads become surrounded by scar tissue and are difficult to remove. We usually remove the beads at 3–6 weeks. To remove the beads, part of the incision is opened, and the strand of beads is found, and as atraumatically as possible, gently teased from the wound. The sides of the cavity are curetted of organized haematoma, if indicated specimens are sent for culture. The walls of the cavity are carefully inspected for necrotic bone that may have been missed in prior debridements. Reconstruction of the defect can now proceed with a soft-tissue transfer, or more frequently cancellous bone grafting.

Absorbable implants

Absorbable implants in the management of dead space have the theoretical advantage that they would not require a second procedure, because as they were absorbed, soft tissue would fill the cavity. While these implants may be useful in the future, the author has no experience with them.

Antibiotic therapy

Appropriate antibiotic therapy depends on the identification of the pathogenic organisms and determination of their susceptibilities to various antibiotics. In order to determine the pathogenic organisms, the patient is taken off all antibiotics for at least two weeks. Material obtained from sinus tracts, open wounds and percutaneous biopsy is cultured for aerobic anaerobic fungal and acid-fast organisms. All organisms identified are assumed to be pathogenic. This includes organisms commonly considered to be contaminants (e.g. *Staphylococcus epidermidis* and *Diptheroides*).

Once the organisms and their susceptibilities to various antibiotics are determined, the appropriate antibiotic is administered. The most common method of administration is systemic intravenous infusion. Local administration via polymethylmethacrylate beads or an infusion pump is an effective method of antibiotic delivery and has several advantages, the most important of which is that local concentrations of antibiotic are very high, while systemic concentrations are very low. Regardless of the method of administration, the antibiotic concentration at the site of the infection must be high enough to kill, or at least inhibit, the bacteria. Systemic levels of potentially toxic antibiotics are monitored by determining peak and trough serum concentrations. Peak concentrations are from peripheral blood obtained 30 minutes after administration of the intravenous antibiotic. Trough levels are determined from peripheral blood obtained just prior to antibiotic administration. The trough level is adjusted by altering the interval of time between administration of the antibiotic. The peak level is adjusted by altering the amount of drug administered.

Therapeutic levels are considered to be four times the mean inhibitory concentration (MIC) of the pathogenic bacteria. The aminoglycosides and vancomycin have significant nephrotoxicity, and are excreted by the kidney. They must be monitored carefully, because initial subclinical toxicity will result in increasing concentrations of drug and permanent severe damage of the kidney. The penicillins, cephalosporins, clindamycin and quinolones usually do not require peaks and troughs as they are less toxic. However, a CBC, albumin, BUN and creatinine are obtained every week to monitor bone-marrow suppression, and liver and kidney toxicity.

Bibliography

Agiza ARH, El Kom S (1981) Treatment of tibial osteomyelitic defects and infected pseudarthroses by the Huntington fibular transference operation, *J Bone Joint Surg* **63A**: 814–19.

Cabanela ME (1984) Open cancellous bone grafting of infected bone defects, *Orthop Clin N Am* **15**: 427–40.

Canale ST, Puhl J, Watson FM, Gillespie R (1975) Acute osteomyelitis following closed fractures. Report of three cases, *J Bone Joint Surg* **57A**: 415–18.

Cierny G, Mader J, Pennink JJ (1985) A clinical staging system for adult osteomyelitis, *Contemp Orthop* **10**: 17–37.

Collins DN, Garvin KL, Nelson CL (1987) The use of the vastus lateralis flap in patients with intractable infection after resection arthroplasty following the use of a hip implant, *J Bone Joint Surg* **69A**: 510–16.

Dagher F, Roukoz S (1991) Compound tibial fractures with bone loss treated by the Ilizarov technique, *J Bone Joint Surg* **73B**: 316–21.

Gilbert A (1979) Surgical technique—vascularized transfer of the fibular shaft, *Int J Microsurg* **102**: 100.

Gordon L, Chiu EJ (1988) Treatment of infected non-unions and segmental defects of the tibia with staged microvascular muscle transplantation and bone-grafting, *J Bone Joint Surg* **70A**: 377–86.

Hansen ST Jr (1987) Editorial. The type-IIIc tibial fracture: salvage or amputation, *J Bone Joint Surg* **69A**: 799–800.

Hogeman KE (1949) Treatment of infected bone defects with cancellous bone-chip grafts, *Acta Chir Scand* **98**: 576–90.

Huntington TW (1905) Case of bone transference. Use of a segment of fibula to supply a defect in the tibia, *Ann Surg* **41**: 249–51.

Lindsey RW, Probe R, Miclau T, Alender JW, Perren SM (1933) The effects of antibiotic-impregnated autogenenic cancellous bone grafting on bone healing. *Clin Orthop* 303–12.

Locht RC, Gross AE, Langer F (1984) Late osteochondral allograft resurfacing for tibial plateau fractures, *J Bone Joint Surg* **66A**: 328–35.

Lord CF, Gebhardt MC, Tomford WW, Mankin HJ (1988) Infection in bone allografts. Incidence, nature and treatment, *J Bone Joint Surg* **70A**: 369–76.

May JW Jr, Gallico GG III, Lukash FN (1982) Microvascular transfer of free tissue for closure of bone wounds of the distal lower extremity, *N Engl J Med* **306**: 253–6.

Moore JR, Weiland AJ, Daniel RK (1983) Use of free vascularized bone grafts in treatment of bone tumors, *Clin Orthop* **175**: 37–44.

Paley D, Catagni MA, Argnani F, Villa A, Benedetti GB, Cattaneo R (1989) Ilizarov treatment of tibial nonunions with bone loss, *Clin Orthop* **241**: 146–65.

Papineau LJ (1973) L'excision-greffe avec fermeture retardee délibérée dans l'osteomyelite chronique, *Nouv Presse Med* **2**: 2753–5.

Reckling FW, Waters CH III (1980) Treatment of non-unions of fractures of the tibial diaphysis by postero-lateral cortical cancellous bone-grafting, *J Bone Joint Surg* **62A**: 936–41.

Salibian AH, Anzel SH, Salyer WA (1987) Transfer of vascularized grafts of iliac bone to the extremities, *J Bone Joint Surg* **69A**: 1319–27.

Sudmann E (1979) Treatment of chronic osteomyelitis by free grafts of cancellous autologous bone tissue. A preliminary report, *Acta Orthop Scand* **50**: 145–50.

Taylor GI (1977) Microvascular free bone transfer. A clinical technique, *Orthop Clin N Am* **8**: 425–47.

Weiland AJ, Moore JR, Daniel RK (1984) The efficacy of free tissue transfer in the treatment of osteomyelitis, *J Bone Joint Surg* **66A**: 181–93.

22
Management of non-union

C.M. Court-Brown

The definition of what constitutes delayed union and non-union is surprisingly difficult. Traditionally, surgeons have tended to apply an arbitrary time when examining either X-rays or patients for signs of bone union. Failure to secure either clinical or radiological union by a specific time has led to either a bone-grafting operation or some other procedure designed to encourage bone union. This principle has advantages and disadvantages. Fractures heal at different rates depending on a variety of factors such as the degree of soft-tissue injury, the extent of bone damage, the location of the fracture in whichever bone is involved, the gap between the bone ends, the method of treatment and the age and general health of the patient. Thus, to apply a fixed time limit to a fracture and specify that there is delayed or non-union after this time is a rather naive concept. However, the use of a fixed time limit has encouraged orthopaedic surgeons to think about early bone grafting in the management of fractures and this concept has certainly reduced the incidence of non-union following fractures and has therefore accelerated the patient's return to maximal function.

An illustration of the futility of applying a specific time to bone union is shown in Table 22.1 which details the union times in a population of adult tibial diaphyseal fractures treated by one particular method, namely a reamed intramedullary nail. The closed fractures have been classified using Tscherne's classification (Oestern and Tscherne 1984) and the open fractures by Gustilo's classification (Gustilo and Anderson 1976, Gustilo et al 1984). It is understood that these classification systems are somewhat unsophisticated but they represent accepted clinical classifications in widespread use which currently have not been improved on. Table 22.1 illustrates that the mean time to union in open fractures varies between 14.7 weeks for

Table 22.1 Bone union times for adult tibial diaphyseal fractures treated with a reamed intramedullary nail

Tscherne type	Time to union (weeks)
C0	12.5
C1	16.2
C2	18.7
C3	23.7
Gustilo type	
I	14.7
II	23.5
IIIa	27.2
IIIb (insignificant bone loss)*	38.0
IIIb (significant bone loss)*	74.0

*Significant bone loss is defined as >50% of the circumference and 2 cm in length. This amount of bone loss constitutes a non-union. The data show that the use of a set time on which to base a diagnosis of non-union is illogical as union times differ greatly.

Gustilo type I fractures and 74 weeks in type IIIb fractures associated with significant bone loss. It also illustrates that Tscherne C3 fractures are of a similar overall severity to Gustilo type II and IIIa open fractures, presumably largely because of the similar degrees of periosteal and muscle damage that accompany these fractures.

Classification

There are a number of basic classifications of non-unions. All non-unions can be divided into infected or aseptic non-unions. They can also be divided into hypertrophic (Figure 22.1) and atrophic (Figure 22.2) non-unions. Hypertrophic non-unions show evidence of attempted union and they are thought to follow inadequate bone stabilization. In atrophic non-union there is no

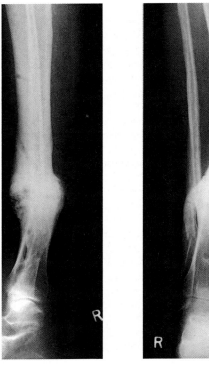

Figure 22.1

A hypertrophic non-union of the tibia following external fixation of a Gustilo type II open fracture. The fixator has failed to hold optimal alignment and the fracture is in valgus and recurvatum.

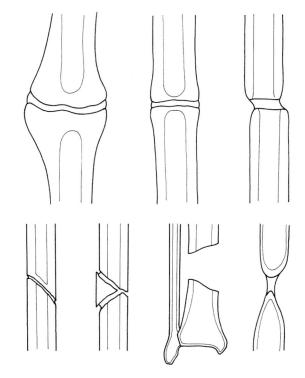

Figure 22.3

The Weber and Cech non-union classification. Non-unions are divided according to their biological reaction. They are either hypertrophic or oligotrophic (top line) or atrophic or with bone loss (bottom line).

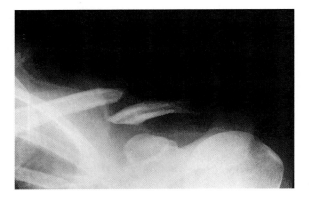

Figure 22.2

An atrophic non-union of the clavicle six months after fracture. There is a considerable gap between the bone ends and no sign of union.

evidence of union and it is likely that these non-unions are caused by deficient or absent vascularity of the bone ends. This simple classification of non-unions does not, however, encompass all the situations that the clinician will encounter although even a simple differentiation between hypertrophic and atrophic non-union will aid the surgeon in treating many non-unions.

Weber and Cech (1976) proposed a classification for diaphyseal non-union which was clinically useful as it included most situations commonly encountered by the clinician. Their classification is shown in Figure 22.3. They recognized the 'elephant's foot' or hypertrophic non-union but pointed out that there could also be an oligotrophic non-union where the bone ends were vital but lack of movement prevented

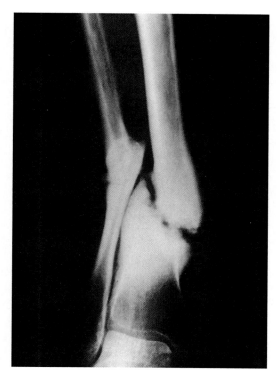

Figure 22.4

A long-standing pseudarthrosis of the distal tibia. Note the sclerosis of the bone ends. Only the fibular union provided stability. The tibial pseudarthrosis was mobile.

the establishment of a classical hypertrophic non-union. This is important in considering non-union following open fractures, as many open fractures will have been stabilized, this preventing excessive fracture movement. Weber and Cech also recognized the union problem associated with butterfly fragments that have a poor blood supply, although this is clearly of more importance in closed than in open fractures. However, they also pointed out that bone defects would, by definition, lead to non-union. This situation is common after Gustilo IIIb fractures and has led most authorities to suggest early bone grafting for these severe injuries.

The classification of non-union is complicated by the use of the terms non-union, pseudarthrosis and synovial pseudarthrosis. These are often

used synonymously, but Milgram (1991) has pointed out that the terms 'non-union' and 'pseudarthrosis' (Figure 22.4) have different meanings as they describe different parts of the non-union process. Milgram analysed a number of extra-articular and intra-articular non-unions. He showed that the radiographic appearance of a typical long-bone non-union was that the zone between the fracture ends lacked mineralization. Microscopically, the zone was shown to consist of vascularized fibrous tissue with a variable degree of chondroid differentiation between the bone ends. In 19 of his 41 cases he documented the presence of microscopic clefts. These originated peripherally from the periosteal soft tissues. As the non-unions healed, the clefts appeared to become bridged along their margins by mineralized callus. However, in cases where the non-union persisted, the clefts appeared to propagate and form a single dominant cleft; this happened in eight of his 41 specimens. Milgram theorized that the clefts lead to progressively more motion at the fracture non-union sites and he referred to these unstable non-unions with microscopic evidence of a dominant cleft as a 'pseudarthrosis'. He also pointed out that, while these non-unions might contain a few millilitres of non-viscous fluid, microscopic examination demonstrated a lack of true synovial lining cells and for this reason the term 'synovial pseudarthrosis' should not be used.

Milgram also pointed out that the entity of delayed union could not be defined by a morphological study of the tissue. He suggested that a delayed union was not a clinical entity but merely represented a slowly healing fracture that might or might not unite. This observation is in accord with the clinical data presented in Table 22.1.

Rosen (1992) has classified non-unions according to their location and presenting characteristics. Figure 22.5 shows a classification of non-unions based on Rosen's classification, but including the essentials of the Weber and Cech classification (1976) and Milgram's work (1991); it illustrates the kernel of the non-union problem as a fibrous non-union which may be intra-articular, metaphyseal or diaphyseal in location. The fibrous non-union may progress to become a pseudarthrosis and it is suggested that, while both fibrous non-unions and pseudarthroses can

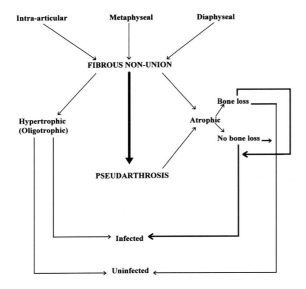

Figure 22.5

A classification of non-union. It takes into account the location, type and infection status of the non-union. The heaviest arrow represents the transition between fibrous non-union and pseudarthrosis and the less heavy darker arrows point out that infected non-unions are usually atrophic.

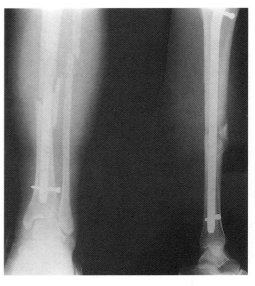

Figure 22.6a

A tibial diaphyseal fracture treated by a reamed intramedullary nail. Note the fracture distraction which is maintained by the static lock. This X-ray was taken 18 weeks after fracture, and an exchange nailing was subsequently performed.

be atrophic, only a fibrous non-union can be said to be hypertrophic. Obviously hypertrophic non-unions, atrophic non-unions without bone loss and atrophic non-unions with bone loss can all become infected.

Aetiology

Most non-unions are caused by infection, excessive movement at the fracture site or avascularity of the bone ends, this being a particular problem in severe open fractures. However, there are other well-documented causes of non-union which can be affected by the surgeon's choice of treatment and his or her skill in carrying out the chosen treatment method. It has been known for many years that soft-tissue interposition in a fracture site will prevent fracture reduc-

tion and fracture union. It has also been understood for a long time that fracture distraction causes non-union. This was well appreciated by both Watson-Jones (1976) and Bohler (1936), two proponents of non-operative fracture management. Bohler, in particular, advocated that no more than 5 lb weight should be used in the traction management of tibial fractures in case fracture distraction occurred. The deleterious effect of fracture distraction secondary to intramedullary nailing has been pointed out by Court-Brown et al (1995).

Grieff (1979) showed that an increasing fracture gap in plated rabbit tibial osteotomies resulted in different tissues being laid down at the bone ends. Obviously, the type of fixation employed by the surgeon may interact with the size of a fracture gap and if a surgeon chooses a plate or external fixator of high rigidity and leaves a fracture gap, non-union may well ensue.

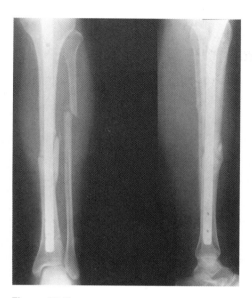

Figure 22.6b

Seventeen weeks after exchange nailing the non-union has closed but remains, and is probably now oligotrophic. Note the persistent fibular non-union.

The use of dynamic external fixation and intramedullary nailing will compensate for a fracture gap to an extent, but obviously significant gaps between the bone ends may interfere with bone union (Figure 22.6).

Court-Brown and McQueen (1987) pointed out the relationship between fracture union and compartment syndrome in a retrospective study of the management of tibial diaphyseal fractures in Edinburgh over a 20-year period. They showed that in patients over 18 years of age, the association of a compartment syndrome and subsequent fasciotomy significantly prolonged time to union. This did not occur in younger patients and the authors theorized that the effect was due to impairment of the vascular supply to the bone during the period of raised compartment pressure. Subsequent prospective studies have confirmed the association between increased compartment pressure and bone union and animal work has suggested that if compartment pressure is raised for a prolonged period, there is interference with bone vascularity and bone healing (McQueen 1995).

Incidence

The incidence of non-union in open fractures is difficult to determine accurately. Much has been written about the problem but many studies present retrospective analyses of heterogeneous fractures treated by a variety of different techniques often by surgeons of varying experience. Thus the fact that one particular surgeon or group of surgeons has a certain non-union rate means little and may merely represent their experience at avoiding infection or employing early bone-grafting techniques. However, it is reasonable to suggest that the incidence of both infected and aseptic non-union following open fractures is declining mainly as a result of improved soft-tissue handling and early bone grafting. Surgeons have tended in the past to ascribe their success, or otherwise, to a particular fracture treatment method rather than their ability to use the method properly or to handle the soft tissues adequately. This must be borne in mind when comparing the incidence of non-union in different fracture treatment methods.

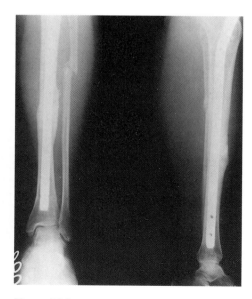

Figure 22.6c

Nine weeks after a second exchange nailing the tibial fracture is united but the fibula has not.

Open tibial fractures

Non-operative management

Unfortunately, it is very difficult to calculate an apparent incidence of tibial non-union following non-operative management by reference to the literature. Much of the literature is now over 25 years old, and quite obviously the criteria that surgeons applied to detail the success or failure of fracture treatment have improved over the years. Brown and Urban (1969) detailed the results of the treatment of 63 open fractures of the tibia in patients injured in combat. These patients were treated late, using long leg casts and less sophisticated plastic surgery techniques. Despite this there were no non-unions. These apparently excellent results are a reflection of different outcome criteria and in no way reflect on their standard of treatment. Nicoll (1964) in his classical paper dealing with the management of 705 tibial fractures had only 35 non-unions, whereas Haines et al (1984) in a consecutive group of non-operatively managed tibial fractures had a 27% non-union rate. It seems, therefore, that there is probably little to be gained from studying older literature; unfortunately, the newer literature usually consists of analyses of patient groups where non-operative management has been reserved for less severe open fractures, with operative management, usually in the form of external skeletal fixation or plating, employed for type II or III open fractures. It is very difficult to compare these series with series of fractures uniformly treated with internal or external fixation. The other problem with the older literature is that surgeons often adopted the policy that the fracture would heal if left long enough. Thus while 20 weeks is often used to define 'delayed union' (Nicoll 1964, Slätis and Rokkanen 1967, Oni et al 1988), true non-union is often only diagnosed after one year in a cast, at which time joint and patient functions have reached their nadir. This philosophy is, unfortunately, fairly common. Den Outer et al (1990) documented a 32% incidence of delayed union in tibial fractures at 20 weeks but only operated on two out of 94 patients for delayed union. It is, therefore, impossible to give figures for the incidence of non-union in non-operatively managed open tibial fractures compared with the incidences of non-union recorded for other treatment methods shown in Table 22.2.

External skeletal fixation

Most of the literature regarding the use of external fixation in the management of open fractures has concerned the tibia and, unfortunately, many authors present data with reference to a mixed selection of open fracture types. Table 22.2 shows some of the data that are available. Kenwright et al (1991) had a 6.1% incidence of non-union in all types of open tibial diaphyseal fracture using a dynamic external fixator. Holbrook et al (1989) and Whitelaw et al (1990) reported a non-union incidence of 11% and 18%, respectively, using a static external fixator. Chan et al (1984) analysed type III open tibial fractures and showed a 60% 'delayed' union rate but in recent years the practice of early bone grafting for this type of fracture has meant that outcome is measured in terms of time to clinical union,

Table 22.2 The quoted incidences of non-union following different methods of management of tibial fractures. There is wide variation reflecting different surgical practice

Author	Device	Fracture type	Non-union (%)
Holbrook et al (1989)	External fixation	C,O(GI,II,III)	11
Whitelaw et al (1990)	External fixation	O(GI,II,III)	18
Kenwright et al (1991)	External fixation	O(GI,II,III)	6.1
Court-Brown et al (1990)	IM nailing	C,O(GI)	1.6
Ruedi et al (1976)	Plating	O(GI,II,III)	5.3
Steen Jensen et al (1977)	Plating	C,O(GI,II,III)	0
Bach and Hansen (1989)	Plating	O(GII,III)	7.7

*C, closed; O, open; G, Gustilo grade.

amputation rate and incidence of infection rather than by the incidence of non-union (Blick et al 1989, Court-Brown et al 1990b). Blick et al (1989) examined the role of posterolateral bone grafting and advocated that this technique be performed two weeks after closed tibial fractures or open high-energy tibial fractures that had been closed by delayed primary closure, split-thickness skin graft or rotational myoplasty. Where vascularized free flaps had been used they suggested bone grafting at six weeks. This type of approach is now widespread and has resulted in a considerable reduction in the incidence of non-union.

Intramedullary nailing

There has been recent interest in the management of severe open fractures by intramedullary nailing. As with external fixation, the literature concerned with intramedullary nailing has usually consisted of a heterogeneous collection of fracture types. Also, since the use of widespread intramedullary nailing is a relatively recent phenomenon, many surgeons have applied the principle of early bone grafting that they learned with external fixation to intramedullary nailing and rates of non-union following intramedullary nailing of open fractures are therefore difficult to determine. However, Court-Brown et al (1990a) suggested a 1.6% incidence of non-union following reamed nailing of closed and Gustilo type I open tibial diaphyseal fractures. Unfortunately, although they later applied the technique of reamed intramedullary nailing to more severe open tibial fractures, the use of early bone grafting and exchange intramedullary nailing meant that the only non-unions that they encountered were in those fractures that either had significant bone loss or infection (Court-Brown et al 1991). This is also true of other groups noted for their interest in intramedullary nailing.

Whittle et al (1992) used the unreamed Russell-Taylor nail but practised early bone grafting and overall they reported a 94% incidence of union. Oedekoven et al (1993), using the unreamed AO tibial nail, also achieved excellent union rates but again employed early bone grafting as considered necessary.

Plating

The literature dealing with plating of open tibial fractures is somewhat older, but excellent results appear to have been obtained by Ruedi et al (1976), Steen-Jensen et al (1977) and Bach and Hansen (1989). Bach and Hansen compared plating with external skeletal fixation and preferred the latter although their non-union rate following plating was comparable to other treatment methods.

Open femoral fractures

Such has been the recent dominance of intramedullary nailing in the treatment of both open and closed femoral diaphyseal fractures that most literature relevant to the problem of femoral non-union concerns nailed femora. Grosse et al (1993) reported on 115 consecutive open femoral fractures and detailed only four cases of 'delayed union' with only three of the fractures requiring bone grafting. Lhowe and Hansen (1988) reported on 67 patients with open femoral fractures and found that only three patients required bone grafting, two of these being due to the presence of a major segmental defect. Wiss et al (1991) treated 56 patients with open femoral fractures secondary to gunshot wounds and recorded only two 'delayed unions' and no requirement for bone grafting at all. It is therefore obvious that open femoral fractures, providing adequate soft-tissue debridement is performed, are associated with a very low incidence of non-union.

Open upper limb diaphyseal fractures

Open upper limb diaphyseal fractures are also associated with a low incidence of non-union. Plating remains the commonest treatment option for fractures of the diaphyses of the radius, ulna and humerus. Moed et al (1986) showed that with good surgery excellent results could be achieved with primary plating of open fractures of the forearm. They documented 57 patients treated by immediate internal fixation and had only an 8.9% incidence of non-union. Humeral diaphyseal fractures are also associated with a low incidence of non-union.

Thus, it is clear that diaphyseal non-union following open fracture treatment is mainly a problem of the tibia and it is with regard to this bone that the treatment of non-union will be discussed. However, the general principles of treatment pertain to all non-unions regardless of their location.

Treatment

The two mainstays of the treatment of non-unions are the alteration of the biomechanical environment of the fracture and the use of bone grafts. In addition, there has been much interest in the use of electrostimulation for the management of fibrous non-union and more recently percutaneous bone marrow grafting, bone morphogenic protein and L-dopa are among other modalities that have been examined.

Hypertrophic or oligotrophic non-union associated with excessive fracture site motion usually follows non-operative fracture management or, as shown in Figure 22.1, may be associated with failure of operative management. Danis (1949) showed that compression of these non-unions resulted in fracture healing without the requirement for bone grafting or the necessity to take down the fracture site. The use of AO compression plates in the management of non-unions was highlighted by Muller and Thomas (1979). They concluded that aseptic hypertrophic non-union required plate stabilization and bone grafting was only needed if the non-union required to be taken down to correct a co-existing malunion. Rosen (1979) agreed with these findings but also demonstrated an 83% success rate with plate stabilization of infected non-unions. However, he did suggest that further surgery was often required in infected fractures after the initial stabilization procedure.

Although hypertrophic non-unions may occur after open fractures, the presence of significant soft-tissue damage associated with the use of internal or external skeletal fixation ensures that the majority of non-unions that occur after significant open fractures are in fact atrophic and a proportion of these may well be infected.

The treatment of stable atrophic non-union associated with open fractures is by bone grafting. There are a number of different methods of bone grafting, but the most commonly used type of graft is the cortico-cancellous autograft popularized by Phemister (1947). In this technique, cortico-cancellous bone slivers are removed from the anterior or posterior iliac crests and applied around the non-union site which does not require to be taken down. The technique is usually associated with bone petalling or shingling, this consisting of the raising of osteoperiosteal fragments with a sharp osteotome or chisel.

The technique of cortico-cancellous bone grafting is usually straightforward. Where possible, tibial cortico-cancellous bone grafts are most easily inserted through an anterior approach. However, it should be borne in mind that the skin over the subcutaneous anterior border of the tibia is often damaged at the time of the original injury and the surgeon may be unwilling to insert bone graft through this damaged area. An alternative technique is the use of posterolateral bone grafting as advocated by Jones and Barnett (1955). In this technique, the posterior compartment of the leg is entered and the posterior surface of the posterolateral intermuscular septum is followed to the fibula. The muscles are then stripped away from the posterior surface of the intermuscular septum and the tibial non-union is visualized. The success of this procedure is well documented (Freeland and Mutz 1976, Reckling and Waters 1980) and its use is recommended in aseptic atrophic non-union of the tibia associated with the use of plates and external fixators in particular. Reckling and Waters (1980) pointed out that more than one bone-grafting procedure may be required to achieve fracture union.

The treatment of aseptic non-union in nailed tibial fractures may involve the use of cortico-cancellous bone grafting as already described, but before this procedure is contemplated the technique of exchange intramedullary nailing may be used in all open tibial fractures except those IIIb fractures associated with significant bone loss.

Exchange intramedullary nailing

Exchange nailing refers to the practice of removing an intramedullary nail, reaming the medullary canal to a larger size and inserting a second appropriately sized nail (Figure 22.6). The technique has two applications. It can be used as part of the treatment protocol for the management of bone infection and infected non-unions (Court-Brown et al 1992). It can also, however, be used for the treatment of aseptic non-union of nailed tibial fractures. In the management of infected non-unions, exchange nailing permits intramedullary stabilization of the diaphyseal non-union after reaming of the infected endosteal membrane. This technique is used in conjunction with soft-tissue resection, bone resection and bone-grafting techniques and is described in more detail in Chapter 21.

Aseptic non-unions are more common than infected non-unions and the use of exchange nailing in aseptic non-union will be described in some detail. Court-Brown et al (1995) examined the use of primary reamed intramedullary nailing in the management of 557 tibial diaphyseal fractures between August 1986 and June 1992: 438 of these fractures were closed and 119 were open. The distribution of these fractures is detailed in Table 22.3. Thirty-three of the fractures which progressed to aseptic non-union were subsequently treated by exchange nailing. The average age of this group was 36.3 years (range 17–66 years). There were 25 males and eight females.

The numbers of different Tscherne and Gustilo fracture types that developed aseptic non-union is also detailed in Table 22.3. Overall, 3.5% of closed tibial diaphyseal fractures went on to non-union. In the open group, 7.1% of Gustilo type I and type II fractures developed an aseptic non-union with 21.7% of Gustilo IIIa fractures and 38.5% of type IIIb fractures without significant bone loss also showing evidence of aseptic non-union. All of the Gustilo type IIIb fractures associated with a bone loss of >50% of the circumference and 2.5 cm of cortical length developed non-union.

Exchange nailing is a straightforward procedure. The patient is set up on the nailing table in the same manner as for a primary nailing procedure (Court-Brown et al 1990a). The original nail and cross screws are removed and the intramedullary canal is reamed to accommodate a nail of at least 1 mm greater diameter than the original nail. The extent of reaming is dictated by the amount of endosteal bone that is brought up by the reamers. Once the endosteal membrane is removed and new endosteal bone is seen on the end of the reamer bit, a new nail can safely be inserted. Cross screws are rarely required because of the stable nature of the fibrous non-union that exists at the time of exchange nailing.

Table 22.3 illustrates that the technique is a successful one. All of the exchange nailing

Table 22.3 Details of the incidence of aseptic non-union and the requirement for exchange nailing following primary reamed intramedullary nailing of the tibia. The closed fractures are divided into Tscherne grades and the open fractures into Gustilo types and subtypes

Fracture type	Number	Uninfected fractures	Aseptic non-unions		Exchange nailings	Bone grafting
			Number	%		
Closed						
CO	38	38	0	0	0	0
C1	261	256	8	3.1	8	0
C2	110	109	6	5.5	6	0
C3	29	29	1	3.4	1	0
TOTAL	438	432	15	3.5	15	0
Open						
GI	29	28	2	7.1	2	0
GII	30	27	2	7.1	2	0
GIIIA	23	23	5	21.7	5	0
GIIIB$_1$	15	13	5	38.5	5	1
GIIIB$_2$	12	11	11	100	4	11

*GIIIB$_1$, Gustilo IIIB fractures with insignificant bone loss; GIIIB$_2$, those with significant loss.

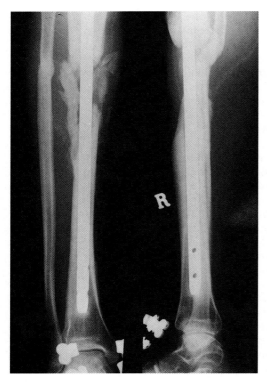

Figure 22.7

A Gustilo IIIb fracture treated by primary nailing and an early latissimus dorsi free flap. Bone grafting was performed at 6 weeks. Five months later there is good incorporation, except anteriorly. A second graft was required to achieve sufficient stability to allow nail removal.

debate in the literature as to the extent of cortico-cancellous bone grafting that can be performed. We have, however, bone grafted up to 12 cm of bone loss using cortico-cancellous autograft although clearly the incorporation of this amount of bone graft takes a considerable time. Figure 22.7 illustrates the use of cortico-cancellous autograft and a reamed intramedullary nail in the management of significant bone loss.

The only complication that appeared to be specific to exchange nailing was superficial infection of the nail entry wound. In primary tibial nailing, Court-Brown et al (1990a) documented the incidence of wound infection at 1.6%. However, in exchange nailing, the same unit found the incidence of superficial wound infection to be 12.1%. The reason for this difference is difficult to determine as the local soft-tissue vascularity is satisfactory.

The success of exchange nailing in the management of aseptic tibial diaphyseal non-union suggests it should be routinely used for all closed fractures and for all open fractures up to Gustilo type IIIa in severity. It is useful in Gustilo type IIIb fractures where the extent of bone loss is <2 cm in length and involves <50% of the bone circumference. For greater areas of bone loss, it is recommended that early cortico-cancellous grafting be used, this being done as soon as the soft tissues around the fracture site are stable, usually at about six weeks.

procedures in the closed fractures were successful and no bone grafting was required for the management of an aseptic tibial diaphyseal non-union during this study period. Similarly all of the Gustilo types I, II and IIIa fractures healed with exchange nailing. There was, however, only an 80% success rate in Gustilo type IIIb fractures associated with bone loss of <50% of the circumference and 2 cm of cortical length. Where there was bone loss of greater than this amount, exchange nailing was uniformly unsuccessful and cortico-cancellous bone grafting was required. There is some

Sequential external fixation and intramedullary nailing

One technique which is allied to exchange nailing of the tibia is the use of primary external skeletal fixation and secondary intramedullary nailing. This technique is detailed in Chapter 7 with information regarding the technique being detailed in Table 7.8. There are a number of reasons for using sequential external fixation and intramedullary nailing. It may be a planned treatment regime but the surgeon may elect to use intramedullary nailing as treatment for non-union following primary external fixation. This can be a successful technique but its use and results will not be discussed further in this chapter and the reader is referred to Chapter 7.

Alternative grafting techniques

Recently, there has been considerable interest in the use of allografts mainly as treatment for tumours and failed arthroplasties associated with bone loss. The use of bone transport and vascularized grafts detailed in Chapter 19 has meant that most cases of post-traumatic bone loss can be treated without the use of allografts. However, autograft harvesting is not without a degree of morbidity and the possibility exists of using homografts or heterografts for non-unions. Leung (1989) summarized the current usage of these grafts in the management of trauma but at present the use of cortico-cancellous autografts must be advocated in the treatment of non-unions. The alternative grafting techniques for the management of bone loss are summarized in Chapter 19.

Partial fibulectomy

A particular technique applicable to hypertrophic tibial non-union is partial fibulectomy. This technique consists of the treatment of hypertrophic or oligotrophic non-unions by resection of between 1 and 2 cm of fibula. There is some debate about the amount of fibula that should be resected. DeLee et al (1981) advocate resection of 2.5 cm of fibula on the grounds that resection of less than this might result in fibula union before tibial union was achieved. However, this situation is rare and 2.5 cm constitutes a significant length of resection. The author has found the resection of approximately 1 cm to be adequate in most cases.

Sorensen (1969) suggested a number of advantages to fibular resection. It allows the correction of a malposition in a mobile non-union, it avoids opening the fracture site and it does not interfere with the potential for internally fixing and grafting the tibial non-union if union fails to occur following partial fibulectomy. The technique was analysed in 51 patients by DeLee et al (1981) and they showed a 77% success rate. Failure was usually associated with the presence of a pseudarthrosis rather than a fibrous non-union. Further analysis of the data indicated that all but two of the partial fibulectomy failures were in open tibial fractures and it is probable

that the technique of partial fibulectomy is more applicable to low-energy tibial fractures associated with hypertrophic non-union than high-energy fractures which may be associated with atrophic non-unions.

Fibular non-union

Böstman and Kyro (1991) and Shen and Shen (1993) have both drawn attention to the problem of non-union of the fibula following tibial fractures (Figure 22.6). Böstman and Kyro estimated the frequency of fibular non-union to be 5.4% with Shen and Shen suggesting that the incidence was 4.5%. Böstman and Kyro observed that fibular non-union did not occur following non-operative management, a fact that they attributed to the overlap associated with non-operative treatment. They also recorded that rigid tibial fixation was associated with atrophic fibular non-union, whereas flexible tibial fixation tended to be associated with hypertrophic non-union. They felt that fibular non-union was a benign problem but Shen and Shen suggested that hypertrophic non-union of the fibula, which they found in three of their four cases of fibular non-union, could be symptomatic and should be treated by local fibular resection. Böstman and Kyro took a contrary view, pointing out that fibular union might take several years to occur and overall they felt that the subjective symptoms experienced by their patients were relatively mild. Where a symptomatic atrophic fibular non-union exists, bone plating and cortico-cancellous grafting is the treatment of choice.

Surgical stabilization of infected non-unions

The role of stabilization of non-operatively managed hypertrophic non-unions has already been discussed as has the role of exchange intramedullary nailing in those non-unions treated originally by the use of an intramedullary nail. However, there are a number of other situations where the surgeon may contemplate changing the method of fracture fixation as an adjunct to bone grafting (Figure 22.7). This frequently arises in the management of infected non-union associated with the use of either a plate or an intramedullary nail where external skeletal fixation is frequently perceived to be better because it does not involve metal crossing the infected non-union site. There is little to justify this view in situations where the infected non-union has been adequately treated but many surgeons favour the use of external fixation in general and the small wire Ilizarov in particular (Morandi et al 1994). The treatment of infected non-union is discussed extensively in Chapter 21), but the basic principles are straightforward. It is accepted by most traumatologists that infected non-union should be treated by fracture stabilization, aggressive debridement of both soft tissues and bone to remove all infected material, then re-establishment of the soft-tissue envelope using appropriate flap cover and subsequent bone grafting or bone transport.

The use of adjunctive external skeletal fixation has been suggested by many workers (Krempen et al 1979, Hedley and Bernstein 1983, Green et al 1984, Marsh et al 1992, Morandi et al 1994). Other workers have advocated the use of intramedullary nails (Christensen 1973, Clancy et al 1982, Warren and Brooker 1992, Alho et al 1993). It is probable that, as with primary fracture management, it is the overall philosophy that is important rather than the type of fracture fixation. The principal disadvantage of external fixation is the length of time that the patient needs to wear the fixator to allow for the maturation of the bone graft. Failure to keep the fixator on for an adequate period may result in fracture malposition and subsequent malunion. External fixation is also labour intensive, with small wire fixators in particular being associated with a high incidence of pin track sepsis and other complications. There is, however, concern that the use of intramedullary nailing in infected or potentially infected situations may lead to a pan-diaphyseal osteomyelitis which may be impossible to eradicate. However, Court-Brown et al (1992) showed that this was not the case and infected non-union of open tibial fractures could be treated by intramedullary nailing. Their suggested protocol for the management of infected non-union associated with the use of a primary intramedullary nail was based on the presence of a pyogenic collection and an established sinus. The protocol is shown in Figure 22.8. Currently, it is the author's view that intramedullary nailing combined with appropriate soft-tissue and bone debridement is the treatment of choice for infected diaphyseal non-union, with external fixation being reserved for infected metaphyseal non-union.

Other treatment methods

Because of the morbidity associated with the harvesting of bone grafts, the difficulty of bone grafting large segment defects and the relative complexity of using small wire fixators and bone transport methods, surgeons have been seeking other ways of treating non-unions and filling bone defects.

In the 1980s there was considerable interest in the treatment of non-union with electricity. In 1981, Bassett et al reported on 125 patients who completed electromagnetic treatment for non-union with an 87% success rate. Other authors also suggested that electromagnetic stimulation had a place in the management of non-unions (Sharrad et al 1982). However, the place of electromagnetic therapy in the management of non-union remains very controversial and, even where good results are obtained, it is often difficult to separate the use of electromagnetic fields from the other treatment modalities employed at the same time. Prolonged immobilization is required and patient rehabilitation is therefore often difficult. Whatever the true place of electromagnetic therapy in the treatment of non-unions, interest in this technique has waned and it is now impossible to recommend its use.

The use of bone-marrow injections to treat non-unions is an obvious step. Bone marrow contains osteo-progenitor cells and Healey et al (1990) report satisfactory new bone formation in the treatment of non-union. Their patients had had tumour resection and some had had other graft reconstructions. They emphasized that their results had been achieved in the face of a number of clinical problems and they advocated further trials. Paley et al (1986) have shown success in the laboratory situation and only time will tell if bone-marrow injection is going to provide a useful clinical method of treating non-unions.

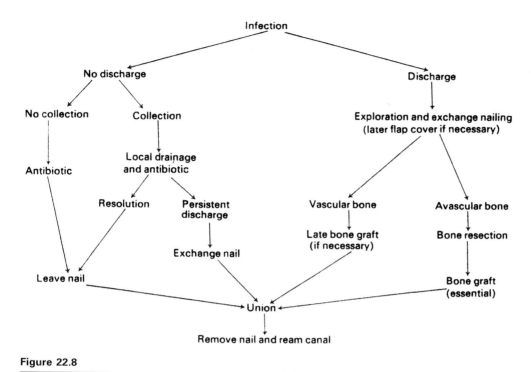

Figure 22.8

Protocol for the management of infection associated with an intramedullary nail (Court-Brown et al 1992).

Similarly, bone morphogenic protein has been used to induce bone formation when implanted in extraskeletal and skeletal defects in laboratory animals. Johnson et al (1988) illustrate the use of human bone morphogenic protein in the augmentation of bone grafts used to treat resistant femoral non-unions. They were clear that they could not distinguish between the use of the graft and the bone morphogenic protein but felt that there was an additive effect. Later work (Johnson et al 1990) showed similar results in the treatment of distal metaphyseal tibial non-unions.

In a recent study, Sciadini et al (1994) have examined diaphyseal defects made in dog radii. The defects were filled with autogenous cancellous bone or demineralized bone matrix, 50% of which were activated by bone morphogenic proteins. At six weeks the cancel-lous bone graft and bone morphogenic protein activated demineralized bone matrix grafts showed radiographic evidence of union whereas the demineralized bone matrix graft without bone morphogenic protein did not. This result was similar at three months and biomechanical analysis of the healed defects showed that the mineralized bone matrix grafts without bone morphogenic protein were weaker. The authors felt that their early results indicated that the rate of healing and strength of healed bone in demineralized bone matrix grafts augmented with bone morphogenic protein were comparable to that of standard cancellous autografts and, if this is shown to be true in further long-term studies, the implications are that cancellous or cortico-cancellous autografting may be superseded by new techniques.

Table 22.4   A suggested protocol for the management of diaphyseal non-unions. The success of reamed nailing in the treatment of atrophic non-unions justifies its use without ancillary bone grafting. If it is unsuccessful, bone grafting should be employed. The management of infected non-union depends more on adequate soft-tissue and bone resection than on the type of stabilization used. The management of metaphyseal and intra-articular non-unions is not dissimilar, although obviously intramedullary fixation is impossible. These are usually atrophic and rely on plates and screws or external fixation to stabilize the non-union. Bone graft should be used

Non-union type	Primary treatment	Suggested treatment
Aseptic		
Hypertrophic	Non-operative	Reamed nail if fracture aligned
		Closed dynamic external fixation if malaligned
	Plate	Reamed nail
	External fixation	Reamed nail if fracture aligned
		Increase rigidity of frame if fracture malaligned
	Unreamed nail	Reamed nail
	Reamed nail	Exchange reamed nail
Atrophic	Non-operative	Reamed nail if aligned
		External fixation and bone graft if malaligned
	Plate	Reamed nail
	External fixation	Reamed nail if aligned
		Bone graft if malaligned
	Unreamed nail	Reamed nail
	Reamed nail	Exchange reamed nail
		(If reamed nailing fails to unite fracture, bone graft later)
Infected	Non-operative	Thorough soft tissue and bone debridement
	Plate	removing all infected material (repeat as
	External fixation	necessary). Stabilize with external fixator or
	Unreamed nail	intramedullary nail, flap cover if required and
	Reamed nail	close bone defect as for bone loss
Bone loss	Non-operative	Stabilize fracture with intramedullary nail or
	Plate	external fixator depending on location. Defect
	External fixation	closed by bone graft, vascularized bone graft
	Unreamed nail	or bone transport. Sometimes primary shortening
	Reamed nail	with later bone lengthening may be used.

Pritchett (1990) examined the use of L-dopa in the management of non-union. He treated 25 adults with atrophic non-union and reported an 84% success rate. However, he made the mistake of defining long-bone non-union according to a rigid timetable and he suggested that tibial non-union occurred after 20 weeks. This is clearly not always the case, and it is certainly possible that some of his fractures healed spontaneously in an acceptable time.

Buchholz et al (1987) summarized the use of hydroxyapatite tricalcium phosphate as a bone-graft substitute. They showed incorporation into bone in the post-traumatic situation, but the usefulness of these compounds was limited by their brittle mechanical structure and the lack of osteo-inductive properties.

Protocol for the management of non-union

It is obvious that the surgeon must differentiate between infected and aseptic non-unions and between hypertrophic and atrophic non-unions when considering management. He or she must also recognize the presence of bone loss which currently should be treated by early bone graftings although bone morphogenic protein-impregnated bone substitutes may prove useful in the future.

A suggested protocol for the management of diaphyseal non-union is presented in Table 22.4. It is suggested that aseptic hypertrophic non-unions are best treated by increasing the rigidity of the fracture and nowadays this is probably best achieved by using an intramedullary nail or a closed dynamic external fixator. Aseptic atrophic non-unions are probably best treated with an intramedullary nail if they are aligned or a dynamic external fixator supplemented by bone graft if the fracture is overlapped but otherwise not malaligned. Significantly malaligned non-unions should be taken down and then fixed by an appropriate method, using an intramedullary nail. As has already been illustrated, the use of reamed nailing may well stimulate union and only if this fails need bone grafting be undertaken.

The management of infected non-unions has been discussed. Regardless of the initial method of fracture management, the treatment of non-union involves adequate soft-tissue and bone debridement followed by stabilization which nowadays is probably best achieved with an external fixation device or an intramedullary nail. The management of bone loss is discussed in Chapter 19.

References

Alho A, Ekelund A, Stromsoe K, Benterud JG (1993) Nonunion of tibial shaft fractures treated with locked intramedullary nailing without bone grafting, *J Trauma* **34**: 62–7.

Bach AW, Hansen ST (1989) Plates versus external fixation in severe open tibial fractures: a randomised trial, *Clin Orthop* **241**: 89–94.

Bassett CAL, Mitchell SN, Gaston SR (1981) Treatment of ununited tibial diaphyseal fractures with pulsing electromagnetic fields, *J Bone Joint Surg (Am)* **63A**: 511–23.

Blick SS, Brumback RJ, Lakatos R, Poka A, Burgess AR (1989) Early prophylactic bone grafting of high energy tibial fractures, *Clin Orthop* **240**: 21–41.

Bohler L (1936) *The Treatment of Fractures* (John Wright: Bristol).

Böstman O, Kyro A (1991) Delayed union of fibular fractures accompanying fractures of the tibial shaft, *J Trauma* **31**: 99–102.

Brown PW, Urban JG (1969) Early weight-bearing treatment of open fractures of the tibia, *J Bone Joint Surg (Am)* **51A**: 59–75.

Bucholz RW, Carlton A, Holmes RE (1987) Hydroxyapatite tricalcium phosphate bone graft substitutes, *Orthop Clin N Am* **18**: 323–34.

Chan KM, Leung YK, Cheng JCY, Leung PC (1984) The management of type III open tibial fractures, *Injury* **16**: 157–65.

Christensen NO (1973) Kunstcher intramedullary reaming and nailing fixation for non-union of fracture of the femoral tibia, *J Bone Joint Surg (Br)* **55A**: 312–18.

Clancy GJ, Winquist RA, Hansen ST (1982) Nonunion of the tibia treated with Kuntscher intramedullary nailing, *Clin Orthop* **167**: 191–6.

Court-Brown CM, McQueen MM (1987) Compartment syndrome delays tibial union, *Acta Orthop Scand* **58**: 249–52.

Court-Brown CM, Christie J, McQueen MM (1990a) Closed intramedullary tibial nailing: its use in closed and type I open fractures, *J Bone Joint Surg (Br)* **72B**: 601–12.

Court-Brown CM, Wheelwright EF, Christ J, McQueen MM (1990b) External fixation for type III open tibial fractures, *J Bone Joint Surg (Br)* **72B**: 801–4.

Court-Brown CM, McQueen MM, Quaba AA, Christie J (1991) Locked intramedullary nailing of open tibial fractures, *J Bone Joint Surg (Br)* **73B**: 959–64.

Court-Brown CM, Keating JF, McQueen MM (1992) Infection after intramedullary nailing of the tibia: incidence and protocol for management. *J Bone Joint Surg (Br)* **74B**: 770–4.

Court-Brown CM, Keating J, Christie J, McQueen MM (1995) Exchange intramedullary nailing. Its use in aseptic tibial non-union, *J Bone Joint Surg (Br)*. In press.

Danis R (1949) *Théorie et Pratique de L'ostéosynthèse* (Masson: Paris).

DeLee JC, Heckman JD, Lewis AG (1981) Partial fibulectomy for ununited fractures of the tibia, *J Bone Joint Surg (Am)* **63A**: 1390–5.

Den Outer AJ, Meeuwis JD, Hermans J, Zwaverling A (1990) Conservative versus operative treatment of diaphyseal non-comminuted tibial shaft fractures, *Clin Orthop* **252**: 231–7.

Freeland AE, Mutz SB (1976) Posterior bone-grafting for infected ununited fracture of the tibia, *J Bone Joint Surg (Am)* **58A**: 653–7.

Green SA, Garland DE, Moore TJ, Barad SJ (1984) External fixation for the uninfected angulated nonunion of the tibia, *Clin Orthop* **190**: 204–11.

Grieff J (1979) Bone healing in rabbits after compression osteosynthesis: a comparative study between the radiological and histological findings, *Injury* **10**: 257–67.

Grosse A, Christie J, Taglang G, Court-Brown CM, McQueen MM (1993) Open adult femoral shaft fractures treated by early intramedullary nailing, *J Bone Joint Surg (Br)* **75B**: 562–5.

Gustilo RB, Anderson JT (1976) Prevention of infection in treatment of 1025 open fractures of long bones: retrospective and prospective analysis, *J Bone Joint Surg (Am)* **58A**: 453–8.

Gustilo RB, Mendoza RM, Williams DM (1984) Problems in the management of type III (severe) open fractures: a new classification of type III open fractures, *J Trauma* **24**: 742–6.

Heines JF, Williams EA, Hargaden EJ, Davies DRA (1984) Is conservative treatment of displaced tibial shaft fractures? *J Bone Joint Surg (Br)* **66B**: 84–8.

Healey JH, Zimmerman PA, McDonnell JM, Lane JM (1990) Percutaneous bone marrow grafting of delayed union and non-union in cancer patients, *Clin Orthop* **256**: 280–5.

Hedley AK, Bernstein ML (1983) External fixation as a secondary procedure, *Clin Orthop* **173**: 209–15.

Holbrook JL, Swiontkowski MF, Sanders R (1989) Treatment of open fractures of the tibial shaft. Ender nailing versus external fixation, *J Bone Joint Surg (Am)* **71A**: 1231–8.

Johnson EE, Urist MR, Finerman GAM (1988) Bone morphogenic protein augmentation grafting of resistant femoral non-unions: a preliminary report. *Clin Orthop* **230**: 257–65.

Johnson EE, Urist MR, Finerman GAM (1990) Distal metaphyseal tibial nonunion, *Clin Orthop* **250**: 234–40.

Jones KG, Barnett HC (1955) Cancellous bone grafting for non-union of the tibia through the postero-lateral approach, *J Bone Joint Surg (Am)* 1250–60.

Kenwright J, Richardson JB, Cunningham JL (1991) Axial movement and tibial fractures, *J Bone Joint Surg (Br)* **73B**: 654–9.

Krempen JF, Silver RA, Sotelo A (1979) The use of the Vidal–Adrey external fixation system, *Clin Orthop* **140**: 122–30.

Leung PC (1989) *Current Trends in Bone Grafting* (Springer Verlag: Berlin).

Lhowe DW, Hansen ST (1988) Immediate nailing of open fractures of the femoral shaft, *J Bone Joint Surg (Am)* **70A**: 812–20.

Marsh JL, Nepola JU, Meffert R (1992) Dynamic external fixation for stabilisation of nonunions, *Clin Orthop* **278**: 200–6.

McQueen MM (1995) Acute compartment syndrome. Its effect on bone blood flow and bone union. MD Thesis, University of Edinburgh.

Milgram JM (1991) Non-union and pseudarthrosis of fracture healing. A histopathological study of 95 human specimens, *Clin Orthop* **268**: 203–13.

Moed BR, Kellar JF, Foster RJ, Tile M, Hansen ST (1986) Immediate internal fixation of open fractures in the diaphysis of the forearm, *J Bone Joint Surg (Am)* **68A**: 1008–16.

Morandi M, Watson JT, Coupe K (1994) *Infected Tibial Intramedullary Nail: A Single Stage Reconstruction Procedure with the Ilizarov Method* (Orthopaedic Trauma Association: Los Angeles).

Muller ME, Thomas RJ (1979) Treatment of non-union in fractures of long bones, *Clin Orthop* **138**: 141–53.

Nicoll EA (1964) Fractures of the tibial shaft: a survey of 705 cases, *J Bone Joint Surg (Br)* **46B**: 373–87.

Oedekoven G, Claudi B, Frigg R (1993) Treatment of open and closed tibial fractures with unreamed interlocking nails, *Orthop Traumatol* **2**: 115–28.

Oestern HJ, Tscherne H (1984) Pathophysiology and classification of soft tissue injuries associated with fractures. In: Tscherne H, Gotzen L, eds, *Fractures with Soft Tissue Injuries* (Springer-Verlag: Berlin) 1–9.

Oni OOA, Hui A, Gregg PJ (1988) The healing of closed tibial shaft fractures, *J Bone Joint Surg (Br)* **70B**: 787–90.

Paley D, Young MC, Wiley AM, Fornasier UL, Jackson RW (1986) Percutaneous bone marrow grafting of fractures and bony defects: an experimental study in rabbits, *Clin Orthop* **208**: 300–12.

Phemister DB (1947) Treatment of ununited fractures by onlay bone grafts without screw or fixation and without breaking down of the fibrous union, *J Bone Joint Surg (Am)* **29A**: 946–60.

Pritchett JW (1990) L-Dopa in the treatment of nonunited fractures, *Clin Orthop* **255**: 293–300.

Reckling FW, Waters CH (1980) Treatment of non-unions of fractures of the tibial diaphysis, *J Bone Joint Surg (Am)* **62A**: 936–41.

Rosen H (1979) Compression treatment of pseudarthroses, *Clin Orthop* **138**: 154–66.

Rosen H (1992) Nonunion and malunion. In: Browner BD, Jupiter JB, Levine AM, Trafton PG, eds, *Skeletal Trauma* (WB Saunders: Philadelphia).

Ruedi T, Webb JK, Allgower M (1976) Experience with the dynamic compression plate (DCP) in 418 recent fractures of the tibial shaft, *Injury* **7**: 252–7.

Sciadini MF, Dawson JM, Johnson KD (1994) *Bone Healing in a Canine Model of a Segmental Defect: Demineralised Bone Matrix Allograft ± Bone Morphogenic Protein Versus Autograft* (Orthopaedic Trauma Association: Los Angeles).

Sharrad WJW, Sutcliffe ML, Robson MJ, Maceachern AG (1982) The treatment of fibrous non-union of fractures by pulsating electromagnetic stimulation, *J Bone Joint Surg (Br)* **64B**: 189–93.

Shen WJ, Shen YS (1993) Fibular nonunion after fixation of the tibia in lower leg fractures, *Clin Orthop* **287**: 231–2.

Sorensen KH (1969) Treatment of delayed union and non-union of the tibia by fibular resection, *Acta Orthop Scand* **40**: 92–104.

Slätis P, Rokkanen P (1967) Conservative treatment of tibial shaft fractures, *Acta Clin Scand* **134**: 41–7.

Steen Jensen J, Wang Hansen S, Johannsen J (1977) Tibial shaft fractures: a comparison of conservative treatment and internal fixation with conventional plates or AO compression plates, *Acta Orthop Scand* **48**: 204–12.

Warren SB, Brooker AF (1992) Intramedullary nailing of tibial nonunions, *Clin Orthop* **285**: 236–43.

Watson-Jones R (1976) *Fractures and Joint Injuries* (Churchill Livingstone: Edinburgh).

Weber BG, Cech O (1976) *Pseudarthrosis* (Huber: Bern).

Whitelaw JP, Wetzler M, Nelson A, Segal D, Fletcher J, Hadley N, Sawka A (1990) Ender rods versus external fixation: the treatment of open tibial fractures, *Clin Orthop* **253**: 258–69.

Whittle AP, Russell TA, Taylor JC, Lavelle DG (1992) Treatment of open fractures of the tibial shaft with the use of interlocking nailing without reaming, *J Bone Joint Surg (Am)* **74A**: 1162–72.

Wiss DA, Brien WW, Becker V (1991) Interlocking nailing for the treatment of femoral fractures due to gunshot wounds, *J Bone Joint Surg (Am)* **73A**: 598–606.

23

Amputation and late management of the severely injured limb

S.P. Makk, M. Vornanen and D. Seligson

Such has been the importance of amputation surgery over the centuries that it could reasonably be claimed that a history of its practice is representative of the history of surgery. A short history of amputation surgery is presented in Chapter 1. Its first use was probably as a punishment, religious rite or primary treatment of severe open fractures and it remained a common method of management, particularly for open fractures of the femur and tibia, until comparatively recently. It is in the past 30 years or so that surgeons have moved from amputation as a primary treatment method to a last resort when other treatment methods have failed.

The challenge to the modern traumatologist lies not in the availability of reconstructive techniques; rather in being able to choose when reconstructive efforts may provide an appropriate alternative to amputation in producing a functional result for a patient that surpasses that of primary amputation. Furthermore, the surgeon has to understand the meaning and symbolism of limb loss and must be able to treat equally the patient with aggressive 'modern' technologically-challenging limb salvage and the patient with limb ablation.

Patient assessment

Triage of patients with badly damaged extremities should follow protocols such as that defined by the American College of Surgeons in the Advanced Trauma Life Support (ATLS) course to rule out other life-threatening conditions (Brothwell and Moller-Christensen 1963, Gregory et al 1985, McAndrew and Lantz 1989). Thirty per cent of patients with open lower-limb fractures are polytrauma patients and 10–17% have associated life-threatening conditions (Gustilo 1982, Lange et al 1985, Caudle and Stern 1987, Gustilo et al 1990). Patient-related factors which favour primary amputation as a treatment for mangled extremities versus salvage include advanced age, short life expectancy, unstable psychiatric background, occupation and patient desires. Underlying chronic metabolic diseases such as diabetes mellitus, or immunological dysfunction decrease the chance of a successful limb salvage. Pre-existing limb deformity or morbidity may cause a tendency towards primary amputation as well (Chan et al 1984, Hansen 1987, Lange 1989, McAndrew and Lantz 1989).

There are, however, several factors that must be considered in a broad scope prior to proceeding with limb salvage (Seligson and Henry 1991). These include the possibilities of joint stiffness, post-traumatic arthrosis, neuralgia and other alterations of sensation, chronic venous and lymphatic stasis, chronic wound drainage and abnormalities of limb length and alignment. These and other morbidities must be evaluated in terms of a patient's age, socioeconomic status and occupation and then be correlated with the site(s) and complexity of the injury. There is too little emphasis on the length, morbidity and cost of treatment and poor documentation of the accurate longterm incapacity caused by injury (Lange 1989, Purry and Hannon 1989, Tsai et al 1988). The patient with an extremity fracture may have coexisting behavioral disorders ranging from alcohol or substance abuse to overt psychosis (Kuhn et al 1989). If treatment aggravates a co-morbidity to produce a dysfunctional individual, then treatment has failed. Goal-setting discussions with the patient and family must include the question of the limb as well as a comprehensive overview of all phases of rehabilitation, including eventual return to work (Augeneder et al 1989, Seligson and Henry 1991).

Esterhai et al (unpublished work) made a comparison between amputees and limb salvage patients and documented a prevalence of negative attitudes and residual bitterness because of limb loss. It is becoming apparent that the restoration of a severely injured limb to one that is noninfected, healed and functional after an open fracture is an historical goal that has progressively become the expectation during our lifetime (Seligson and Henry 1991).

The acute condition of a patient with a mangled extremity including the severity of other injuries, the presence and duration of shock, the length of warm ischaemia time and the presence of a compartment syndrome all assume important roles in the acute decision-making process of whether to amputate or to proceed with limb salvage (Lange 1989, McAndrew and Lantz 1989).

It is important to assess the physical reserve of the injured patient. This takes into account the quality of the injures person's health, general muscle tone and condition and how severely these reserves would be taxed by limb salvage in contrast to amputation. The same injury in a patient with ruptured diaphragm and severe liver laceration (high injury severity score) is amputated while in a patient without complex polytrauma, an attempt at salvage may be appropriate (McAndrew and Lantz 1989). Not only must the responsible physician assess the patient with injury vis-à-vis amputation, but also the circumstances must be evaluated. Frequently, these considerations may not be discussed. They concern the time of night, facilities available, alertness of the operating team and even geopolitical circumstances. Everything which is said will be remembered by all who participate in the care of the patient because of the significance of limb loss. When presented thoughtfully, the words that are used help to heal.

Limb assessment

Initial assessment of a severely injured extremity should be undertaken after life-threatening conditions have been addressed. The examination should include colour, capillary refill, pulses, the condition of the tissues (skin, subcutaneous tissue, muscles, bone), neurological status (sensory and motor), degree of contamination, degree of crush, the size of the wound and compartment pressure status. Open fractures should be taken to the operating room within eight hours for irrigation and debridement and fracture stabilization with vascular re-anastomosis when required (Gustilo 1982). Appropriate X-rays and angiographic studies, or open-vessel exploration, should be performed. Indications for angiography include an ischaemic extremity, knee dislocation, high-energy fracture pattern and massive soft-tissue injury in areas of risk (Chapman 1980, Gustilo 1982, Gustilo et al 1990, O'Meara 1992).

Heatley described anatomical characteristics which predispose severe compound tibia fractures to amputation and these include a minimal medial soft-tissue sleeve, the vessels having a fixed point at the distal end of the popliteal artery and vulnerability of the nerves to direct contusion or traction injury (Heatley 1988).

The most widely utilized classification system for open fractures in the United States is that described by Gustilo et al (Gustilo and Anderson 1976; Gustilo et al 1984). This system is described in detail in Chapter 2. This system emphasizes wound length rather than depth of injury and is not predictive for limb salvage. Caudle and Stern (1987) examined the prognostic value of the Gustilo classification in a review of 62 type III lower-extremity fractures. They found that type IIIA fractures had a 27% incidence of nonunion with no deep infections or secondary amputations. Type IIIB fractures had a nonunion rate of 43%, a 29% deep infection rate, and a 17% rate of secondary amputation. Type IIIC fractures had a 100% complication rate with an amputation rate of 78%. It is really much clearer to state that compound fractures with vascular injury have a poor prognosis. Jargon tends to obscure the message and makes physicians look as foolish as Dr Sganarelle in Molière's Le Médicin malgré lui.

The classification system of Allgöwer popularized in Europe stresses the mechanism of the compound fracture. A Grade I fracture has small wound associated with compounding by a bony spike perforating the skin—the so-called 'inside–out' fracture. A grade II is a fracture with the wound caused by direct trauma from without ('outside–in'). Severe wounds with neurovascular bundle involvement are classified as grade III (Allgöwer 1971, LaDuca et al 1980, Seligson and Henry 1991).

This system has been replaced by other grading systems which classify compound fractures by depth (as with burns) and complexity (Cauchoix et al 1975, Oestern and Tscherne 1984, Seligson and Henry 1991).

In our view, there are really two major groups: simple and difficult compound fractures (Seligson and Henry 1991). Simple compound fractures require debridement and irrigation and then are treated basically as closed fractures with the expectation that healing will occur in the usual time. Complex fractures, on the other hand, have special characteristics—loss of bone or soft tissue, periosteal stripping, marked contamination or arterial injury—which require individualized therapeutic management including tissue grafting, compartment release or arterial repair (Lange et al 1985, Gustilo et al 1987, Seligson and Henry 1991). Difficult fractures have a high incidence of delayed healing, chronic infection and amputation and they frequently require resource-intensive therapy (Clancey and Hansen 1978, Lange et al 1985, Lange 1989).

Goals and decisions

The goal of limb salvage in a severely injured lower extremity is to create a limb that is functionally superior to one that is amputated, fitted with a prosthesis and rehabilitated (Chen et al 1981, Shaw 1983, Lange et al 1985, Swartz and Jones 1985). Often the fundamental goals of limb salvage are obscured by the armamentarium of orthopaedic, vascular and plastic surgical techniques available for reconstructive endeavours (Aldea and Shaw 1986, Hansen 1987, Heatley 1988). As Samuel D Gross stated (Gross 1862, Aldea and Shaw 1986),

The cases which may reasonably require and those which may not require interference with the knife are not always so clearly and distinctly defined as not to give

rise, in very many instances, to the most serious apprehension . . . that, while the surgeon endeavors to avoid Scylla, he may not unwittingly run into Charybdis, mutilating a limb that might have been saved, and endangering life by the retention of one that should have been promptly amputated.

Other goals include achieving bony union and avoiding infection. The major determinants of treatment outcome are the initial soft-tissue injury and loss, the amount of wound contamination, fracture stability and the presence of neural or vascular injury. Potential local complications with limb salvage include delayed primary, or secondary, amputation, osteomyelitis, delayed union, non-union, limb deformity, limb shortening, chronic lymphoedema and chronic ulceration due to the loss of protective sensation with posterior tibial nerve injuries (Hicks 1964, Chan et al 1984, Hansen 1987, Dellinger 1988, Heatley 1988, Gustilo et al 1990, Helfet et al 1990, Howard and Makin 1990). The systemic complications of failed limb salvage include not only loss of life from sepsis, thromboembolism and drug side effects, but also loss of job, poor general health, drug and alcohol abuse, as well as social and sexual problems.

Microsurgical reconstructive techniques have made it possible to attempt limb salvage in even the most extreme cases. It is imperative to remember, though, that prolonged salvage attempts may destroy a person physically, psychologically, socially and financially. Failed limb salvages may lead to devastating complications and prolonged rehabilitation. It has also been shown that if a patient is not back at work by two years, there is virtually no chance that he or she will return to work at all (Hansen 1987, Heatley 1988, Purry and Hannon 1989, Helfet et al 1990).

The role of amputation in severe open lower-extremity fractures can be separately analysed in three recent studies of tibial fractures with vascular impairment. Caudle and Stern (1987) studied 22 fractures of which 13 had primary amputation. Seven of the remaining nine had delayed amputations and the remaining two patients were having complications and were considering amputation (Caudle and Stern 1987, Heatley 1988).

Lancaster et al (1986) performed 11 primary and two delayed amputations in 15 type IIIc fractures for an overall amputation rate of 87% (Lancaster et al 1986).

Lange et al (1985) performed five immediate and nine delayed amputations in 23 type IIIc fractures for an overall amputation rate of 70%. They found that poor outcomes for limb salvage correlated with crush injury mechanisms, segmental fracture patterns and a delay of revascularization of >6 hours. In this series, 'successful' limb-salvage patients were still frequently disabled and suffered complications (Lange et al 1989, Lange 1989).

These studies demonstrate that reconstructive efforts in severely mangled extremities are difficult at best. The numbers are small and were analysed retrospectively without statistical analysis yet they generally reflect high amputation rates for severe limb injuries at multiple facilities with a >50% delayed amputation rate which reflects the inability of surgeons to make correct decisions for primary amputation acutely (Lange 1989).

Georgiadis et al (1993) examined the long-term outcomes and quality of life in patients who had an open fracture of the tibial diaphysis associated with severe soft tissue loss. They compared 16 patients who had had limbs salvaged using microvascular free flap techniques with 18 patients who had had an early below-the-knee amputation. The patients who had had limb salvage procedures carried out had significantly more complications (5 subsequently had an amputation, mostly because of infection), more operative procedures and a longer stay in hospital than the patients who had had an early below-knee amputation.

As far as the long-term functional results were concerned, the patients who had had a successful limb salvage procedure took significantly more time to achieve full weight bearing, were less willing or able to work and had higher hospital charges than the patients who had been managed with an early below-knee amputation. They also had significant ankle and subtalar joint stiffness. The authors emphasized the importance of adopting a total care philosophy in the management of patients who have had limb salvage procedures. They stressed the importance of an interactive programme of hospital treatment, physical rehabilitation and vocational retraining. It was the view of Georgiadis et al that these measures would shorten the time of rehabilitation, improve function and enrich the quality of life after limb salvage, but they also stressed that in the future the prognosis for patients who had an early below-knee amputation was also likely to improve because of advances in modern prosthetics.

Boudurant et al compared primary versus delayed amputation following severe open tibial fractures. They included 43 cases of which 14 primary and 23 secondary amputations were performed. Delay in choosing the option of amputation was associated with statistically significant increases in hospital stays, hospital costs, number of operations, overall disability and a 20.7% increase in mortality secondary to sepsis from the injured extremity (Boudurant et al 1988). Delayed amputation is often performed for extremity infection and is associated with more proximal amputation levels than primary amputation (Lange 1989). It becomes intuitively obvious that the attitude of 'save all extremities at all costs' indeed causes increased morbidity and mortality and that true surgical heroism may lie in being able to properly select the indications for primary amputation in severely injured extremities (Hansen 1987, Heatley 1988).

There are several guidelines in the surgical literature for determining indications for primary amputation versus extremity salvage in severely injured limbs (Hennen 1838, Gustilo 1982, Howe et al 1987, Johansen et al 1990, O'Mears 1992).

Gustilo recommends primary amputation when there is complete neurovascular loss associated with crushing injury, severe bone and/or soft-tissue loss with an intact neurovascular system that makes reasonable function unlikely, and an intact or repairable vascular system associated with a complete loss of function and sensation of the nerve without the possibility of repair (Gustilo 1982, 1987, O'Meara 1992).

Lange et al describe complete anatomical disruption of the posterior tibial nerve in adults and a crush injury with warm ischaemic time >6 hours as absolute indications for primary amputation in Gustilo type IIIc fractures. Their relative indications include serious associated polytrauma, severe ipsilateral foot trauma, and an anticipated protracted course of rehabilitation. Primary amputation is indicated if either absolute or two or three relative indications are met (Lange et al 1985). This protocol envelops fairly objective absolute indications and rather subjective relative indications which require acute judgement by the treating surgeon(s).

Drost et al in their outcome study of combined orthopaedic and vascular trauma, found that impaired sensory or motor neurological function and/or serious soft-tissue loss with combined injury to lower extremity vascularity at, or distal to, the popliteal artery increased the chances of residual function disability or subsequent amputation (Drost et al 1989).

Several authors have attempted to develop grading systems that evaluate objective criteria in attempts to predict when to attempt limb salvage and when to amputate (Gregory et al 1985, Howe et al 1987, Heatley 1988, Helfet et al 1990, Pozo et al 1990). These include the Predictive Salvage Index of Howe et al (1987), the Mangled Extremity Syndrome Index of Gregory et al (1985), the Mangled Extremity Severity Score of Helfet et al (1990) and Limb Injury Scoring of Pozo et al (1990) (LaDuca et al 1980, Gregory et al 1985, Howe et al 1987, Helfet et al 1990).

These grading systems were each developed with relatively small numbers of patients utilizing multiple variables which were retrospectively reviewed. They are, therefore, difficult to interpret on a per-patient basis and they tend to be subjective. Objective predictive scales which are prospectively tested are yet to be developed to accurately assist surgeons in making good clinical determinations of whether to attempt limb salvage or to amputate (Hansen 1987, Lange 1989).

Decision-making

What then is the guidance for treating difficult limb fractures? There are, in our view, no indices, scales or objective tests that can make what must be a human and—above all—a humane decision. Neither the patient, who is most probably intubated, nor the family, who have their own conflicts and pressures, can make the decision. It is ultimately the physician who has the best overall view of the possibilities and consequences. Our services are engaged for precisely that reason; surgery is a healing art, not a science. So the first recommendation is to find the practitioner with the most *experience* and get that person to the bedside. It does not, as has been suggested, require 'courage' to amputate, only experience (Heatley 1988). The decision is influenced not only by the objective assessment criteria that have been discussed, but by the gestalt generated by the situation. Subtle factors—the patient's grooming, the tone of a relative's voice, the skills of on-call team members—are the signs that wiser hands integrate into the decision-making process.

If experience is the first rule for limb salvage or amputation, the second is *timing*. Amputations are either primary (done as the first procedure after injury), delayed primary (done within five or six days at the second or third debridement) or secondary (done weeks or months after the original injury). Primary amputation is a more obvious and preferred option when difficult extremity injuries present in epidemic proportions such as during war. Delayed primary amputation is usually an accepted alternative when a sensible and competent effort has failed. An initial revascularization which repetitively fails would be an example. 'Everything possible' has been done and the outcome will not be substantially different from immediate primary amputation. In both of these settings, emphasize that the damage was done 'on the road' not at the bedside. The most difficult cases are those in which extensive reconstruction which will inevitably produce a dysfunctional limb is failing. Settings such as mechanical difficulty with limb lengthening, repetitive failure of free flaps, and colonization with resistant organisms are those in which secondary amputation should be considered. For physicians, the most difficult decisions will be faced in coming decades as well-meaning attempts at cost containment in health care may exert pressures in directions yet not anticipated in this professional decision. Ultimately, basic humane values must be the leading consideration and not administrative mandates.

Techniques of amputation

It is beyond the scope of this book to describe the techniques of amputation of surgery in any detail. These have a long pedigree and are well described in the major orthopaedic and surgical texts. Amputations following trauma, however, differ in certain respects from amputations carried out electively. The most obvious differences are that the skin flaps available to the surgeon may well be determined by the amount and distribution of the soft tissues available after debridement. In addition the amputation stump may well be contaminated or the surgeon may be unsure about the viability of the muscles left after amputation. Obviously under these circumstances it is wise to leave the amputation stump open just as the wound should be left open after debridement of an open fracture. It is recommended that a relook procedure is carried out 36 to 48 hours after the amputation to see if further soft tissue or bone resection is required.

The level of amputation is of considerable importance. Obviously this will vary with the location of the open fracture but, as Chapter 3 illustrates, it is very likely that the surgeon will most often be faced with an open tibial fracture and will have to make the choice between an above-knee or below-knee amputation. It is now well understood that the energy involved in walking with a below-knee amputation is much less than that with an above-knee amputation. Thus the surgeon should always attempt to carry out a below-knee amputation if this is possible. However, this should not be attempted in the face of non-viable soft tissue and bone merely to gain length. This is tantamount to performing an inadequate debridement and may well lead to infection and other complications.

Until recently the choice facing the surgeon was whether to carry out an above- or below-knee amputation, the latter only being possible if a sufficient length of viable bone surrounded by adequate soft tissue existed below the knee. Recent innovations in surgical technique have, however, extended the surgeon's ability to perform below-knee amputations and these merit description.

The most important recent advance in traumatic amputation surgery has been the ability to use the skin of the sole of the foot to cover the amputation stump (Figure 23.1). This has the twin advantages of allowing the surgeon to create a longer amputation stump as well as giving the patient heel skin to 'walk-on' in the prosthesis. Obviously the skin of the foot must

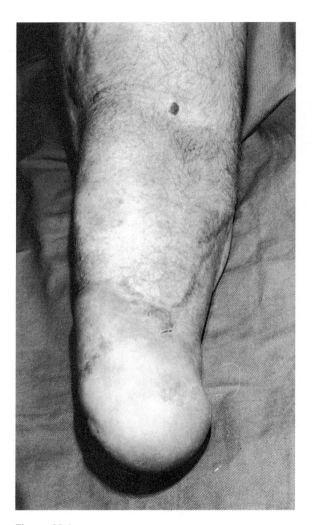

Figure 23.1

A below-knee amputation stump which has been lengthened by the application of the sole of the foot to the stump. This serves to lengthen the stump but also to provide tougher skin and, if the neurovascular pedicle is intact, sensate skin.

be intact to permit this type of surgery; if it is, the surgeon has two options. Firstly, the skin can be transferred with an intact neurovascular supply. This technique has the advantage of transferring sensate skin to the amputation stump. If this is not possible, the second option is that the skin of the sole of the foot can be transferred using a free flap technique – as was

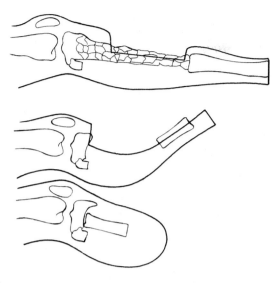

Figure 23.2

The turn up technique used for stump lengthening. This technique is only possible if there is a viable posterior soft tissue flap and a section of viable distal tibia. The comminuted middle third of the tibia is resected and the intact segment of the distal third turned up to the proximal tibia.

done in the patient illustrated in Figure 23.1. Indeed, if the surgeon is skilled in free flap transfer a number of donor sites can be used to supply soft tissue to facilitate the reconstruction of a viable below-knee amputation. Kasabian et al (1991) describe 22 cases of traumatic below-knee amputations with inadequate soft tissue cover salvaged with microvascular free flaps. They describe 24 flaps in 22 patients, using a parascapular free flap in 11 patients, a foot fillet in 6 patients and a latissimus dorsi free flap in 4 patients. One patient each had a lateral thigh, tensor fascia lata or groin flap performed.

The authors stress the complexity of this type of surgery. Their 22 patients required a total of 107 operations, although the complications of surgery appear not to have been all that severe. They stated that most of their patients had excellent results with good joint function. There seems no doubt that this type of approach should be adopted where possible in patients whom otherwise might have had an above-knee amputation.

Another unusual but useful technique in the preservation of length of a below-knee amputation stump is the turn-up technique, whereby a length of viable distal tibial diaphysis can be salvaged and turned upwards on a viable posterior soft tissue flap to facilitate a longer

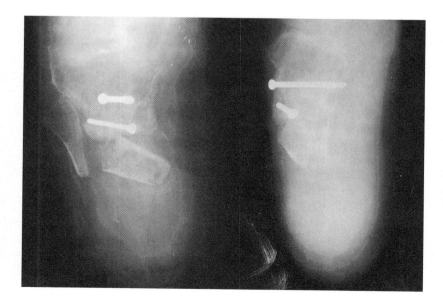

Figure 23.3

X-rays of a turn up amputation stump in a 20-year-old male who had a Gustilo type IIIc fracture as a result of a road-traffic accident. The distal fragment displaced but despite this the stump length that was gained was beneficial. It is however recommended that the distal fragment be plated to the proximal tibia to prevent this problem. The proximal screws were inserted at the original operation shortly after the accident.

below-knee stump. This technique is illustrated in Figure 23.2 and an example of such a flap is shown in Figure 23.3. Obviously this technique is only possible when the posterior soft tissues of the leg are intact.

References

Aldea PA, Shaw WW (1986) The evolution of the surgical management of severe lower extremity trauma, *Clin Plast Surg* **134**: 549–69.

Allgöwer M (1971) Weichteilprobleme und infektionsrisko der osteosynthese, *Langenbecks Arch Chir* **329**: 1127–36.

American College of Surgeons, Committee on Trauma, *Advanced Trauma Life Support Student Manual* (American College of Surgeons: Chicago).

American College of Surgeons, Committee on Trauma, *Early Care of the Injured Patient*, 3rd edn (WB Saunders: Philadelphia).

Augeneder M, Boszotta H, Sauer G (1989) Zur Behandlung der offenen Unterschenkelfraktur mit dem fixateur Externe, *Unfallchirurgie* **92**: 531–6.

Boudurant FJ, Cotler HB, Buckle R (1988) The medical and economic impact of severely injured lower extremities, *J Trauma* **28**(8): 1270–3.

Brothwell C, Moller-Christensen V (1963) Medicohistorical aspects of a very early case of mutilation, *Danish Med Bull* **10**: 21.

Cauchoix J, Duparc J, Boulez P (1975) Traitement des fractures ouverts de jambes, *Med Acta Chir* **83**: 811.

Caudle RJ, Stern PJ (1987) Severe open fractures of the tibia, *J Bone Joint Surg* **69A**: 801–7.

Chan KM, Leung JCY, Leung PC (1984) The management of type III open tibial fractures, *Injury* **16**: 157–65.

Chapman MW (1980) The use of immediate internal fixation in open fractures, *Orthop Clin N Am* **11**(3): 579–91.

Chen ZW, Meyer VE, Kleinhert HE (1981) Present indications and contraindications for replantation as reflected by long-term functional results, *Orthop Clin N Am* **12**: 849.

Clancey GJ, Hansen ST (1978) Open fractures of the tibia, *J Bone Joint Surg* **60A**: 118–22.

Dellinger EP, Miller SD, Wertz MJ (1988) Risk of infection after open fracture of the arm or leg, *Arch Surg* **123**: 1320–6.

Drost TF, Rosemurgy AS, Proctor D (1989) Outcome of treatment of combined orthopedic and arterial trauma to the lower extremity, *J Trauma* **29**(10): 1331–5.

Georgiadis GM, Behrens FF, Joyce MJ et al (1993) Open tibial fractures with severe soft tissue loss, *J Bone Joint Surg* **75A**: 1431–41.

Gregory RT, Gould RJ, Peclet M (1985) The mangled extremity syndrome (MES): a severity grading system for multisystem injury of the extremity, *J Trauma* **25**(12): 1147–50.

Gross SD (1862) *A Manual of Military Surgery or Hints on the Emergencies of the Field, Camp and Hospital Practice* (JB Lippincott: Philadelphia).

Gustilo RB (1982) Management of open fractures and complications, *Instr Course Lect* **31**: 64–75.

Gustilo RB (1987) Current concepts in the management of open fractures, *Instr Course Lect* **36**: 359–66.

Gustilo RB, Anderson JT (1976) Prevention of infection in the treatment of 1025 open fractures of the long bones—retrospective and prospective analysis, *J Bone Joint Surg* **58A**: 453–8.

Gustilo RB, Mendoza RM, Williams DN (1984) Problems in the management of type III (severe) open fractures: a new classification of type III open fractures, *J Trauma* **24**(8): 742–6.

Gustilo RB, Gruninger RP, Davis T (1987) Classification of type III (severe) open fractures relative to treatment and results, *Orthopedics* **10**(12): 1781–8.

Gustilo RB, Merkow RL, Templeman D (1990) Current concepts review: the management of open fractures, *J Bone Joint Surg* **72A**: 299–304.

Hansen ST (1987) The type IIIc tibial fracture, *J Bone Joint Surg* **69A**(6): 799–800.

Heatley FW (1988) Severe open fractures of the tibia: the courage to amputate, *Br Med J* **296**: 229.

Helfet DL, Howey T, Sanders R (1990) Limb salvage versus amputation, *Clin Orthop* **256**: 80–6.

Hennen J (1838) *Principles of Military Surgery* (Carey & Lea: Philadelphia).

Hicks JH (1964) Amputation in fractures of the tibia, *J Bone Joint Surg* **46B**: 388–92.

Howard PW, Makin GS (1990) Lower limb fractures with associated vascular injury, *J Bone Joint Surg* **72B**: 116–20.

Howe HR, Poole GV, Hansen KJ (1987) Salvage of lower extremities following combined orthopedic and vascular trauma—a predictive salvage index, *Am Surg* **53**(4): 205–8.

Johansen K, Daines M, Howey T (1990) Objective criteria accurately predict amputation following lower extremity trauma, *J Trauma* **30**(5): 568–72.

Kasabian AK, Colen SR, Shaw WW et al (1991) The role of microvascular free flaps in salvaging below-knee amputation stumps: a review of 22 cases, *J Trauma* **31**: 495–501.

Kuhn WY, Bell RA, Netscher RE (1989) Psychiatric assessment of leg fracture patients: a pilot study, *Int J Psych Med* **19**: 145–54.

LaDuca JN, Bone LL, Seibel RW (1980) Primary open reduction and internal fixation of open fractures, *J Trauma* (1980) **20**: 580–6.

Lancaster SJ, Horowitz M, Alonzo J (1986) Open tibial fractures: management and results, *South Med J* **79**: 39.

Lange RH (1989) Limb reconstruction versus amputation decision making in massive lower extremity trauma, *Clin Orthop* **243**: 92–9.

Lange RH, Bach AW, Hansen ST (1985) Open tibial fractures with associated vascular injuries: prognosis for limb salvage, *J Trauma* **25**: 203–8.

McAndrew MP, Lantz BA (1989) Initial care of massively traumatized lower extremities, *Clin Orthop* **243**: 20–9.

Oestern HJ, Tscherne H (1984) Pathophysiology and classification of soft-tissue injuries associated with fractures. In: Tscherne H, Gotzen L, eds, *Fractures with Soft Tissue Injuries* (Springer-Verlag: New York) 1–9.

O'Meara PM (1992) Management of open fractures, *Orthop Rev* **21**(10): 1177–85.

Pozo JL, Powell B, Andrews BG (1990) The timing of amputation for lower limb trauma, *J Bone Joint Surg* **72B**: 288–92.

Purry NA, Hannon MA (1989) How successful is below-knee amputation for injury? *Injury* **20**: 32–6.

Seligson D, Henry SL (1991) Treatment of compound fractures, *Am J Surg* **161**: 693–701.

Shaw WW (1983) Microvascular free flaps: the first decade, *Clin Plast Surg* **10**: 3.

Swartz WM, Jones NF (1985) Soft tissue coverage of the lower extremity, *Curr Prob Surg* June.

Tsai TM, Werntz JR, Kirkpatrick DK (1988) Free tissue transfer in type III open lower extremity fractures, *Surg Rounds Orthop*, 17–23.

United States Army (1970) *Orthopedic Surgery in the Zone of the Interior: Surgery in World War II* (Medical Department, United States Army, Office of the Surgeon General: Washington, D.C.).

Wangensteen OH, Smith J, Wangensteen SD (1967) Some highlights in the history of amputation reflecting lessons in wound healing, *Bull Hist Med* **41**: 97.

Zimmerman LM, Vieth I, *Great Ideas in the History of Surgery* (Williams & Wilkins: Boston).

24
Open fractures in children

J.E. Robb

Conventionally, children's fractures are discussed separately from adult fractures. There are many good reasons for this but the surgeon should not lose sight of the fact that many aspects of the management of open fractures in children and adults are similar. The same classifications and treatments are available for both soft-tissue and bony injuries and to minimize repetition a number of the aspects of the management of open fractures in children will not be discussed fully in this chapter. Thus the reader is referred to Chapter 5 for a discussion on pre- and per-operative wound assessment and management. Chapters 14–18 deal with the management of soft-tissue defects and although there are slight differences in the soft-tissue surgery between adults and children, much of the philosophy and many of the surgical techniques are very similar. In addition, the management of the complications of fracture is very similar in children and adults. The goals of fracture management in children and adults are also the same. It is no longer acceptable for the surgeon to merely achieve union in a fracture but the patient must be returned to maximal function. The surgeon should always remember that a child left with unnecessary deformity or joint stiffness will be handicapped for his or her lifetime.

There are a number of obvious differences between child and adult fractures. Children's bones retain the capacity for growth and physeal fractures are not uncommon (Hanlon and Estes 1954, Mann and Rajmaira 1990, Peterson et al 1994). Ligaments often insert into an epiphysis so that force applied to the epiphysis is transmitted to the physis producing a fracture rather than the ligamentous injury which is more common in the adult. Physeal damage may produce growth arrest and additionally non-physeal fractures may produce bone overgrowth,

a phenomenon with which adult traumatologists do not have to contend.

Periosteum is thicker and stronger in children than in adults, giving rise to different fracture patterns. Fracture patterns in children comprise compression or torus fractures, incomplete tension/compression or green-stick fractures and physeal fractures (Figure 24.1). In addition to these fractures, older children display fracture morphology which is similar to that seen in adults. This is detailed in the AO classification (Muller et al 1987).

Other differences between adults and children centre around the speed with which children's fractures heal and their capacity for remodelling. Thus, paediatric traumatologists may accept more residual bone deformity than would be acceptable in adults provided the residual deformity lies within the plane of motion of the adjacent joint, that there is sufficient growth potential left and the fracture lies close to the physis. Surgeons should remember that there is minimal remodelling in rotational deformities.

Open fractures in children are less common than in adults and when they do occur they may well be associated with other injuries. Head injury, facial damage and intra-abdominal injuries are not uncommon in children and they not infrequently have parenchymal lung damage in the absence of sternal or rib fractures because of the elasticity of the rib cage.

Fracture classification

The classifications listed in Chapter 2 apply to children as well as adults. The only fracture classifications which are not applicable to adults are those that classify physeal fractures. The most commonly used classification of physeal

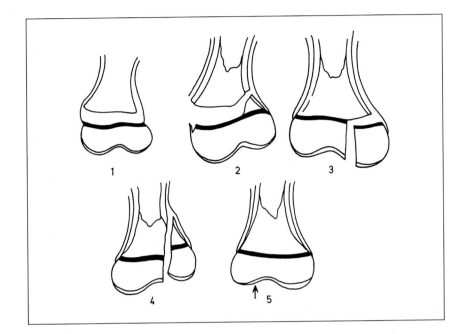

Figure 24.1

The Salter Harris classification of physeal fractures.

fractures is that of Salter and Harris (1963). This is illustrated in Figure 24.1.

Epidemiology

Epidemiological data regarding open fractures in children are remarkably scarce and there is no detailed analysis of the incidence of different open fractures in children. There are, however, a number of papers which discuss fracture epidemiology in children and extrapolation of their data allows some conclusions to be drawn about the incidence of certain open fractures.

It is popularly assumed that, in general, open fractures in children are less common than in adults. This is true but a review of the literature suggests they are not as uncommon as has been assumed in the past. Mann and Rajmaira (1990) analysed 2650 physeal and non-physeal long-bone fractures and detailed an overall incidence of open fractures of 2.1%, with Cheng and Shen (1993) finding that 2.2% of 3350 paediatric fractures were open. If the equivalent figures for fractures are extrapolated from the data

presented in Chapter 3, it appears that the incidence of open fractures of the diaphyses and metaphyses of adult long bones is 3.2%. Mann and Rajmaira (1990) indicated that open physeal fractures in their series were extremely rare, with an incidence of only 0.3%. However, they had a 2.9% incidence of open fractures for non-physeal fractures, these presumably mainly corresponding to diaphyseal fractures in adults. In an earlier paper, Hanlon and Estes (1954) had supplied enough data to estimate incidences of open fractures of the hand and foot at 7.8% and 5.1%, respectively. When the figures of these two papers are taken together, it is possible to provide some comparative data for certain paediatric fractures. These data are compared in Table 24.1 with the equivalent data presented in Chapter 3 for adults. There would appear to be a different epidemiological pattern between adults and children. Although Table 24.1 lists open paediatric tibial fractures as having an incidence of 8.1%, other authorities have suggested lower incidences of 4.6% (Hanlon and Estes 1954) and 3.4% (Shannak 1988). It would appear that the incidence of open long-bone fractures is certainly less in children than in adults, but the little evidence that exists suggests that open fractures of the foot and hand may well be more common.

Open physeal fractures were rarely encountered by Mann and Rajmaira (1990). They documented only two tibial physeal fractures, giving an incidence of 0.3%. However, Peterson et al (1994), in a larger study of physeal fractures, documented an incidence of open physeal fractures of 2.1%.

Pre- and per-operative assessment

This is described in Chapter 5. The surgeon should, however, be aware of the fact that there may be co-existing injuries in children who present with open fractures. Careful examination looking for other musculoskeletal and soft-tissue injuries should be undertaken. The surgeon should approach the examination of a multiply injured child in a systematic fashion as governed by ATLS principles.

As with adults, it is vital that the surgeon carry out an adequate debridement and not leave dead or dubious soft tissue or bone in the wound. If necessary, repeated debridements should be performed until all devitalized tissue has been removed. Again, as in adults, there is no excuse for leaving an open wound in a child and it is mandatory that all open fractures should be surgically explored. Failure to do this will eventually give rise to major problems.

Fracture fixation techniques are the same in children as in adults and it is interesting to note that over the last decade or so paediatric surgeons have become more aware of the benefits of fracture fixation. However, casting techniques are probably still used more commonly in open fractures in children than in adults.

Fracture treatment

The general principles of managing severe open long-bone fractures in children are very similar to those applied to adults in that surgeons now tend to avoid the use of traction and casts.

However, the presence of open physes has meant that most surgeons have advocated external skeletal fixation or plating for long-bone injuries rather than intramedullary nailing, which has become very popular in the management of adult open long-bone fractures.

As in the management of adult fractures paediatric traumatologists have found open fractures of the tibia to be most difficult and time-consuming to treat. Buckley et al (1990) examined the treatment of 42 open diaphyseal or metaphyseal fractures in children of which 12 were Gustilo type I, 18 were type II and 12 were type III. Of these fractures 4 were IIIb fractures and 2 were IIIc fractures. All of the open tibial fractures were treated by irrigation and debridement, with 20 being externally fixed and 22 immobilized with a plaster cast. The treatment method selected largely depended on the severity of the fracture, with external fixation being used for the more severe injuries. They documented their results well and showed that the type I fractures healed in an average of 16 weeks, the type II and type IIIa fractures united in 17.2 weeks on average and the type IIIb fractures united in 35.1 weeks. The type IIIc fractures united in an average of 56.7 weeks. It is of considerable interest that these figures are very similar to the union times for open adult tibial fractures. Their complications were few. They only encountered one case of osteomyelitis in a IIIb fracture and the delayed union incidence was 14%, again comparable to results gained in adults. Four of their patients had tibial lengthening of >1 cm. All these patients were treated with external fixation and restoration of anatomical limb lengths.

Cramer et al (1992) examined 40 open tibial diaphyseal fractures in children over an eight-year period. There were seven type I open fractures, the remainder being either type II or type III in severity. They documented their treatment well and showed that 12.5% of the patients required flap cover, with 37.5% requiring split-skin grafting to gain soft-tissue closure. Chapter 13 showed that in the adult open tibial fractures treated in Edinburgh, 22.5% required split-skin grafting and a further 32.4% of patients required flap cover. Thus it would appear that in open tibial fractures children have a lower requirement for flap cover. Cramer and her co-workers also documented that four of the patients with Gustilo type IIIc fractures required below-knee amputation and of the remaining 36 patients, 14 (39%) had union problems. Hope and Cole (1992) reviewed 92 children with open tibial fractures of whom 22 had type I fractures, 51 had type II fractures and 19 had type III fractures. Again, delayed union and non-union problems were not uncommon and there was a 21% incidence of osteomyelitis in the type III fracture group. They found that older children were more liable to union problems and they also noted that external fixation appeared to be associated with non-union, although in a retrospective uncontrolled series it is unlikely that cast management and external fixation were used to treat equivalent fractures and it is inadvisable to draw more than general conclusions about the effect of external fixation on bone union.

All of these papers were retrospective and spanned a considerable number of years. The general conclusion is that Gustilo type I open fractures can be treated by a cast but that other more severe fractures need external fixation. It is clear that in all these papers the surgeons have become more aware of the problems of treating open tibial fractures during the period of the study and have adopted external fixation and more sophisticated methods of soft-tissue closure. It is also quite obvious that the treatment methods and results for the management of open tibial fractures in children are very similar to those for adults. Schranz et al (1992) examined the use of external fixation in children. They sensibly suggested that unilateral fixators were adequate for both femoral and tibial open fractures and in tibial fractures they advocated a unilateral configuration with two pins in each fragment as shown in Figure 24.2.

Open femoral fractures

Table 24.1 indicates that open femoral fractures in children are uncommon, having an incidence of about one-fifth of that of adult open tibial fractures. It is probable that many surgeons work in hospitals that serve a population of about 250 000 patients (BOA 1992). Extrapolation of the data presented in Chapter 3, assuming a 1:4 rota and an incidence of open femoral fractures of one-fifth of the adult incidence, means that the average surgeon will encounter an open femoral

Table 24.1 Comparative incidence of some open fractures in adults and children. Paediatric data from Hanlon and Estes (1954) and Mann and Rajmaira (1990)

Fracture	Adults (%)	Children (%)
Humeral diaphysis	5.7	0.4
Forearm diaphysis	9.3	5.5
Hand	4.2	7.8
Femoral diaphysis	12.1	2.4
Tibial diaphysis	21.6	8.1
Foot	3.1	5.1

fracture in a child every five years. It is obvious that he or she will find it difficult to gain the necessary expertise to handle these fractures proficiently.

There are two reasons for considering internal or external fixation in open femoral fractures in children. Not only is it desirable to adequately stabilize severe open femoral fractures, but there is a strong association between open femoral fractures and head injury. Buckley et al (1994) working in a specialist paediatric trauma centre noted that 26% of children with open femoral fractures had an associated head injury. In addition, 9% had an associated chest injury and 6% had an abdominal injury. Femoral fractures are frequently difficult to manage in a cerebrally irritated child and internal or external fixation is indicated.

Nowadays, the standard method of management of both open and closed femoral fractures in adults is the interlocking intramedullary nail. Its use is detailed in Chapter 6. However, its use in children is currently being debated by paediatric traumatologists. O'Malley et al (1995) have described avascular necrosis of the femoral head due to injury to the posterior superior branch of the medial circumflex artery, which lies in close proximity to the piriform fossa. Raney et al (1993) have also recorded premature trochanteric epiphysiodesis and, as a rule, the passage of nails across physes should be approached with caution.

Galpin et al (1994) examined the use of reamed Grosse Kempf nail as well as unreamed flexible Rush and Enders nails in the management of femoral fractures in children. They stated that trochanteric arrest was not associated

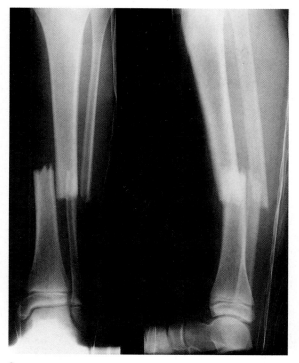

a

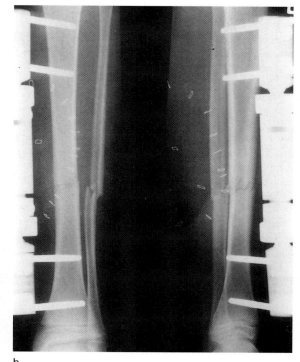

b

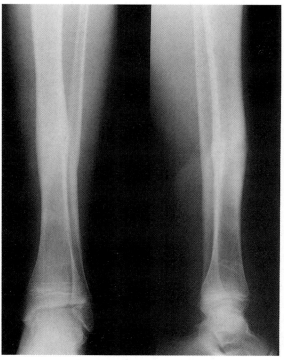

c

Figure 24.2

A Gustilo type II open tibial fracture treated by immediate external fixation with a fasciocutaneous flap being carried out at 48 hours. (a) An AO type A 3.3 fracture of the tibia and fibula. (b) A unilateral external frame was applied and fasciocutaneous flap was used to cover the defect at 48 hours after the initial fracture. (c) The result at one year. There was no functional deficit.

with the use of non-reamed nails but in 5 of 22 patients treated with a reamed intramedullary nail, there was some evidence of physeal damage although there was no functional deficit noted on final examination of the patient. They documented that 80% of the patients had equal leg lengths at final follow-up, a further 14.3% had a discrepancy of 1 cm and the remainder had overgrowth of up to 3 cm. They only encountered two malunions, neither of which required corrective surgery.

Beaty et al (1994) examined 31 femoral shaft fractures treated with interlocking intramedullary nails. They noted few complications, with an average leg length discrepancy of 0.51 cm (range −1.8 cm to 3.2 cm). The average difference in the articulotrochanteric distance between the injured and uninjured limbs was −0.04 cm (range −1.7 cm to 1.5 cm). The neck shaft angle between the injured and uninjured side differed by <1° (range −10° to 10°) and the functional deficit was minor. This group advocated the use of intramedullary nails in patients aged between 10 and 16 years and they noted that they had gradually extended their indications for the use of intramedullary nails in children. They, like Galpin et al (1994), stressed the importance of not damaging the blood supply by extending the dissection onto the neck of the femur and they also emphasized the need to leave the nail 1 cm proud of the bone to facilitate later nail removal.

Other surgeons have advocated different management techniques for open femoral fractures. Kregor et al (1993) examined the role of plate fixation in both closed and open femoral fractures in children. In their six open fractures they noted very few complications, with minor limb length discrepancy and only one malunion being seen. Kirschenbaum et al (1990) and Schranz et al (1992) both advocated external skeletal fixation. Kirschenbaum and his co-workers did not encounter malunion and only 1 of 10 patients with severe femoral fractures showed a significant leg length discrepancy. Schranz and his colleagues treated nine femoral fractures and had excellent results. They stressed the advantages of unilateral external fixation utilizing three pins in each femoral fragment.

It seems reasonable to advocate the use of either plating or external fixation for open femoral fractures. Intramedullary nailing may prove to have a place but as demonstrated earlier only paediatric trauma centres specializing in the management of the severely injured child may get enough experience in femoral nailing to minimize potential complications. Both plating and external skeletal fixation are straightforward techniques and are probably preferable. Analysis of the literature suggests that while limb length discrepancy may be a problem following accurate fracture reduction with plating or external fixation, few patients seem to have a functional problem. External fixation is a particularly useful technique in the management of the head-injured child as the fixator can be applied quickly with minimal trauma.

Open fractures of the upper limb

There is virtually no literature dealing with the management of open diaphyseal fractures of the upper limb in children. Table 24.1 suggests that open humeral diaphyseal fractures are extremely rare but that open fractures of the diaphyses of the radius and ulna are more common. In the absence of evidence to the contrary it seems reasonable to treat these fractures in a similar way to fractures of the lower limbs with severe fractures of the upper limb diaphyses being treated with external fixation and the less severe fractures being treated according to the preference of the surgeon, this usually being with cast management.

Gunshot injuries

Gunshot wounds to the extremities in children are an increasing problem particularly in the United States. Both Letts and Miller (1976) and Stucky and Loder (1991) have detailed an increasing incidence of these injuries. In the earlier Canadian series of Letts and Miller (1976), the commonest weapon used was a shotgun but in the more recent report from Detroit, 60% of the children were injured by a hand gun, with only 12% having shotgun injuries.

Stucky and Loder recognized four different types of radiological pattern in their 85 patients. Twenty-eight (32.9%) patients showed radiological evidence of bullet fragments without a fracture and 24 (28.2%) showed a fracture without evidence of both fragments. A further 16 (18.8%) had both the fracture and retained bullet fragments, and the remaining 17 (20.1%) had neither evidence of a fracture nor retained bullet fragments. Thus 40 (47%) of the group had open extremity fractures after gunshot injuries. Predictably, there were a number of associated injuries affecting the chest and abdomen. Only one patient had a significant vascular injury but eight patients had severe nerve damage. In the rural population of Manitoba, Canada, the average age of the children with shotgun wounds was nine years but in the urban population detailed by Stucky and Loder the average age of the children was 12.3 years. These authors point out that most paediatric gunshot injuries occur in children older than 11 or 12 years of age and that there is a rapid yearly increase from age 12 until 16 or 17 years of age. There is usually a marked male preponderance, Stucky and Loder reporting that 83% of their injuries were in boys.

Treatment of a gunshot extremity has been documented in other chapters. It is basically the same as for the adults in terms of debridement and soft-tissue management although the fracture fixation methods in children may differ somewhat in adults, and as suggested previously in this chapter, it is recommended that external skeletal fixation be used where possible.

Lawnmower injuries

There has been recent interest in lawnmower injuries in both adults and children, particularly in the United States. It has been estimated that 75 000 lawnmower-related injuries occur annually in the United States and that the estimated annual costs of these injuries is 253 million (Dormans et al 1995). Lawnmower injuries tend to affect children under 16 years of age and adults over 44 years of age (Anger et al 1995). Children either operate lawnmowers or fall off the back while being given a ride by another operator. Push mowers are also implicated, with injuries being sustained as the mower passes over the child's foot. Dormans et al (1995) examined 16 children with 18 lower-extremity injuries caused by lawnmowers. The average age of the children in this series was only 4 years and 9 months and the injuries that they sustained were extremely severe. There was an average of 4.9 operations per patient and 14 (78%) of the limbs eventually required an amputation, most of which were either below-knee or Syme's amputations. Seven patients (43.6%) required split-skin grafting and three (18.6%) needed flap cover. This group divided the lawnmower injury into two types, shredding and paucilaceration types. Their shredding type was most common with 16 of the 18 limbs falling into this category. Only two such injured limbs were saved, and both appeared to

have poor long-term results. The two paucilaceration patients did well.

Vosburgh et al (1995) examined 32 children who had foot and ankle injuries in lawnmower accidents. The average age of this group was older at eight years. Again, the level of injury was severe with 14 patients requiring toe amputation and five patients more proximal amputations. A particular problem was damage to the heel or plantar surface of the foot. Nine patients had no problems, the remainder showing hyperkeratosis at the junction of the normal plantar surface and the graft. A total of 12 patients required split-skin grafting and two patients had free flaps performed.

Anger et al (1995) reported on 33 open injuries of the foot over a seven-year period. Twenty-two were from push mowers, nine resulted from the use of ride-on mowers and two were from self-propelled mowers. Fifteen of the patients were children with an average age of 10 years. A total of 40 open fractures in the whole patient group were treated, these being fractures of the proximal middle and distal phalanges as well as fractures of the metatarsal. One open calcaneal fracture was seen in the series. A total of 20 amputations were performed. These authors stressed the contaminated nature of these wounds, with an average of 3.1 organisms per patient being cultured. A wide variety of different organisms were reported.

There is no doubt that lawnmower injuries in children can be extremely severe. The most severe injuries were noted in the paper by Dormans et al (1995) and this presumably correlates with the young age of their patients. In older children, the lawnmower presumably passes over less of the body but foot and ankle injuries can ensue. As with other open fractures, a successful management of these injuries requires participation by both orthopaedic traumatologists and plastic surgeons.

Soft-tissue management

The management of the soft tissues associated with open fractures in children is very similar to the management in adult patients and is well detailed in Chapters 15 to 17. Although information about the requirement for free-flap cover in

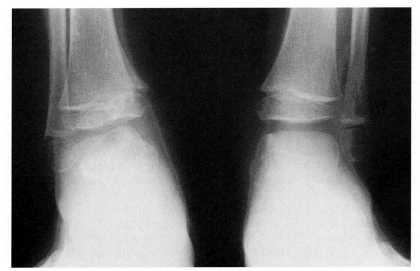

a

Figure 24.3

A bony bar complicating an open Salter Harris type IV epiphyseal fracture of the distal tibial epiphysis. (a) Injured and non-injured sides showing the bridge and varus inclination at the ankle. (b) The bony bar (illustrated by arrow) shown in the sagittal plane using MRI imaging. (c) The bony bar (illustrated by arrow) shown in the coronal plane using MRI imaging.

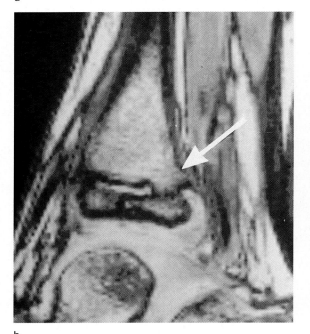

b

c

children who have open fractures is scarce, it would appear that the requirement for free flaps is less than in adult fractures (Cramer et al 1992). However, the other feature that becomes clear on analysis of the literature dealing with paedi- atric open fractures is that surgeons are becoming more aware of the importance of good soft-tissue cover and it is likely that the use of local flaps and free flaps will assume a greater importance. Thus it is important that any surgeon who is dealing with the problems of soft-tissue deficit in children be skilled in the use of both local and free flaps. Generally surgeons will use the same criteria for choosing between local flaps and free flaps in children as in adults. However, consideration should be given to the cosmetic aspects of using local flaps. As pointed out in Chapter 16 local flaps are not as cosmetically attractive as well applied free flaps and this should be considered when planning flap cover in a child. However, the cosmesis should only be one factor which is taken into consideration when planning flap cover.

Complications

Complications of open fractures in children can be devastating and are minimized by adequate primary management. However, even in the best of hands complications will occur and problems such as bone infection, non-union, malunion and compartment syndrome should be dealt with as detailed in the chapters dealing with the equivalent complications in adults. There is no significant difference in the treatment of these complications between children and adults. The indications for amputation in children are very similar to those in adults and as with adults all attempts should be made to conserve limb length and in particular to preserve the knee joint. Surgeons should give consideration to the use of the plantar skin to cover a below-knee amputation stump and the use of turnup flaps should be considered where possible as described in Chapter 23.

Post-traumatic physeal arrest is obviously a complication which is unique to children. In general, Salter Harris type I, II and III fractures have a good prognosis for subsequent growth provided the blood supply remains intact, but the high-energy nature of open physeal fractures suggests that the prognosis for open fractures is worse. Salter Harris type IV fractures carry a poor prognosis unless the plate is anatomically reduced and type V fractures carry the worst prognosis (Langenskiold 1981). The age of the child at the time of injury will also influence outcome; the younger the child, the more serious the outlook. The commonest site for a post-traumatic physeal bar is in the distal femur followed by the proximal and the distal tibia. The bar can result in progressive angular deformity and limb shortening and requires resection and the possibility of subsequent repeated osteotomies and limb lengthening (Figure 24.3).

References

Anger DM, Ledbetter BR, Stasikelis PJ, Calhoun JH (1995) Injuries of the foot related to the use of lawn mowers, *J Bone Joint Surg (Am)* **77A**: 719–25.

Beaty JH, Austin SM, Warner WC, Canale ST, Nichols L (1994) Interlocking intramedullary nailing of femoral-shaft fractures in adolescents: Preliminary results and complications, *J Pediatr Orthop* **14**: 178–83.

British Orthopaedic Association (1992) *The Management of Skeletal Trauma in the United Kingdom* (BOA, London).

Buckley SL, Smith G, Sponseller PD, Thompson JD, Griffin PP (1990) Open fractures of the tibia in children, *J Bone Joint Surg (Am)* **72A**: 1462–9.

Buckley SL, Gotschall C, Robertson W, Storm P, Tosi L, Thomas M, Eichelberger M (1994) The relationship of skeletal injuries with trauma score, injury severity score, length of hospital stay, hospital charges, and mortality in children admitted to a regional paediatric trauma centre, *J Paediatr Orthop* **14**: 449–53.

Cheng JC, Shen WY (1993) Limb fracture patterns in different paediatric age groups: a study of 3350 children, *J Orthop Trauma* **7**: 15–22.

Cramer KE, Limbird TJ, Green NE (1992) Open fractures of the diaphysis of the lower extremity in children, *J Bone Joint Surg (Am)* **74A**: 218–32.

Dormans JP, Azzoni M, Davidson RS, Drummond DS (1995) Major lower extremity lawn mower injuries in children, *J Pediatr Orthop* **15**: 78–82.

Galpin RD, Willis RB, Sabano N (1994) Intramedullary nailing of pediatric femoral fractures, *J Pediatr Orthop* **14**: 184–9.

Gustilo RB, Anderson JT (1976) Prevention of infection in the treatment of 1025 open fractures of long bones: Retrospective and prospective analysis, *J Bone Joint Surg (Am)* **58A**: 453–8.

Hanlon CR, Estes WC (1954) Fractures in childhood—A statistical analysis, *Am J Surg* **87**: 312–20.

Hope PG, Cole WG (1992) Open fractures of the tibia in children, *J Bone Joint Surg (Br)* **74B**: 546–53.

Kirschenbaum D, Albert MC, Robertson WW, Davidson RS (1990) Complex femur fractures in children: Treatment with external fixation, *J Pediatr Orthop* **10**: 588–91.

Kregor PJ, Song KM, Routt ML, Sangeorzan BJ, Liddell RM, Hansen ST (1993) Plate fixation of femoral shaft fractures in multiply injured children, *J Bone Joint Surg (Am)* **75A**: 1774–80.

Langenskiold A (1981) Surgical treatment of partial closure of the growth plate, *J Paediatr Orthop* **1**: 3–11.

Letts RM, Miller D (1976) Gunshot wounds of the extremities in children, *J Trauma* **16**: 807–11.

Mann DC, Rajmaira S (1990) Distribution of physeal and nonphyseal fractures in 2650 long-bone fractures in children aged 0–16 years, *J Paediatr Orthop* **10**: 713–16.

Muller ME, Nazarian S, Koch P, Schatzker J (1987) *The Comprehensive Classification of Fractures of Long Bones* (Springer-Verlag: Berlin).

O'Malley DE, Mazur JM, Cummings RJ (1995) Femoral head avascular necrosis associated with intramedullary nailing in an adolescent, *J Pediatr Orthop* **15**: 21–3.

Peterson HA, Madmok R, Benson JT, Ilstrup DV, Melton LJ (1994) Physeal fractures: part I. Epidemiology in Olmsted County, Minnesota, 1979–1988, *J Paediatr Orthop* **14**: 423–30.

Raney EM, Ogden JA, Grogan DP (1993) Premature trochanteric epiphysiodesis secondary to intramedullary femoral rodding, *J Pediatr Orthop* **13**: 516–20.

Salter RB, Harris WR (1963) Injuries involving the epiphyseal plate, *J Bone Joint Surg* **45**: 108–15.

Schranz PJ, Gultekin C, Colton CL (1992) External fixation of fractures in children, *Injury* **23**: 80–2.

Shannak AO (1988) Tibial fractures in children: Follow-up study, *J Paediatr Orthop* **8**: 306–10.

Stucky W, Loder RT (1991) Extremity gunshot wounds in children, *J Pediatr Orthop* **11**: 64–71.

Vosburgh CL, Gruel CR, Herndon WA, Sullivan JA (1995) Lawn mower injuries of the pediatric foot and ankle: Observation of prevention and management, *J Pediatr Orthop* **15**: 504–9.

Index